NUTRITION AND OUR OVERPOPULATED PLANET

This monograph draws attention to the intimate relationship between nutrition, population and the task of feeding the masses. Our planet has become so congested that interdependence between nations in almost all spheres of human activity is not only desirable but essential. In this context the consequences surrounding the continued increase in population of developing nations, housing more than three-fourths of humanity, cannot remain the sole concern of those countries alone. It is becoming evident that the overpopulated and overcrowded countries cannot feed their growing numbers from their own resources. If this rate of growth continues it is doubtful whether they will be able to control by themselves the social, economic and political consequences which may follow.

This text focuses special attention on the nutritional needs of special age groups in order to describe ways in which they can obtain the maximum nutritive value from their existing food resources. Since the animal sources of food are scarcer and more expensive, the vegetable sources of food when used in combination, can be as effective for good health as such animal products as meat, dairy products and poultry. Education on the nutritional value of foods is important for the vulnerable sections of our society, i.e. the pregnant women, the infants, the preschool children and the lactating mothers. Emphasis has also been placed on the nutritional needs of the adolescent and adult under normal and special conditions such as stress and physical performance.

Nutrition and Our Overpopulated Planet

By

SOHAN L. MANOCHA

Yerkes Regional Primate Research Center
Emory University
Atlanta, Georgia

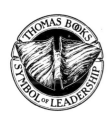

CHARLES C THOMAS • **PUBLISHER**
Springfield • *Illinois* • *U.S.A.*

Published and Distributed Throughout the World by

CHARLES C THOMAS • PUBLISHER

Bannerstone House

301–327 East Lawrence Avenue, Springfield, Illinois, U.S.A.

© *1975, by* CHARLES C THOMAS • PUBLISHER

ISBN 0-398-03180-0 cloth   0-398-03181-9 paper

Library of Congress Catalog Card Number: 74 5206

With THOMAS BOOKS *careful attention is given to all details of
manufacturing and design. It is the Publisher's desire to present books
that are satisfactory as to their physical qualities and artistic possibilities
and appropriate for their particular use.* THOMAS BOOKS *will be true
to those laws of quality that assure a good name and good will.*

Library of Congress Cataloging in Publication Data

Manocha, Sohan L
    Nutrition and our overpopulated planet.

    1. Nutrition.   2. Food supply.   3. Population.
I. Title. [DNLM: 1. Nutrition.   2. Nutrition
disorders.   3. Population growth.   QU145 M285n 1974]
TX353.M29   338.1'9   74-5206
ISBN 0-398-03180-0
ISBN 0-398-03181-9 (pbk.)

Printed in the United States of America

CC-II

Directed toward thinking people of all socioeconomic strata in all countries, rich and poor, this monograph attempts to highlight the nutritional requirements of various age groups and the relationship between the available food supply and the number of mouths laying claim to it. The ultimate solution to the present dilemma of population and food supplies lies in halting explosive population growth, implementing programs of nutrition education, developing more equitable distribution of food supplies both between and within societies and reorienting our concept of a balanced diet based on more complete usage of varieties of food products of vegetable and animal origin, including unconventional synthetic foods. Educated laymen will find the chapters on nutritional needs of the various age groups as well as the causes and effects of obesity and malnutrition both interesting and useful in helping to improve their concept of a balanced diet. Students of sociology, anthropology, nutrition, medicine, biology, political science and history will find this book both valuable and informative.

Doctor Manocha, a noted authority in the field of nutrition, has authored another book on the subject entitled MALNUTRITION AND RETARDED HUMAN DEVELOPMENT also published by Charles C Thomas. *Pediatric Herald* has this to say about it: " . . . there is so much important information in this volume that it can and should be recommended to all interested in eradicating malnutrition throughout the world."

o
H. Bourne
and an eminent
his 65th Birthday

PREFACE

The real implications of the shrinkage in the size of our world are not yet quite apparent to most of the human beings all over the world. They still seem to live in their own little worlds, unimpressed by what happens beyond their national borders. This reflects a false sense of security. The truth is that people living in one part of the world cannot remain unaffected by the events happening elsewhere. An energy crisis in one country affects the lives of individuals living in another. A famine or drought in one area will have repercussions in the lives of people living elsewhere. In this context, the consequences of a rapid increase in the human population in the developing nations cannot remain the sole concern of those countries only. Significant improvements in medical, public health, and social services over the last few decades have drastically reduced mortality rates without changing those of fertility.

Today we have 80 percent of the net growth in human numbers being contributed by the poorer countries of the world. India alone adds fourteen million babies every year. The result is an unprecedented population explosion which threatens to further degrade the quality of human life. It is becoming evident that the overpopulated, overcrowded countries cannot feed their growing numbers from their own resources. If this rate of growth continues, it is doubtful if they will be able to control by themselves the social, economic and political consequences that may follow. There is widespread, chronic undernutrition among the children of the poor. A citizen of a developing country uses as little as 450 pounds of grain per year, while the per capita consumption in the United States is more than one ton. This gap widens each year.

In order to earn cash from the rich countries, the poorer ones sell away precious food items which could go a long way towards improving the dietary standards of their own people. India sells to the West a significant quantity of seafood to earn some foreign exchange. Until the Peruvian anchovy fisheries failed, Peru and Chile exported fish meal to the United States in quantities that could have met the entire animal protein requirements of their countries.

Yet, in the United States, the fish meal was fed to chickens and other animals. Animals in the developed countries eat a better, more nutritionally balanced diet than two thirds of the human population in the poorer nations. The imbalance between the rich and poor countries is all the more glaring in in terms of consumption of resources. The United States, with 6 percent of the population, consumes more than 33 percent of the world's resources. The western countries of Europe and Russia are also continuously running a race with the United States in increasing their share of resource consumption. Over the last few decades, the developed countries have used more resources than the entire world in a million years! At this point in history, overpopulation of humans in one part of the world and excessive use of material resources in the other have brought the human species to a point where a rational decision has to be made in order to maintain some decent standard of quality of human life. The population dilemma is real. We cannot close our eyes to it. Whatever it takes—free contraceptives, abortions, delayed marriages, or mandatory sterilization—human numbers must be stabilized. What is at stake is the supreme position of the human in the animal kingdom as an intelligent, progressive, and forward-looking species. I sincerely hope that we or our future generations may not see the day when the strain of intolerable overcrowding, coupled with widespread malnutrition and material misery, may force us, like lemmings, into some form of mass self-destruction.

This monograph brings to attention the intimate relationship between nutrition, population and the task of feeding the masses. It also emphasizes the need for the knowledge of nutrition for special age groups. We must learn to get the maximum nutritive value from our food resources. Infants and preschool children are vulnerable groups. Feeding them in an adequate manner should be our prime concern because the shape of tomorrow's world depends largely on how we raise our children today. Emphasis is also made on the nutritional needs of the adolescent and adult under normal and special conditions such as stress, physical performance, pregnancy and lactation. Special attention has been paid to the nutritional needs of the latter group.

This monograph is directed to the thinking people of all socio-economic stratas in all countries, rich and poor. From our first breath to the last, we depend on nutrition for sustenance, and it is only fitting that we must know the nutritional requirements of various age groups as well as the relationship between available food and the number of mouths that lay claim to it. It is hoped that the educated layman will find the chapters on nutritional needs of the various age groups, as well as the causes and effects of obesity and malnutrition, interesting and useful in helping to improve his or her concept of a balanced diet. The author sincerely hopes that the students of sociology, anthropology, nutrition, medicine, biology, political science and history will also find the book interesting and informative.

S. L. MANOCHA

ACKNOWLEDGMENTS

It is one of the most pleasant tasks in this venture to get the opportunity to extend my heartfelt thanks to a few individuals whose help went a long way in producing this book. My grateful thanks are due to Dr. G. H. Bourne, informal discussions with whom inspired the writing of this monograph. To Dr. K. K. Vijai, I am very thankful for his critical evaluations of the rough pages of the manuscript and his valuable suggestions. To Mr. Otto Schaler, chief population and health branch AID, Washington, D.C., I am deeply thankful for his many useful suggestions. Special thanks go to Mrs. Peggy Plant, who with meticulous, painstaking care and deep interest, typed the manuscript, to Mrs. Nellie Johns, who helped me greatly in the library work, and to Mrs. Michel Bowen Adams for her painstaking care in correcting the galleys.

Thanks are also due to Dr. Carlin Pinkstaff, Dr. T. R. Shantha, Dr. P. V. Rao, Mr. William Bouris and Miss Manorma Pandit, for their reading of different parts of the manuscript and for making helpful corrections. It is also a pleasure to acknowledge the help of Mrs. Helen C. Wells for her artwork and Mr. Frank Kiernan for his help in photography and format. To the various authors, whose material I have quoted in the text at appropriate places, I extend my gratitude. I must also express my deepest appreciation to my wife, Swaran, and children, Anuj and Atul, without whose cooperation, patience, and sweetness I could not spend countless evenings and weekends in isolation to pour my thoughts on this book.

Finally, it is a great pleasure and privilege to acknowledge the assistance of the following authors and publishers, whose material has gone a long way towards improving the text and the contents of this volume: the U.S. Department of State for Figure 1; The Sciences, The New York Academy of Sci-

ences for Figure 2; Dr. D. Meadows and The Universe Books
for Figures 3 and 4; Dr. Ernst Jokl and Charles C Thomas
for Figure 5; Prof. S. Chandrasekhara for Table I; Dr. D. B.
Jelliffe for Table II; Dr. E. M. Widdowson for Table III;
Drs. R. MacKeith and C. Wood and J. A. Churchill, London,
for Table IV; Dr. C. H. Robinson and The Macmillan Co.
for Table V; Food and Nutrition Board, National Academy
of Sciences, National Research Council for Tables VI and
VIII; Dr. I. McDonald for Table VII; Drs. A. M. Thomson
and F. E. Hytten and S. Karger for Table IX; Dr. R. M. Hill
and C. V. Mosby Co. for Table X; Prof. Jean Mayer for Table
XI; Population Reference Bureau Inc. for Appendix I; and
Dr. P. L. Altman and The Federation of American Societies
for Experimental Biology for the material in Table IV and
Appendices II and III.

The author acknowledges with appreciation the help of
Grant No. RR-00165 from the Animal Resources Branch of
the National Institutes of Health to Yerkes Regional Primate
Research Center.

S.L.M.

TABLE OF CONTENTS

Nutrition and
Our Overpopulated
Planet

CHAPTER 1

NUTRITION AND OUR OVERPOPULATED PLANET

PATTERN OF HUMAN POPULATION GROWTH

MAN ENTERED the cosmic scene about a million years ago and soon demonstrated his ability to survive and flourish in spite of the dangers from predators and wild animals. Endowed with the largest brain size of all the creatures in the animal kingdom, man systematically began to master this planet. He successfully killed his enemies, the wild animals, and domesticated a large number of them to serve him and provide food for him. However, there were certain types of animals which he could not master until recently, and which always seemed to control his numbers in spite of his fertility. These animals are the organisms which cause such epidemics as cholera, plague, tuberculosis, small-pox, and a host of diseases which took a heavy toll of human life throughout its history. The infectious diseases proved a major factor in the growth and genetic composition of populations because they eliminated a high proportion of those attacked before or during the reproductive period (Allison, 1973).

There is a variety of guessworks and estimates about the number of human beings in the prehistoric era, but there is a consensus of opinion that up to the mid-Seventeenth Century, about 300 years ago, the human population was not more than half a billion. This is indeed a very slow rate of growth starting from about a million, in the year 300,000 B.C. (Table I). It is estimated that the human population at

3

the beginning of the Christian era was around 250 million people; it took about 1,650 years to double this number to half a billion people. It was mainly because the laws of nature that governed the population numbers of other animals applied, to a great extent, to humans as well. The birth rate was high but the death rate was almost equally high, with the result that the net addition to the population was insignificant.

In the middle Seventeenth Century the world population was growing at the rate of approximately 0.3 percent annually. However, during this period some extremely important changes were taking place in man's understanding of the universe. The most important was man's understanding of the numerous organisms that were responsible for killing large numbers of children in their early period of life, as well as those which afflicted the adults. The science of medicine had started to show maturity, with the result that human lives which were needlessly wasted began to be saved. Man started proliferating faster, and by the year 1830 he touched the first billion mark. After that, it took him less than 100 years to double this number. The human population touched two billion by the year 1925.

Thereafter, it took the humans only 35 years to add another billion to their numbers and by 1960 the human population reached the three billion mark. It was a matter of great achievement for the human species to be able to master this planet in a manner reflected by its rate of proliferation. During the same time, most mammalian species dwindled in their number unless they had the patronage and the protection of man.

In modern times, the death rate has been drastically reduced and the net growth rate is over 2.0 percent, which means that it will need only 35 years to double the population. In countries where the growth rate is 3 percent, it takes only 25 years to double their numbers. From this it is evident that over the last few hundred years of human existence, not only the population in terms of numbers has been growing exponentially, but the rate of growth has also been growing.

TABLE I

GROWTH OF HUMAN POPULATION FROM 1 MILLION B.C. TO A.D. 2000
Man enters the cosmic scene—a little over a million years ago

Approximate period or year		Total population
B.C.	1,000,000	125,000
	300,000	1 million (and the following numbers are in millions)
	25,000	5
	8000	10
	1000	100
A.D.	1	250
	1500	300
	1650	565
	1700	623
	1750	728
	1800	906
	1830	1,000 (first billion)
	1850	1,194
	1900	1,608
	1920	1,811
	1925	2,000 (second billion)
	1930	2,015
	1940	2,249
	1950	2,509
	1960	3,008 (third billion)
	1970 (estimate)	3,500
	1975 (projection)	4,000 (fourth billion)
	2000 (projection)	6,000 to 7,000

From S. Chandrasekhra, *Infant Mortality Population Growth and Family Planning in India* (Chapel Hill, University of North Carolina Press 1972).

Meadows, *et al.* used the word "super-exponential" to describe this kind of growth rate (Meadows, 1972) (Fig.1). This super-exponential growth has been possible mainly because of man's control over nature and his environment and because of countless innovations in the health sciences which alleviated suffering, prolonged life, postponed death and increased the expectation of life at birth from about 25 years in 1750 to more than 74 years in advanced countries today (Chandrasekhra, 1972).

However, the question arises: Is it really an achievement to conquer the checks and balances that nature has provided for most of the species to keep their population at a certain level so that it does not disturb the ecological balance of this planet? Starting from a 3 billion number in 1960, man threatens to reach 6 or 7 billion before the end of this century.

Is this uncontrolled proliferation a mark of triumph over nature, or is it a race towards ultimate suicide when the limited room on this planet will simply not be able to accommodate another hungry mouth? At the present time, every time the clock ticks, day or night, there are additional hungry mouths to lay claim to our scarce food resources. Every day we add more than 170,000 people to the existing population; that is, every year about 130 million babies tip-toe their way into our world. A maximum of 60 million persons of all age groups say good-bye, leaving us with a net addition of some 70 million to the existing population. "This is population explosion—par excellence!" (Chandrasekhra 1972).

POPULATION DILEMMA OF THE MODERN WORLD

Although the population explosion is a global phenomenon, the rate of population growth varies from continent to continent, country to country, and region to region. In most countries belonging to the developed regions, the population growth has greatly slowed down and some, like West Germany, East Germany, and Luxembourg, have actually stabilized their populations. Reduced birth rates in the industrialized countries are the result of a long historical process which has led to a drastic reduction in the rate of mortality and has promoted a voluntary birth control among all sections except the very poor (Woodham, 1971). In the developing countries, on the other hand, the mortality rate has significantly dropped without any change in the birth rate with the result that over the last two decades there has been a phenomenal increase in their populations. Eighty percent (55 million out of a total of 70 million) of the annual increase in the human population takes place in the developing countries. India alone is adding 13 million persons a year, which is more than the entire population of the Australian subcontinent. A small country like Mexico is adding more to the world population than the United States. The Philippines add more people each year than does Japan. Brazil adds to its existing population 2.6 million people every year, and this presents an interesting contrast with the Soviet Union

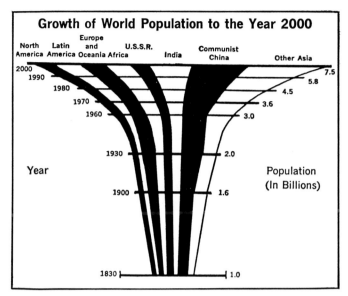

Figure 1. Growth of world population to the year 2000.

which adds 2.9 million yearly to its population (Brown, 1973). (See Appendix I)

It is only natural then that there is an ever-increasing demand for larger and larger quantities of food in the developing countries because they have to feed significantly more hungry mouths with each passing year. The result is that most of their economic growth or increased food output is eaten away by the growing populations with little progress in raising the per capita consumption, which is extremely low as compared to the developed countries.

It has been estimated that by the turn of the Century, 85 percent of the world population growth will occur in Africa, Asia and Latin America. In the year 2000, these areas will have 80 percent of all the world population. Whereas the population in the developed countries is likely to increase by about 50 percent, the population in the developing countries where food is scarce will increase by more than 100 percent (Williams, 1966). Asia and the Far East have experienced a unique degree of population explosion, but this has not always been the case. During the period of 1800 to 1900, the population grew by about 50 percent, which is quite comparable to what happened over the rest of the world. However, the Twentieth Century witnessed a sudden explosion of population in Asia which was brought about by the declining death rate and an unaffected birth rate. The net result is that during the 100 years between 1900 and 2000, the population of Asia and the Far East is expected to increase by as much as 400 percent. This phenomenon has been aided by traditional sociocultural set-ups of these old societies. Certain social factors that have a strong sway on the minds of these traditional cultures have not only contributed to this kind of growth, but are not likely to be helpful in reducing this growth rate in the near future. The agrarian pattern of economic set-up still persists and the family is still the primary producing unit. The network of kinship obligation remains unaltered and there is no satisfactory substitute for the children as a source of old age security. Production methods are still labor intensive and larger families still think of extra children as additional income.

Contraceptive distribution programs or contraceptive education can only help prevent unnecessary pregnancies, but unless some drastic changes take place in the mode of living, the desired number of living children per couple is going to continue to be high (Hawley, 1973). An average family norm in most of the developing countries is still five or more children. This type of demographic growth has led to certain changes in the composition of the population. Approximately 20 percent of the population is under five years old, and for the majority of the countries fully 50 percent of the population is under 15 years of age. In West Africa, between the 1960 to 1970 decade, the population under 15 years of age grew from 45 to more than 50 percent (Sai, 1973). The youth population between the ages of 15 and 24 in Asia is expected to be 90 million higher in 1980 than in 1970. As existing educational and training facilities in most developing countries are inadequate to meet current demands, this increase will have serious implications for the countries in which high rates of underemployment and unemployment already prevail. The children who will enter the youth ages are already born and deserve the immediate attention of government administrations and planners. (Asian Student, 1972).

It is this pattern of growth that is likely to determine the shape of things and the destiny of a vast majority of human beings in the future. More than two thirds of the population is crowded in Asia, with China and India topping the list. Whereas not much reliable data is available from China because of its close political set-up, the conditions in India are to some extent a reflection of the situation in most of the developing countries in Asia, Africa and Latin America. India has only 2.4 percent of the total land area, but houses 14 percent of the world's population. The land area is likely to stay the same but the percentage of human numbers is changing unfavorably.

The overpopulation or overcrowding of the Asian subcontinent is nothing new. Even in the prehistoric times the population was considerable in Asia as compared to the rest of the world. Asia is the cradle of ancient civilization and as time passed, it became the cradle of larger and larger numbers of human beings. According to various estimates, the population of India was between 100 and 140 million around 300 B.C., (Davis, 1959; Nath, 1929) and it stayed almost the same up to the year 1600. Moreland estimated the Indian population at the death of Emperor Akbar in 1605 to be around 100 to 130 million (Moreland, 1920). It is clear from these figures that India has been the home of large sections of the human race from ancient times. In 1600, the world population was around 500 million and India housed more than 20 percent of this population. During this period, the number of births and deaths was approximately equal and the population did not rise significantly. However, starting from the medieval ages, the population of India showed a steady increase. The number of births significantly exceeded the number of deaths, reaching the present stage of 21 million births and eight million deaths, leaving a net of 13 million people to add to the already very large pool of human numbers.

Between 1951 to 1961, India added 78.1 million people to its population and between 1961 to 1971, it added 108 million people, adding up to a gigantic figure of 550 million by 1971. In other words, between 1951 and 1971, India added to its population, the numbers roughly equivalent to the total population of the United States of America at that time. With the present rate of declining death rate and a somewhat stationary birth rate, it is very likely that the population of India may reach one billion before the turn of the Century, which means that the total human population of 1830 will be jammed in a single country comprising only 2.4 percent of the land area of this planet. While all this explosion is going on, there is no reason to think that the average Indian is very much aware of the 13 to 14 million more Indians who will be inhabiting his subcontinent a year from now (Sai, 1973).

It is indeed irrelevant to engage at this point in human history in an argument of whether or not our planet now has more human beings than it can afford to provide a decent living. The majority of the existing populations live in a substandard fashion. We are swamped by socio-economic and political problems caused directly by our overcrowded situation. Our social standards have been significantly lowered, and increasing the *people input* during the next 26 years, before we greet our next century will only aggravate our existing problems. Now is the time when we should seriously plan for our future growth, not only for our sake, but for our future generations as well. A vigorous and imaginative planning in the field of population may not help us substantially now, but it will certainly give us some time to work for their solutions in the future (Pion, 1971).

The findings of the Commission on Population and American Future can be quite illustrative of the socio-economic consequences of a growing population. In 1972, with 2.3 children per family, the U.S. population was 209 million.

If this figure is reduced to 2 children per family, the U.S. population in the year 2000 will be an ideal 271 million, but it will jump to 322 million in the same period if the family norm is changed from 2 to 3 children. In the year 2020, with a 2 child family norm, the U.S. population will grow to 307 million, but with a 3 child family norm it will jump to 447 million, which poses a real population dilemma for the country.

Let us examine the socio-economic consequences of average 2 and 3 children families in the United States by the year 2000. With a 2 child family norm, there will be 75 million people under 18 years of age, 167 million between 18 and 64, and 29 million over 64. There will be 62 dependents per 100 people. All would get better education than they get today. Water shortages may be apparent in one third of the country, but there will be little pressure on food prices because of population. The average family income will be more than $20,000, and per capita income will be 15 percent higher than today.

Now, let us measure the same socio-economic parameters of a 3 child family norm in the year 2000. The population will be 322 million, out of which 114 million will be under 18 years of age, 179 million between 18 and 64, and 29 million over 64. There will be 80 dependents per 100 people. The population will never stabilize; instead, it would double in 45 years. Only 7 percent of all students would receive a better education than now. One half of the country would be short of water. The price indices would be 40 to 50 percent higher because of the greater cost of producing food on low quality land. The per capita income will not rise. Between 1990 and 2000, 44 million new workers will be looking for jobs. Because of the greater percentage of young people in the population, there will be a heavy pressure on the outdoor recreation facilities (Commission on Population and American Future). It is evident, therefore, that decreasing average family size from three to two will reduce expenditures for education, health, and other services by billions of dollars and would provide more options for resource utilization (Lebowitz, 1973a). The conclusions arrived at by the U.S. Commission on Population Growth are very enlightening.

> In the case of the larger population—with less land per person and more people to accommodate—there are fewer alternatives, less room for diversity, less room for error. To cope with continued growth, technology must advance; life styles must change. Slower population growth offers us the difference between choice and necessity, between prudence and living dangerously (U.S. News and World Report).

Applying these living standards to the entire human population all over the world may be appropriate and absurd at the same time. It is appropriate because the above account gives a clear picture of consequences of the addition of one extra child to the 2 child family norm. It is absurd because 80 percent of the population cannot yet think of the material standards enjoyed by the industrialized countries, and because their family norm at the present time is 5 children or more. It is going to require gigantic efforts to reduce, not only the size of the average family, but also to improve the quality of their life by providing the blessings of material happiness. It is generally agreed that the developing countries, left to themselves, will never be able on their own to bridge this gap between themselves and the richer nations of the world. It has to be global human effort to raise the quality of human life all over the world. The former Secretary-General of the United Nations, U. Thant, expressed his fears in these words.

> I don't wish to seem overdramatic, but I can only conclude from the information that is available to me as Secretary-General, that the members of the United Nations have perhaps ten years left in which to subordinate their ancient quarrels and launch a global partnership to curb the arms race, to improve the human environment, to diffuse the population explosion, and to supply the required momentum to development efforts. If such a global partnership is not forged within the next decade, then I very much fear that the problems I have mentioned will have reached such staggering proportions that they will be beyond our capacity to control.

An exhaustive study of the limits to growth on this

planet was conducted by Meadows, *et al.* under the auspices of the Club of Rome. This group investigated, with computer models, the limits to exponential growth of capital and population, as well as technology, as related to limits to growth and concluded that:

> 1. If the present growth trends in world population, industrialization, pollution, food production, and resource depletion continue unchanged, the limits to growth on this planet will be reached sometime within the next one hundred years. The most probable result will be a rather sudden and uncontrollable decline in both population and industrial capacity.
>
> 2. It is possible to alter these growth trends and to establish a condition of ecological and economic stability that is sustainable far into the future. The state of global equilibrium could be designed so that the basic material needs of each person on earth are satisfied and each person has an equal opportunity to realize this individual human potential.
>
> 3. If the world's people decide to strive for this second outcome rather than the first, the sooner they begin working to attain it, the greater will be their chances of success. (See page 83 for more details.)

NUTRITION STATUS AS RELATED TO POPULATION GROWTH

State of Nutrition—Its Impact on Human Welfare

Throughout human history, man has suffered miseries because of lack of food to eat. There have been numerous famines which resulted in the deaths of millions of people. In 436 B.C., the Roman Empire was in the grips of a terrible famine and thousands of starving Romans threw themselves into the Tiber River. Between 108 B.C. and 1911 A.D., as many as 1,828 famines have been reported from China. Between 10 A.D. and 1846 A.D., 201 famines have been reported from the British Isles. India has suffered a great many famines. In 1770, a severe famine in Bengal wiped out one third of the entire population (Paarlberg, 1973). The modern world, with its technology and mass communications, has made mass deaths due to starvation somewhat improbable. There have been droughts and crop failures, cyclones and political upheavals during the last two decades in many parts of the world, but deaths due to starvation have been rare.

In 1965 to 1967, India experienced the worst drought in a century, yet massive food shipments from the United States prevented deaths by starvation. In 1971, Bangla Desh went through a political upheaval and 10 million destitute refugees crossed into India, and yet there were no deaths by starvation. In 1972 to 1974, six African countries suffered untold miseries due to starvation and yet not many died. All this does not mean that we have conquered hunger. As a matter of fact, due to the phenomenal growth in population, there is more hunger today than was ever experienced by mankind. It is not in the form of starvation and death. It is in the form of chronic undernutrition, which leaves a person so much debilitated that he succumbs to minor infections. Hunger prevents millions of children from achieving their growth and achievement potential. In nations where large numbers suffer from undernutrition, socio-economic and cultural development is greatly hurt. While some progress is being made to grow two blades of grass where one grew before, the addition to food output is eaten away by a pouring stream of new arrivals. Consequently, the nutrition status of more than two thirds of the human population is less than satisfactory.

About 60 percent of the human population, most of which belongs to the underdeveloped or developing countries of the world, is undernourished or inadequately fed. Not only do these humans not get adequate amounts of proteins, vitamins and minerals essential for body building growth and physical well-being, but they fail to get adequate numbers of calories in order to meet their energy needs. Most countries in Africa and Asia provide less than 2,000 calories per capita and a sizeable proportion of their population is in real terms perpetually hungry (Fig. 2). If this is the case today with a world population of less than 4 billion, we must give serious thought to the problem of human nutrition during the next three decades when the numbers are

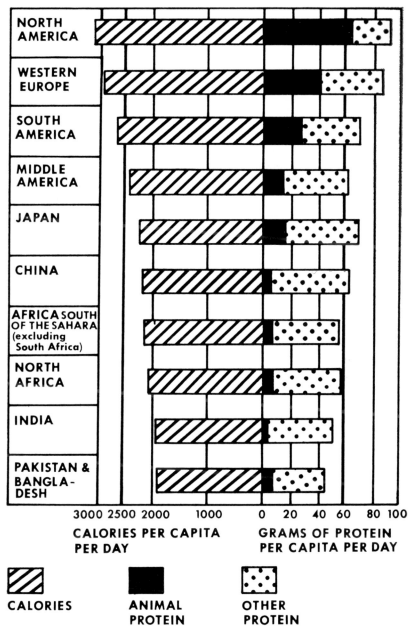

Figure 2. A comparative picture of the diets of rich and poor nations. If 2,500 calories and 60 grams of protein per capita per day is considered a desirable food intake for an adult male, more than two thirds of the present population is undernourished. Can we improve the dietary standards of the existing population if, at the same time, we continue adding approximately 70 million extra hungry mouths every year?

likely to double at the present rate of 2 percent per year (Allison, 1973).

The world food panel of the United States President's Science Advisory Committee (Bennett, 1969) rightly concluded as early as 1967 that hunger and malnutrition and the so-called population explosion are not the primary issues of the developing countries. They are, in fact, the symptoms of an underlying malady — *lagging economic development*. The panel strongly urged all the rich nations to extend to the poor nations a commitment for long range, coordinated action, dedicated to the systematic solution of a series of interrelated problems, none of which can be solved in isolation from its cousins. Until that is done, the situation is likely to continue to worsen steadily and the poorer nations will never be able on their own to come out of the present mess in which they find themselves.

It is a strange paradox that the agriculture in the developing countries accounts for a large fraction of the gross national product and accounts for more than half the total labor force, yet for the majority the standard of living today is lower than it was ten years ago. (Berg, 1973; Berg and Muscat, 1972). In these countries, the annual per capita availability of grain is around 400 pounds, most of which is directly consumed by the people in the form of food in order to supply their energy and protein needs. In the developed countries, the annual per capita availability of grain is extremely high — as much as one ton per person per year in the U.S.A. and Canada, out of which only 150 pounds per person per year are utilized as food and the rest is fed to the animals from which meat, milk, eggs, etc., are obtained as food. These are the needs of affluence. It has been estimated that the grains are utilized directly as food until the per capita income approaches $500 per year, whereupon it begins to decrease, but simultaneously the need for feed grain increases at a much faster rate to get the animal products for food. "The agricultural resources — land, water, fertilizer— required to support an average North American are nearly five times those of an average Indian, Nigerian or Colombian (Brown, 1973). In the United States, the demand for the food grains has been sharply rising over the last three decades. This is indicated from the rise in per capita consumption of beef from 55 pounds in 1940 to 117 pounds in 1972. Poultry consumption rose from 18 pounds to 51 pounds during the same period.

With a population of close to 600 million people, India needs about 125 million tons of food grain to meet the annual needs at the present level of food consumption, which by any standard is unsatisfactory. In 1971, the production was around 108 million tons, but dropped to 100 million tons in 1972 due to drought. The population during the same period rose by 14 million people. In 1985, India's population is likely to be 800 million requiring at least 170 million tons of food grains to feed them at the present level of nutrition. What if a severe drought or natural calamity strikes the subcontinent at that time causing a shortage of 40 million tons of food grains? Probably the entire food reserves of the world would not be able to avert a catastrophe. It is likely that the shadow of famine will continue to threaten the Indian subcontinent if adequate population control measures are not instituted now.

In spite of the population growing at a fast rate in the developing countries, the food situation over the last two decades has been fairly stable, if not comfortable. This has been mainly because of the surpluses of some of the major exporting countries such as the U.S.A., Canada, Australia and Argentina. But, unfortunately, things have changed in 1972 to 1973, and are not likely to improve in 1973 to 1974 because Russia and China have emerged as extra major buyers in addition to the traditional customers. Food deficits are now a world-wide phenomenon. Even the U.S. citizens are feeling a pinch in their budget due to soaring food prices. In this context, it has become a very costly affair for the traditionally deficient developing countries to import food.

Governments of developing countries will find this year that the soaring prices of food grains and freight rates have driven their imported

food bills up by 60 percent or roughly $2 billion, a drain on foreign
reserves which, should it continue, threatens to retard economic development and make the gap between rich nations and poor grow
faster still. Much besides the threat of famine, therefore, hinges upon
the ability of developing countries to make crop yields grow faster
than people (Wade, 1973).

The inevitable questions come up. Can these poor countries feed their ever-increasing numbers? Can the developed
countries afford to be satisfied with stabilizing their own numbers and letting the developing countries suffer from their
economics of chronic food shortages and increasing numbers of mouths laying claim to their limited food supplies?
In this small interdependent world, can the human numbers
swell beyond a certain limit in one part without affecting
the fortunes of those living in more comfortable homes?
These are some of the questions that we must try to answer.
As things stand today, most of the overcrowded countries
have adapted so well to overcrowding, living on a subsistence
diet and accepting a certain amount of death among their infants as normal, that they don't feel that they are the ones
who are overcrowding the planet. Although the officialdom
of the government of India and some other countries recognize the need for curtailing the astronomical growth rate,
they seem to be least alarmed about it. They exhibit a growing sense of optimism that they can produce food faster than
the rate of population growth. For example, an Indian official would tell you that India has doubled its output of food
during the last twenty years and this rate of growth is likely
to be accelerated as the "Green Revolution" (production of
larger quantities of food by scientific farming utilizing modern irrigation facilities and fertilizers) is extended to all
parts of the country. A Philippino or another representative
of Southeast Asia will give similar figures. They will politely
tell you that, although we are not complacent about it, there
is no need to be alarmed because the food production is keeping pace with the growth in population, and every new arrival
will have ample to eat.
However, few knowledgeable people feel that way. Dr.

Chandrasekhra, the former Minister of Health and Family Planning of the government of India, is more pragmatic. Discussing the Indian situation, he believes that "there is no reason to believe that conditions have improved. If anything, because of the enormous increase in the country's population without any comparable increase in resources, educational and health facilities, or the monthly income of poor rural families, the malnutrition of mothers and children in India today must be a little worse." In India, while the total food output doubled, from 50 million tons to 100 million tons, between 1950 and 1970, the per capita net availability of food grains increased by only 18 percent. Even this increase did not put an average Indian in the category of a person who satisfies his daily nutritional needs from the point of view of quality as well as quantity. Whereas the minimum requirement of nutritional intake is 18 ounces per day, the average Indian, with his spectacular doubling of food output, gets only 14.4 ounces, which is 82 percent of his needed caloric requirements. The vulnerable groups (pregnant and nursing mothers and children) get the largest share of such a scarcity. Most of the increased food output goes to feed the new arrivals, while maintaining or slightly lowering the living standards of the existing population.

Yet, when we pose the question of whether we can feed the growing numbers, we just don't think in terms of providing them bread, rice or beans; we are also thinking in terms of an enlightened citizenry who is capable of widening the horizon of human knowledge and pushing ahead the growth of *human civilization*. Chandrasekhra, while calculating the needs of the 13 million population which, at present, is being added annually by India to its population, stressed that "to provide for the net annual addition of some 13 million, the country needs resources to the tune of 126,500 schools, 372,500 teachers, 5.9 million housing units, 188 million meters of cloth, 12,545 quintals of food, 4 million jobs, etc." When a country fails to provide these needs the result is that there is a "high percentage of illiteracy, inadequate housing facilities, urban deterioration, rural blight, overcrowding and pollution of a primitive kind, dislocation at individual and group levels, and a general air of distemper and dissatisfaction (Chandrasekhra, 1972).

Can Agricultural Technology Feed the Growing Human Population?

Optimism and confidence are the essential qualities that make the human species the dominant one in the animal kingdom. We cannot give ourselves to despair. The human ingenuity in producing food has shown itself in ample measure in spite of the unchecked population growth. There is every reason to believe that as long as man maintains his grasp on the technology and keeps on improving it, he is not going to starve. It will not be surprising that, as the use of technology in agriculture widens, especially in the developing countries, the human population will be better fed than ever before. The Malthusian forecasts have not come true so far, and may not come true in the future. With the growing use of technology, most of the developing countries are gaining confidence in their ability to produce extra food. An increasing amount of food is becoming available from the increased use of fertilizers, genetically improved crops, and higher yielding varieties of cereals and other food grains. At this stage, some of the most populous countries of Asia, Africa and Latin America are using a very small fraction of fertilizers as compared to Japan and industrialized countries of the West, and therefore possess a great potential for increases in food output on the same area which is under cultivation at present.

There are a number of other advances in agriculture that have yet to be applied on a large scale. Every one of these advances could prove a major breakthrough in its own right. For example, the identification of necessary trace elements and their incorporation into fertilizers and feeds has opened vast areas not only in plant cultivation, but in animal husbandry as well. Selective breeding of plants and animals has led to the development of varieties of species which could provide increased yields as well as greater resistance to infection. Aside from better nutrients, machines can be put to use to do the work which humans cannot do as well. Already in the field of poultry production, computers are programmed "to calculate the cheapest method providing a diet of known energy and known content in ten essential amino acids, total protein, and other nutrients, automatically set the controls that will mix basic staples providing the cheapest adequate poultry diet (Mayer, 1972).

The application of agricultural science and technology is progressively increasing in most countries these days. As a matter of fact, scientific research in the field of agriculture is much more advanced than what is being applied in the field. Pilot research projects of great promise are in progress which can produce food in vast quantities. Petroleum products are being used to produce fatty acids and proteins. Some of the plants such as algae, which hitherto were considered useless, are showing great promise as food. The unconventional modes of food production will become familiar (for details, see the next chapter). The oceans are an almost inexhaustible supply of foodstuffs at the disposal of man. Taking algae as an example, with proper fertilization and removal of the finished products, the efficient mode of photosynthesis by the algae can be put to maximum use and as little as one square meter may produce enough to meet the nutritional needs of one human being. Protein from petroleum is now becoming a reality and so are concentrated protein isolates from vegetable and animal sources which, at present, are not considered as foods.

Even in terms of production of traditional foods, if new agricultural technology is more extensively used, the increase in per acre yield will be economically more attractive than the cost of bringing new lands under cultivation. This is also understandable from the point of view of limits to expanding the area under cultivation, as more and more land will be needed for social needs such as roads, schools, hospitals, residential and industrial purposes. In addition to increasing the yield per acre, growing more than one or two crops per year on the same land will be easy. Multiple cropping is not a new concept. It has been used for centuries, but modern research has produced varieties that can be harvested with more than traditional yields in lesser time, occasionally half as much time as may be needed for that particular crop. This can facilitate raising one more crop than is possible with the traditional method of multiple cropping. For example, a new high-yield variety grain, IR-5, a Philippine developed rice, has cut the growing time of the most popular high-yielding variety, IR-8, from 120 days to 90 days. This is in comparison to 180 days required by the traditional varieties, which means that two crops instead of one can be raised in the same period of time (Dalrymple, 1971).

Thus there are optimists who do not see any catastrophic danger in the ever-increasing world population or the rate at which it is growing at present. They feel that food technology and industrial science will always keep pace with the human numbers. Luce, while commenting on the challenge of the future, maintained that it is physically and technically possible to produce enough food for all in every nation. "We have opened the door into a universe of boundless energy and our problems, which are problems of abundance, can be solved by education and in particular political education, because good government promotes material welfare" (Luce, 1966). Bogue similarly expressed great optimism in man's ability to produce large quantities of extra food so as to chase away scarcity, hunger and undernutrition within a decade or two (Bogue, 1969).

Before we are carried away by the prospects of producing unlimited quantities of food by the use of technology, we must assess the present situation in a realistic manner. Agricultural technology in its advanced form, which can no doubt help, is in the hands of developed countries, which are quite comfortable in their food supply as far as their own needs are concerned. It will be self-defeating if those who own the technology at present should grow extra food and give it or sell it to those who cannot produce adequate food. It will create socio-economic and political upheavals of the greatest magnitude. The need is to transfer the technology to places where the extra food is needed. Let us think for a moment about the cost of transportation in the event food is transferred from a surplus country such as the United States to a needy country in Asia. Besides the sea transportation through huge ships, the cost of grain can be doubled in those countries where means of overland transport is minimal, if porters are used to carry the food for 75 miles, even at the lowest possible wages (Clark, 1963). The ability of the developing countries to pay for imported food is so severely limited that any outflow of capital from their countries is likely to have a crumbling effect on their economies. The ultimate solution to the problem of undernutrition in the developing countries is only by raising their own agriculture to a level that they can produce enough food for themselves. It will not be an easy task to introduce the agricultural technology at a scale demanded by the extra food needs.

The shortage of food in the developing countries can be overcome to a great extent if the agricultural technology used in the developed countries is introduced on a mass scale. It is estimated that the food producing capacity of the earth is many fold more than has been exploited at present. Let us analyze, however, a few factors that could be formidable in realizing our goals. The first requisite is an abundant supply of water. The developing countries depend too much on the rains and do not have an adequate irrigation system which would assure a continuous supply of water for the crops. The failure of monsoon rains in 1965 to 1967, 1971, and 1972 in India created unprecedented drought and huge quantities of food grains had to be imported in order to avoid starvation and famine. Thus an irrigation system is essential to increasing food producing capacity on a constant basis. The development of the irrigation system requires the technology as well as capital investment to build dams, harness the rivers and dig new canals.

The second requisite in order to augment food production in the developing countries is the use of mechanical energy. Most developing countries do not have good sources of mechanical energy (gas and petroleum). Too much depen-

dence on imported sources of energy cannot be conducive
in the long run. These countries need to develop their indig-
enous sources of mechanical energy. Agriculture is still
carried on by harnessing draft animals for tilling the soil.
Mechanically driven tractors need to replace the muscle
power.

The third requisite is the use of agricultural chemicals
in order to improve soil fertility as well as to control pests. If
the nutrients removed from the soil by farming are replaced
by the use of fertilizers, the land will not be depleted and will
continue to produce bumper crops and better yields in order
to meet the needs of the growing populations. The pests
(mainly insects and rodents) eat away or destroy as much as
12 percent of the total food produced in the developing countries. If only these pests can be controlled or eliminated, the
food situation will vastly improve.

Even if these requirements are met, it is quite dangerous to assume that the new technology can double or triple
the food output without any fear of uncertainty. Willett
notes that "even with good irrigation system, multiple cropping requires a high level of managerial skill to coordinate a
series of complex activities; hence it is unlikely that it will
spread quickly to areas where it is not already practiced"
(Willett, 1969). It is not an attempt to override the asser-
tions of those who believe that, if the developing countries
can handle satisfactorily the problems of assured supply of
irrigation, water, fertilizers, new seeds, pesticides, as well
as introduce mechanization in crop handling and storage,
the process of multiple cropping can lead to a substantial increase in food output. Paarlberg stressed that making the
new agricultural technology work for the benefit of man
would require a sustained effort of great magnitude. In addition, "it will require huge increases in adapted production
technology and investments in efficient marketing systems.
Public and private investments in research, teaching and
extension are likewise required as well as the increased participation of private industry in furnishing production req-
uisites and handling the farm output (Paarlberg, 1973).

As things now stand, justified pessimism is coming into vogue. The developing countries are not increasing their agricultural production fast enough. An FAO study indicates that these countries will have to accelerate food production at more than 4 percent per year for the rest of the decade even to continue to feed the population at the present diet level (FAO 1970). Between the years 1962 and 1975, the agricultural production was supposed to increase by 3.4 percent per year. The actual fact is that between 1962 and 1970, the growth rate has been 2.8 percent, dropping from 2 percent in 1971 to 1 percent in 1972. Yields per acre increased only 0.3 percent and much of the growth has been brought about by bringing new land under cultivation. This poor performance is in comparison to 3 percent per acre increase in yield in the developed countries (Pyke, 1968). The United States Department of Agriculture in its report to the President in 1970 made certain projections about the ability of the developing countries to support their populations. Under the assumption that modern technology available in the United States is applied all over the underdeveloped countries and all the land area under cultivation is expanded to the fullest extent, 4.4 billion people can be fed at their present unsatisfactory level of nutrition. However, if the minimal amount of required calories has to be provided, 4.3 billion can be fed and if we want to provide adequate proteins as well, 3.8 billion can be fed (Paarlberg, 1973; U.S.D.A., 1970).

As more and more data regarding the food situation all over the world is analyzed, the optimists have less to say and the pessimists have the sway. The projections of the Food and Agriculture Organization of the United Nations are no less pessimistic. According to these projections, the developing or poor countries of the world, which represent three fourths of the human population, are getting into deeper and deeper trouble as their present growth rate continues. When the population and income factors are combined in these countries, their food demands by 1985 are projected to be 140 percent higher than their 1962 needs, which represents an annual increase of 3.9 percent. However, the actual growth rate has been stable since 1962 at about 2.7 percent. Therefore, a recomputation of the needed per year growth based on 1967 is 4.3 percent, and this gets higher with every passing year (FAO, 1962; FAO, 1970).

This brings us back into the problem of population growth and the ability of the developing countries to feed their populations. At present, the poor nations are gradually compromising the basic human right of the individual and a paramount obligation of the human society, i.e. the provision of nutritionally balanced, adequate quality food for all human beings (Michanek, 1972). A high rate of population growth has a very undesirable effect on the health of the people as well as the economy of the country. The rate of population growth of the developing countries increased from 1 percent in 1900 to 2 percent in 1955, 2.6 percent in 1968, and approximately 2.8 percent in the early 1970's. The annual rate of increase in food output averaged 2.5 percent, which has led to a deterioration of the nutritional status of the populations. Tuncer measured specifically the impact of population growth on the Turkish economy and observed that if the country vigorously implements a program of irrigation, fertilizers, new high-yielding variety seeds and pest control, a credible 3 percent annual increase in wheat production can be achieved. In terms of its availability to the population, if the latter grows by 3 percent, there will be no extra food for anybody and it will stay at the level of 188.2 kg per capita per year. However, if the population increases by 2.6 percent, the approximate current Turkish rate, the per capita availability could go to 215.7 kg by the year 2000, and if the population growth can be brought down to 2 percent, the per capita availability of wheat will be 264.8 kg for the year 2000 (Tuncer, 1968). There can be a significant improvement in nutrition if the population grows at the most desirable rate of 1 percent per year or less. All these calculations, however, depend on the fact that there is no natural or man-made calamity and the food output is continuously increased over the years at the rate of 3 percent.

NEED TO STABILIZE HUMAN POPULATION

It is only fair to say that the problem of overpopulation cannot be solved by technology. We may buy some time developing new strains of wheat or rice to feed the newcomers, but it will not be long before the optimum level of production is reached. Even a century or two is a small period in the life of our planet. A finite world can support only a finite population; therefore, population growth must eventually be brought to zero. Hardin stressed that the most rapidly growing populations on earth today are the most miserable (Hardin, 1968). No one should have the absolute right or the freedom to breed any way he thinks fit and methods mutually agreed upon by the majority of the people have to be adopted to solve the population problem. While describing it as a tragedy of the commons, Hardin described that no technical solution can rescue us from the misery of overpopulation. Freedom to breed will bring ruin to all. While knowing the unpleasant truth about the consequences of overpopulation, we tend to indulge in the luxury of only suggesting conscientious and responsible parenthood instead of taking the hard decision necessary to solve the problem. An appeal to independently acting consciences only leads to the disappearance of all consciences in the long run. If we want to preserve and nurture other more precious freedoms, we can do so by relinquishing the freedom to breed, and that very soon. "Freedom is the recognition of necessity, and it is the role of education to reveal to all the necessity of abandoning the freedom to breed. Only so, can we put an end to this aspect of the tragedy of the commons (Hardin, 1968).

It is now generally agreed that the urge and the ability to plan one's family is the product of economic, social, psychological and other factors. However, when ignorance, illiteracy and poverty are abundant, as is the case in most developing countries, the absence of planned parenthood may be due more to cultural and social factors than to anything else. In the overcrowded countries few pregnancies are really planned, needed or looked forward to. Almost all of them are accidental. Most women do not know how to avoid the future accidental pregnancies because in some of these unadvised pregnancies the mothers are either physically and physiologically unfit to bear any more babies or the family's economy cannot afford the necessary minimum care needed for the new arrival. While we are talking of ignorance, it has been the experience of many that, while it has been easy to sell the prescription for curing a disease, it has not been easy to persuade people to accept the prescribed remedy of the small family norm (Desai, 1973).

The seriousness of the problem in a developing country like India can be imagined from a plea of her Health Minister, Dr. Chandrasekhra, a few years ago.

> Our house is on fire. Don't you see we have already over 520 million people in the country. We add 13 million more every year. At this rate within the next 28 years we will double our population. If we go on producing babies at the rate of one every second and a half, we will make nonsense of our plans. There won't be enough room for everyone. We cannot afford to go on breeding like rabbits. Can we? . . . With unemployment figures which have already soared sky high, and food in perennial shortage, not to mention housing and other civilized amenities, life is fast becoming nasty and brutish, if not short for the overwhelming majority. To continue the drift is to frame an invitation to further humiliation and finally to chaos.

The only way in which India may hope to narrow the ever-widening gap between population growth and agricultural and industrial production is to reduce numbers on the one hand and to increase the production of goods and services on the other. This equation appears quite simple and reasonable on paper, but its implementation requires huge investments for increasing production, and an intensive promotion of family planning on a massive scale. The problems are obvious and formidable. Apart from the sheer magnitude of the task of reaching India's 550,000 villages where 80 percent of the country's population lives, there are enormous problems of motivation and communication. These problems become all the more magnified when we become aware that 70 percent of the people are illiterate and mass communication media are not available. Added to these difficulties is the cultural resistance of not only certain communities, but of the officialdom which is reinforced by the force of custom, tradition, apathy and inertia (Sanyal, 1972).

Limits to Food Production

The primary resource essential for producing food is land. It is certain that our planet is not expanding and we have to develop our strategy of feeding the growing human population within the presently available land. Taking the world as a whole, recent studies indicate that there are almost 3.2 billion hectares (7.86 billion acres) of land which can be put to use for agriculture. At the present time approximately half of this quantity is under active cultivation. The remaining half, although potentially useful for cultivation, is not likely to be made available because of certain reasons. First most of the unused, potentially cultivatable land is located in those countries which have a slow population growth and have enough to feed their existing populations. Secondly, this land is economically not a sound investment because it will need immense capital investment in order to clear, irrigate or fertilize before it is ready to produce food as is the case in some countries in Africa and may not be an attractive proposition as a means of producing more food. Recent costs of developing new land have ranged from 215 to 5,275 dollars per hectare. It has been estimated that the average cost for opening land in unsettled areas is around 1,150 dollars per hectare at 1972 prices (Meadows, 1972). According to an FAO report, opening more land to cultivation is not economically feasible, even given the pressing need for food in the world today (FAO, 1970).

That there are serious limitations in the production of food where it is needed the most or where most of the consumers live is also highlighted by the pattern of human habitation of this planet. One half of the world population lives on only 5 percent of the earth's surface and then there is the lucky 5 percent of the population which has 57 percent of the land to support their needs (White, 1964). Large areas which make up 35 to 40 percent of the total land surface cannot support populations because of aridity, salinity, swampiness, cold or inaccessibility. Of the remainder, about one-sixth is arable, one-third is pasture, and one-half is forest (Christian, 1964).

In the overpopulated countries where the need for extra food is the greatest, not much potentially suitable land is available, even if there is a will to put the required economic input. Over the centuries, especially during the last few decades, most of the available land has already been brought under cultivation. In a country like India further acquisition of land for farming will be an encroachment on the land that may be essential for roads, schools, hospitals, business areas or even residential areas which are necessary for accommodating the present population in a somewhat decent manner. According to the Food and Agriculture Organization of the United Nations, in the whole of Southern Asia, and in some countries of Eastern Asia, the Near East, North Africa and Latin America, there is no scope for expanding the available area (FAO, 1970). The land is already heavily cultivated. The only way of increasing the food supply in these areas is to increase the inputs such as better irrigation, fertilizers and seeds of high-yielding varieties. The recent experience of Brazil, India, Pakistan, Philippines and some other countries has shown that food output can be substantially increased by the sagacious use of fertilizer, irrigation and high yielding varieties of seeds. It has often been called the "Green Revolution" (see next chapter for details). But the question remains: will the "Green Revolution", with limited land resources, feed indefinitely the ever-increasing human population?

The "Green Revolution" has its limitations. First of all, the very success of the "Green Revolution" depends on a huge industrial capacity, which should turn out the needed amount of fertilizer, assure artificial irrigation not dependent on the rain god, and sophisticated scientific research in agriculture. Most of the poor overpopulated countries cannot afford the huge investments required. It has been estimated that in order to achieve the 34 percent increase in world food production from 1951 to 1966, agriculturists increased yearly expenditures on tractors by 63 percent, annual investment in nitrate fertilizers by 146 percent, and annual use of pesticides by 300 percent (Meadows, 1972). Can the developing countries afford to maintain the tempo of added investment at a desired rate? Let us for a moment believe that the "Green Revolution" is a reality and the underdeveloped countries will come up with the capital investments and this will lead to increased food production. But if the population keeps growing (even at a modest rate of 2.0 percent growth it takes only 35 years to double the population), a crisis point is bound to come when the land needed is greater than the land available. The food prices will rise so high that the people of the lower socio-economic groups will be unable to buy adequate quantities of food. The law of diminishing returns will start working on the investment. The demands on the fresh water resources of the earth are even bigger than the demands on the available land. Desalination of sea water in the needed quantities will involve a huge capital cost which may be prohibitive for most of the countries.

At the present time the land under cultivation has been under great agricultural stress, which in turn has put strains on the biological ecosystems of this planet. The "Green Revolution" in the poorer countries of the world cannot be maintained for an indefinite period and it is doubtful that the high yield per acre achieved in the developed countries can be expanded or even maintained for a long stretch of time. Human beings at present are at that juncture in their long history where they have to develop a global strategy in order to maintain and improve the quality of human life on this planet for the present and future generations. The developing countries need to curb their population growth before it is too late even if it means using coercive methods.

On their part, the developed countries should give serious thought to simplifying their diets in order to reduce their per capita claims to the food resources of this earth. Feeding huge quantities of grain to animals to get animal products is indeed a wasteful method of obtaining food when it is scarce for human consumption. The per capita consumption of 2,000 pounds of food grains by a citizen of a developed country, as compared to a per capita consumption of 400 pounds of food grains by a citizen of a developing country, is a luxury which this shrinking world can ill afford. The utilization of vegetable sources of protein by the use of technology is the probable answer so that more food can be spared for human consumption (see Chapter II, "Processed Foods"). Soy proteins are especially suitable to use in the processed food products. These foods can spare the requirements of meat and the need to feed seven pounds of grain to animals in order to obtain one pound of meat. Let us consider some of the factors which limit our capacity to produce abundant food for everybody.

Soil Erosion

The intensity with which the soil has been used for thousands of years, especially in the developing countries, without adequate input, has resulted in wastage of large quantities of otherwise extremely good land. Nature took centuries to create the earth's thin mantle of life-sustaining topsoil and man has destroyed it in a short period of time. The pressure of population on the land is more evident in Asia, where more than half of the human population lives. Not only has excessive land use contributed to soil erosion, but over-grazing by cattle has accelerated the destruction of water-retaining vegetation. This has resulted in the formation of semi-arid and arid zones out of very fertile areas. While lamenting the accelerating soil loss, Brown described that as livestock herds are increased to meet the growing demands for food and draft power, they graze over ever larger areas, stripping the land of its natural cover in many parts of the world (Brown, 1973). With the population expanding at a high level, the need for new agricultural land and for forest products for fuel is increasing while, at the same time, the countryside is being steadily denuded of trees and other protective vegetation cover. While the cover of grass and trees is grazed out by the livestock, much of the earth's land surface is vulnerable to erosion by wind and rain. In some of the overcrowded countries, millions of acres of these unproductive lands are abandoned each year by rural people who are forced to go to urban areas to look for employment in the nonagricultural sectors. This problem during recent years has become quite serious in North Africa, the Middle East, and the Indian subcontinent.

Furthermore, the shortage of other sources of energy is accelerating the process of deforestation. In such countries as India and Pakistan, the people use cow dung for fuel and deprive the land of a natural source of fertilizer. As the demand for food expands, there is no other choice except to resort to using lands of marginal value which are too steep or too dry to sustain cultivation. In numerous cases, the farmers move up the hillsides to fulfill their needs to grow food for their families, but in the process accelerate the erosion process. More and more forests are being removed in the name of extra demand for land to produce food for the ever-increasing populations.

As a result of soil erosion a number of developed countries in Western Europe and Japan are reducing their acreage under crop cultivation. The same is true of other parts such as India, the Middle East, North Africa, the Caribbean, Central America and the Andes countries. A classical example of soil erosion is the continent of North Africa. Once a fertile grainery of the Roman Empire, the soil was eroded by continuous cropping and over-grazing until much of it will not sustain any agriculture and is a waste desert land. Even with a population of 4 billion humans, the ability of this planet to produce adequate food for all is under severe strain.

Can we ignore the writing on the wall if we allow a growth of 2 percent in world population on a continuous basis?

Limits to Availability of Water for Irrigation

The availability of water for irrigation could become the single most important obstacle in increasing the food output beyond a certain stage. Although water is found over most of the earth, it varies greatly in distribution and quality. Even in those areas which have abundant water resources, there is a critical shortage of good potable water. The demand for water can be roughly estimated from the simple fact that more than 10,000 litres of water are needed to grow the daily food of one person. To put it another way, 5,000 tons of water are needed to grow one ton of wheat. Rice takes a lot more. If the population keeps growing constantly as the trend goes, the demand for fresh water will expand beyond belief or availability. Besides the heavy demands of agriculture, water is also needed for the industry, which must produce the machinery and chemicals for agriculture as well as other necessities of human existence.

In recent years, many areas of the world have suffered at the hands of famine, scarcity, infectious diseases, etc., due to too much dependence on rains for raising crops. Most countries in their best production years live on subsistence agricultural economies due to a very heavy load of population and cannot produce adequate amounts of food, if nature in the form of timely rain does not cooperate. The Indian droughts of 1965 to 1967, and 1972 to 1973, are examples of the failure of rains and nonavailability of water for irrigation. In most of the developing countries not more than 20 percent of the cultivated land is irrigated and, unless huge capital is invested, the acreage under irrigation cannot be substantially increased. This brings to light too much dependence by vast populations on rains and the vagaries of nature, which could bring crises of catastrophic and unmanageable proportions. All the technologically developed varieties which yield better quantity and quality of food grains need generous amounts of water as well as fertilizers. Unless and until, therefore, we have the availability of a sufficient quantity of water, it may not be possible to maintain an increased level of food production indefinitely in proportion to the demands of a growing human population. Irrigation projects built at huge costs in order to provide water for agriculture have their own problems and they cannot be depended upon completely. Brown gave some good examples of the irrigation problems facing the developing countries.

In West Pakistan the recently completed $600 million Mangla irrigation reservoir, which originally had a life expectancy of 100 years, is now expected to be nearly filled with silt in half that time. The clearing of steep slopes for farming, progressive deforestation, and overgrazing in the reservoir's watershed are responsible for its declining life expectancy. Effort to expand the area of farmland in one locale is reducing the water for irrigation in another. Farmers moving up the hillsides in Java are causing irrigation canals to silt at an alarming rate. Damming the Nile at Aswan expanded the irrigated area for producing cereals but largely eliminated the annual deposits of rich alluvian silt on fields in the Nile Valley, forcing farmers to rely more on chemical fertilizers. In addition, interrupting the flow of nutrients into the Nile estuary caused a precipitous decline in the fish catch there. Intensive farming in the Philippines with chemical fertilizers is expanding the rice supply but causing freshwater lakes and streams to eutrophy, destroying fish and depriving local villagers of their principal sources of animal protein. One of the most costly and tragic side effects of the spread of modern irrigation in Egypt and other river valleys in Africa, Asia and northeastern South America is the great incidence of schistosomiasis. The debilitating intestinal and urinary disease, produced by the parasitic larvae of a blood fluke that burrows into the flesh of those working in water covered fields, affects a sizeable number of the Egyptian people (Brown, 1973).

In the 1950's, the Soviet Union launched a plan to cultivate nearly 100 million acres of virgin dry lands only to find out that it lacked sufficient precipitation to sustain continuous cultivation. In many countries of the world, extra agricultural land can be made available if only fresh water is available for irrigation. The hope of providing extra water depends on technological innovation and huge capital investments in the area of diversion of rivers towards fertile areas, desalting sea water, and manipulating the patterns of rainfall in order to provide a better share of rain to those agricultural areas which are moisture deficient.

Chemical Pollution

One important by-product of industrialization is the chemical pollution of waters which makes them unfit for agriculture and deprives us of an important source of food rich in proteins, i.e. freshwater fish and other fauna. Increasing food output needs the production and utilization of large quantities of chemical fertilizer. However, in our zeal to produce more foods or conserve more food for human consumption, we are likely to produce severe adverse environmental results which, after a certain stage, may cause the degree of chemical pollution that may irreversibly damage our previously balanced ecology. Brown rightly questions, "We do not know how many species of birds, fish, and mammals must be sacrificed in order to achieve a 5 percent increase in the world's food supply" (Brown, 1973).

Pollution can be categorized in two ways. First, the pollution of our environment, which affects our health and well-being, and second, the pollution of the earth and ocean which obstructs our ability to produce uncontaminated food in larger quantities for our growing population. In the first category, we may include the pollution of air, drinking water, pollution of environment by solid wastes, lead pollution, fluoride pollution, pollution from radiation and chemical mutagens, noise pollution, etc. In combinations, they have deteriorated our environment upon which depends our existence. The major contributors to air pollution in the United States are 110 million automobiles, which throw approximately 70 million tons of carbon monoxides into the air along with significant quantities of other dangerous substances such as sulfur oxides, nitrogen oxides, and hydrocarbons. The share of pulp and paper mills, iron and steel factories, petroleum refineries or chemical plants is no less significant. All added up, approximately 150 million tons of pollutants are added annually to the atmosphere, which is approximately three fourths of a ton for every man, woman and child in the United States (Ehrlich and Ehrlich, 1970).

Air pollution is a major factor in the respiratory ailments which are on the increase in most industrialized countries. As the population grows, it will be more and more difficult to clean our polluted atmosphere. Each new worker adds his share of pollutants into the air. As overcrowding increases, fresh or clean air will become a rarity. We may be able to produce food for our billions, but we may be choked by the unclean air that we will have to breathe. Closely related to air pollution is water pollution, whose solution will become more difficult as the population grows. We have progressively increased our levels of chlorination of the drinking water, but there is evidence that high content of organic matter in water protects viruses from the effects of chlorine. The sewage treatment and processing of solid wastes are becoming, in most urban areas of the world, a problem and a menace. At the rate at which the population is growing, even the most modern facilities will become inadequate within a few years. The problems are most acute in the sprawling urban areas of developing countries such as Calcutta, Bombay, Karachi, Dacca, Singapore and others. Ehrlich rightly remarked:

> As population grows, so does industry, which pours into our water supplies a vast array of contaminants: lead, detergents, sulfuric acid, hydrofluoric acid, phenols, ethers, benzenes, ammonia and so on. As population and industry grow, so does the need for increased agricultural production, which results in a heavier water-borne load of pesticides, herbicides and nitrates. A result is the spread of pollution not just in streams, rivers, lakes and along seashores, but also (and most seriously) in ground water, where purification is almost impossible. With the spread of pollution goes the threat of epidemics of hepatitis and dysentery, and of poisoning by exotic chemicals.

Some of the pollutants such as lead, mercury, fluorides and hydrocarbons reach us in so many different ways. They are present in our drinking water, in our fruits and vegetables and in the air we breathe. At times, the dosage is high and directly harmful. Scientists are beginning to assess the harm that the chlorinated hydrocarbons may have on our physiology over a long period of time. In experimental animals, high doses of DDT cause liver cancers and affect the reproductive physiology by their effect on the sex hormones.

Our ability to increase agricultural production at a scale required by our needs of the growing populations is seriously jeopardized by the pollution process that is inevitable as we try to reach the optimum levels of food production. The human species is trapped by its own innovative genius. If we try to produce food with full commitment to the environmental quality, we are unable to harvest the quantities that are essential to sustain our present numbers, not to mention food for the unending stream of 70 million new mouths that arrive year after year. When we use the technology that helps to produce extra food, we pollute our environment in the process, which puts its own stresses and strains on our quality of life. "World agriculture today is an ecological disaster area (Ehrlich and Ehrlich, 1970).

The use of insecticides and pesticides has progressively increased as strenuous efforts are being made to save food for human consumption. The insects and other pests respond to our chemicals by developing resistance and by evolving mutant species. According to a rough estimate, 10 percent of the food crops all over the world are destroyed by insects. In the developing countries, the losses are even higher because the food lost to pests after the crop is harvested is also significantly high. There is reason to believe that the percentage of crop losses to insects in the United States has remained about the same for the last 20 years, despite the enormously increased use of pesticides during this period. What actually happens may be reflected in the following scenario.

We have developed potent insecticides which have a devastating effect on the insect population. However, our spraying methods do not discriminate between the harmful insects and those which do not hurt our crops and, instead, prey on the harmful insects. After the effect of the insecticide is worn off, the harmful insects again appear on the scene with a difference. This time they do not have their natural enemies. Experimental data from various laboratories indicate, for example, that an insecticide, Azodrin,® used to exterminate ballworms, had a devastating effect on their natural enemies with the result that the ballworm population actually increased.

Similar results have also been obtained by the use of other broad spectrum pesticides. Often, when the target insects appear again, the dose level of the insecticide is increased and over a long period of time it has a disastrous effect on the ecosystems. A classical example of the ecosystem disturbance may be cited here in support of our argument that it does not help to use the highly toxic insecticides indiscriminately. During the period between 1960 to 1963, Endrin and one of its derivatives (potent insecticides) were used to treat cotton and cane crops in the lower Mississippi valley. The residues were washed into the water, which led to the destruction of about 15 million fish in the lower Mississippi. These fish included some of the edible and sought-after species for human consumption such as catfish, menhaden, buffalo fish, sea trout, mullet, drumfish, etc.

These examples demonstrate that there are limits to man's capacity to keep increasing his output of farm products from a given land, even if he is under the compulsion that extra food must be produced to feed the new hungry mouths that have arrived since the last crop was harvested. The indiscriminate use of insecticides and pesticides will kill the target insects and pests, and also leave a track of murder which manifests itself in hurting man's interests at some other point in his food chain. It has been reported that DDT inhibits photosynthesis by marine phytoplankton. Since phytoplankton is the major source of food for the marine animals, it could result in significant reduction in the amount of life in the sea. This could directly hurt man's economic and food interests. Ehrlich warned that at present "no one knows how long we can continue to pollute the seas with chlorinated hydrocarbon insecticides, polychlorinated biphenyls and hundreds of thousands of other pollutants without bringing on a world wide ecological disaster. Subtle changes may already have started a chain reaction in that direction."

We have not estimated as yet the harm done by the residues of insecticides which become a part and parcel of our soil. The earth's soil is not merely dirt. It is quite rich in organisms that have a direct effect on the fertility of the soil, which in turn determines the amount of food we can produce from it.

> In a study of pasture soils in Denmark, up to 45,000 small oligochaete worms, 10 million nematodes (round worms) and 48,000 small arthropods (insects and mites) were found in each square meter. Even more abundant are the microflora of the soil. More than a million bacteria of one type may be found in a gram (0.035 ounce) of forest soil, as well as almost 100,000 yeast cells, and about 50,000 bits of fungus mycelium. A gram of fertile agricultural soil has yielded over 2.5 billion bacteria, 400,000 fungi, 50,000 algae and 30,000 protozoa. (Ehrlich and Ehrlich, 1970).

All these organisms play an important role in the ecology of the soil and make it suitable for growing our food crops. The soil organisms, responsible as they are for soil fertility, are hurt very badly by the continued use of heavy doses of deadly poisons in the form of insecticides. Approximately 39 percent of DDT and 40 percent of deadly insecticides such as Aldrin and Endrin persist in the soil after they have been used (Nash and Woolson). Our ignorance about the interactions of insecticides with the soil life is simply monumental. We have callously ignored the long term effects of these chemicals on the microorganisms that are the friends of mankind. If we keep on deteriorating the environment thoughtlessly, it could ultimately prove fatal to the human species (Ehrlich and Ehrlich, 1970).

The solution lies in carefully planned, short as well as long term, studies of every chemical that we introduce into our environment. To allow researchers time for these studies we must stabilize our population so that we may have some respite from rushing to produce significant quantities of extra food from one harvest to the other. Because we depend on our ecosystem for our food supply and other life support facilities, we have to learn to guard its interests. The preservation of our natural ecology is a better guarantee to feed our populations than a callous disregard of its welfare.

Limits to Technological Innovations

The only hope of feeding the future generations of mankind when their numbers exceed the 5 billion mark (expected in the next decade) is the large scale use of technology in the field of agriculture and aquaculture, and economical ways for the production of animal sources of protein. Some of the advanced countries have already reached their peaks of per acre yields of agricultural products. A further increase will require such heavy inputs that may be economically unfeasible. This is especially true of Japan, the Netherlands and, to a great extent, the United States as well, where increasing the per capita yield could be more expensive than bringing unused land under cultivation. For example, raising rice yields in Japan from the current 5,000 pounds per acre to 6,000 pounds could be a very costly proposition. Raising yields of corn in the United States from 90 to 100 bushels per acre requires a much larger quantity of nitrogen than was needed to raise yields from 50 to 60 bushels. The same is true of soybeans, which are a major source of high quality vegetable proteins.

The United States has been producing three fourths of the world's soybean crop and has been expanding production by increasing the acreage rather than the yield per acre. Unfortunately, the United States' idle land is coming to an end and this could be serious. Fortunately, there is still scope for increasing substantially the per acre yield in the developing countries, where the pressure of population is the most acute. Rice yields in India or Nigeria are still one-third that of Japan. Corn yields in Brazil and Thailand are one-third that of the United States. But these countries do not have the capital resources to generate economically feasible energy, chemical fertilizers, and irrigation systems and tools of mechanized agriculture so necessary to increase the per acre output. The technology is indeed a great blessing, but we must recognize its limitations and work actively to stablize our numbers before we discover to our sorrow that technology could take us only so far.

Technological innovations have led to a phenomenal increase in the production of fish and other marine species, but again there are limitations in this area. The world's oceans can produce only a certain amount of fish per year and if we press too hard, we are likely to disturb the ecological balance which provides us with a certain amount on an indefinite basis. We are already seeing the results of too much fishing in greatly reduced output of anchovies off the Peruvian coast this year. However, as more research is conducted, fish could become a valuable source for large scale supplies of animal protein, but at this time there are so many unresolved technical problems that fish are not likely to become a major source of food for the vast human populations. The story of poultry, beef, eggs and milk is no different. Technology has greatly helped to increase their yield, but as the demand goes, there is no prospect of doubling or tripling their availability in a short time. For example, in beef production, research has not helped to produce more than one calf per cow per year and the grazing capacity of our pasture land is clearly limited. As the demand for animal products grows in the developed as well as developing countries, there is likely to exist a greater shortage of these products. The price of livestock is likely to go so high that only the affluent few will be able to afford it.

LIMITS TO RESOURCES

The earth has been generously endowed with resources. Man, with his superior intellect and innovative imagination, has made good use of them and created for himself a very comfortable life whereby he sleeps comfortably in the coldest or hottest of temperatures, flies thousands of miles within hours and eats a rich variety of foods all the year around. Man is so much enthused by his success in developing a mastery over these rich resources that he has set for himself higher and higher limits to their utilization year after year. The demand for the utilization of the resources is assuming fantastic proportions as human life transforms itself to an industrialized mode of living. This is especially true of the industrialized countries. The 210 million people of the United States own more than 110 million automobiles and approximately 10 million new cars are produced every year. The United States Bureau of Mines has collected data on the known world resources of a number of metals that are the backbone of our industrial civilization, and the manner in which they are used. It shows that the United States alone uses 42 percent of the world's total aluminum, 19 percent chromium, 44 percent coal, 32 percent cobalt, 33 percent copper, 26 percent gold, 28 percent iron, 25 percent lead, 14 percent manganese, 24 percent mercury, 40 percent molybdenum, 63 percent natural gas, 38 percent nickel, 33 percent petroleum, 31 percent platinum, 26 percent silver, 24 percent tin, 22 percent tungsten and 26 percent zinc (U.S. Bureau of Mines, Minerals, Facts and Problems, 1970). The developing countries of the world which have the largest aggregation of human population so far have been at the bottom in the utilization of these precious minerals, but their utilization and demand is steadily increasing as they try to bring their societies into the industrial age. The net result is that the world's usage rate of every natural resource is growing at a much faster rate than the growth in population. With the growing population more people are consuming the resources and the consumption per person per year is likely to increase year after year. It is evident that the economic development based on the industrialization greatly depends upon the availability of these resources. Feeding the growing populations on limited land also depends on the utilization of the natural resources. With the industrialized countries continuously increasing their resource utilization, and more and more developing countries sharing the resources at a progressively increasing rate, it is inevitable that the earth will become poorer in its reserves year after year and may soon become one of the major limits to the growth of world's population (Cheney, 1974). The sooner we realize the limitations of the resources at our disposal and take steps to learn to live with them, the better it is for the future of the industrialized human species (Sokolov, 1973). It is time to heed the warning of the first annual report of the Council on Environmental Quality that

> the quantities of platinum, gold, zinc, and lead are not sufficient to meet demands. At the present rate of expansion . . . . silver, tin and uranium may be in short supply even at higher prices by the turn of the century. By the year 2050, several more minerals may be exhausted if the current rate of consumption continues . . . . Despite spectacular recent discoveries, there are only a limited number of places left to search for most minerals. Geologists disagree about the prospects for finding large, new rich ore deposits. Reliance on such discoveries would seem unwise in the long term.

Even in the short term, the scarcity of these resources is reflected in their unusual increase in prices. The price of mercury, for example, increased 500 percent during the last 20 years (U.S. Bureau of Mines, Minerals Year Book). The price of lead increased 300 percent in the last 30 years (Somerset, 1970). If we maintain the present rates of resource consumption and consider the projected price increases in these rates, the great majority of the currently imported nonrenewable resources will be extremely costly, as well as in limited supply, 100 years from now (Meadows, 1972).

SOCIO-ECONOMIC CONSTRAINTS

Population increases are intimately tied to the economic growth. On the one hand, the economy of a country or region must move forward as the numbers increase or else the mortality rate due to starvation or lack of social and medical services will greatly increase. On the other hand, the numbers tend to decline as economic growth leads to certain degrees of affluence. The birth rates are highest in those countries which have the lowest per capita gross national product. The birth rates are comparatively very low in those countries which have a high rate of productivity. In general as the gross national product rises, the birth rate falls. There is no direct relationship between the two, but indirectly certain socio-economic changes bring about this phenomenon. The most desirable method of slowing down the population growth in the poor countries is, therefore, to improve their economies and the education level of their populations. With a growing economy, the health services improve resulting in lower mortality, better health, lesser sick days and greater productivity. The availability of industrial goods, especially those facilitating family planning methods (condoms, diaphragms, pills, etc.) , increases the effectiveness of the birth control measures. The educational level brings out the social and cultural changes which are necessary to receive the message of the desirability of limiting the family numbers to a desirable number.

But the greatest benefit which is endowed by a growing economy is the realization of the economic value as well as the economic costs of an additional member. The necessity of sheer manpower in terms of quantity decreases in an industrialized society. The latter also brings about health and old age insurances, and parents do not view their children as an insurance policy, and produce only as many as can be properly cared for, loved, fed and trained to take their place in society. There are reasons to believe that an economically well-off family consciously or unconsciously weighs the value and cost of an additional child, as well as his need (Spengler, 1966) . An industrialized and economically prosperous community needs fewer human hands than would be required in an agrarian community. The value of a child in the former is judged more as an object of love, carrier of family name, inheritor of property and, above all, the fulfillment of the unconscious psychological need of seeing your descendant in a good socio-economic position.

There is also a strong relationship between the economic growth of a region and the rate of its population growth. In the early 20th Century, the population growth turned out to be a great asset to a growing economy, especially in the technologically advanced countries. The latter, with their efficient methods of exploitation of natural resources and continuous growth of scientific knowledge, greatly enhanced the economic development of their regions.

However, as the level of education grew and the economy did not need extra labor, certain social forces went into operation to promote voluntary reduction in numbers. This favorable relationship between the economic growth and the additions to population did not materialize in the present day developing countries. These regions continued adding large numbers to their already huge populations without the accompanying economic growth. Improved public health measures reduced the rate of mortality, thereby triggering all the more the rate of population increase. Due to lack of capital accumulation, poor savings, poor rate of exploitation of natural resources and poor state of education, the economic growth of these regions has been extremely unsatisfactory, and has produced major developmental problems. Economic development became stymied as a result of unsatisfactory capital savings (Lebowitz, 1973). The technologically advanced countries became economically richer during the same time the developing countries became poorer. As the population balance tilted in favor of the developing countries, the economic balance tilted in favor of the developed countries, the result being an ever-increasing gap in the economic growth of the two regions.

Let us take a few figures of some countries, collected by the World Bank (*World Bank Atlas*, 1970) that will illustrate this gap in economic growth. In the year 1968, China, with a population of 730 million and a population growth rate of 1.5 percent, had a per capita GNP equivalent to 90 U.S. dollars. The per capita GNP growth rate between 1961 to 1968 averaged 0.3 percent. Another heavily overpopulated country, India, had somewhat similar figures. With a population of 524 million and an annual population growth rate of 2.5 percent (much more than China), it had a per capita GNP equivalent to 100 U.S. dollars. For the sake of comparison, let us take the example of two rich countries. Japan, with a population of 101 million, had an annual population growth rate of only 1.0 percent and had a per capita GNP equivalent to 1,190 U.S. dollars. Her average per capita GNP between 1961 and 1962 grew at a rate of 9.9 percent (10 times that of India). The United States, with a population of 201 million, had a population growth rate of 1.4 percent and a per capita GNP of 3,980 U.S. dollars. (See also Appendix I). All this means that the rich countries get richer and the poor countries get children.

If we assume that the growth rate of population in the poor and rich countries remains the same in the years 1968 to 2000, the disparity between the rich and poor countries will widen to still further in the next 30 years. If the present trends continue based on 1968 dollars with no allowance for inflation, the per capita GNP of China and India in the year 2000 will be equivalent to 100 and 140 U.S. dollars respectively. These figures are in sharp contrast to 23,200 and 11,000 U.S. dollars for the United States and Japan respectively. This clearly shows that "the process of economic growth, as it is occurring today, is inexorably widening the absolute gap between the rich and the poor nations of the world" (Meadows, 1972). The future prospects for improved economies in the face of growing populations are not very bright. Lack of capital and raw materials and economic intrastructure such as energy, transportation and communication systems in proportion to the population will most likely cause the poverty to perpetuate. An average family would spend the largest proportion of its income on food and other basic survival items and the nation would not have the necessary capital to pull them out by their economic bootstraps. This state of affairs will further widen the economic gap between the poor nations and the rich nations of the world. This could prove quite dangerous.

In a social sense, there is always an ideal number of inhabitants within the limits of a certain defined boundary such as city limits. Those boundaries can be kept clean and civic responsibilities can be neatly carried out if the number of people using these facilities is within a desirable range. The social life of the people in terms of mutual respect for each other's rights and privileges can be richer if this number is not allowed to increase beyond a certain optimum. In an overcrowded state, not only do men tend to forget other people's rights, but do not hesitate to violate them out of the sheer necessity of coexistence. As Slater remarked, "because there are too many of us, a man does his neighbors more harm than good, just by staying alive. As numbers increase this will become a more self-evident factor in our lives (Slater, 1972).

The social pressures of overcrowding manifest themselves in a number of ways; particularly serious consequences follow when these tend to change the behavioral patterns of the human beings. Overcrowding results in a general deterioration in the quality of a man, which results in a change in the human attitudes for the worse. The space remains constant and social adjustability of increased numbers within that space results in many pulls and pushes that ultimately break down the social cohesion which binds the whole human civilization. It is the social cohesion among humans that singles them apart from other species of animals.

If it is supposed that nothing is done by us or our succeeding generations to stabilize our numbers and the present rate of growth continues, it would lead to a population of 500 billion by the year 2200, and give the surface of all continents a population density equal to that of Washington, D.C., at present (Mayer, 1972). Even if we are able to feed these numbers, it is doubtful if we can survive the socioeconomic and political consequences of this density, and the chaos that these numbers are likely to bring in their trail. There will be a complete breakdown of social cohesion of the human species long before the above projected figures materialize. The economic and political consequences will still be worse. We will deplete the natural resources of the earth at a rate which will not give it the time to replenish itself. The ecology of this planet will be disturbed to such an extent that all the land, air and water will be subjected to chemical, thermal or radioactive pollution. Describing the present day disturbance of ecology in an industrialized country such as the United States, Mayer explained that we spread 48 billion (rust proof) cans and 26 billion (nondegradable) bottles over our landscape every year. We produce 800 million pounds of trash a day, a great deal of which ends up in our fields, our parks and our forests. Only one third of the billion pounds of paper we use every year is reclaimed. Nine million cars, trucks and buses are abandoned every year and, while many of them are used as scrap, a large, though undermined number is left to disintegrate slowly in our back yards, in fields and woods, and on the sides of highways. The 8 billion pounds of plastics we use every year are nondegradable materials . . . . we are likely to run out of certain metals before we run out of food; of paper before we run out of metals. And we are running out of clear streams, pure air, and the familiar sights of nature (Mayer, 1972).

The economic losses resulting from poor nutrition are no less drastic. If malnutrition and debility result in the death of a person in the prime period of his productive life, the loss has to be computed in terms of the worker's future income, had he lived, especially when the society has already made the investments in him in terms of health, food, clothing, housing, education and other expenditures necessary to enable him to develop a particular skill. Fortunately, the death rate among adults as a result of malnutrition is not very high, but a chronic undernutrition leads to huge losses in productivity which are a direct result of the debility and lack of energy of the labor force (Hammonds and Wunderle, 1972).

If we take India as a typical developing country with a per capita consumption of less than 2,000 calories per day, the economically weaker sections of the society get substantially less than this highly unsatisfactory amount. The caloric shortages among the workers may be as high as 50 percent. The productivity of such a person subsisting on calories only slightly above the needs of the basal metabolism cannot be compared with the productivity of a worker who gets 3,000 or more calories per day. Such losses in productivity are directly reflected in the incomes of the individuals and the families dependent on them. From 1960 to 1970 the per capita income in countries which have two thirds of the world's population grew only 1.5 percent yearly. During the same period, the population grew at the rate of 2.6 percent per year. The food prices have been steadily rising, which means that the per capita availability of food must have gone down.

The poorer sections of the overcrowded societies, who incidently have a larger share of dependent children as well, have been hit the hardest. As explained by Alan Berg (1973a), during the period from 1960 to 1970, in some countries the increments in income were distributed in such a way that the poorer segments of the population received even less than the average share. In Brazil, the poorest 40 percent of the population saw their share of the national income decline during this period by 20 percent. In Mexico, the income share of the poorest 40 percent fell from 14 percent in 1950 to 11 percent in 1969; the already low share of the poorest 20 percent of the population dropped by a third—to 4 percent of the national income. In short, the nutritionally needy portions of the population often have not benefitted from their country's income growth and, in some cases, their living standards may even have deteriorated (Berg, 1973b). The ability of our undernourished worker to get an extra share of the national income is directly dependent on his physical ability to work harder. When the individual income rises, there is an automatic increase in the amount of money the family spends on food, which not only leads to better performance of the earning member, but also the health of the vulnerable members of the family, especially the mother and young children.

The Indian National Institute of Nutrition has observed that youngsters with three or more older brothers or sisters constitute 34 percent of the child population but account for 61 percent of all cases of protein-calorie malnutrition (Berg, 1973a). These children not only need extra food but are unable to utilize properly whatever they get. The infections that often accompany the state of malnutrition lead to significant losses of nutrients (Pollack and Sheldon, 1970; Scrimshaw, 1951; *U.S. News And World Report,* 1972). For example, in a case like typhoid, as much as 15 to 20 gms of body nitrogen are lost per day, resulting, in about 10 to 12 days, in a loss of as much as 625 gms of protein, which could have grave consequences (Shaffer and Coleman, 1909).

The first and foremost benefit from improved nutrition will be savings that the society is spending at the moment to prevent the demise of those who are malnourished. There is a huge waste of natural resources taking place because of premature deaths; investments in medical care, clothing, food and education comprise some of these wasted resources. However, with improved nutrition, there is a general decline in the demand for medical services which helps to reduce needed expenditures (Popkin and Lidman, 1972).

Improved nutrition will provide extra calories which can sustain prolonged physical work and raise the productivity as well as the motivation of the worker. It is estimated that the productivity of an Asian worker is less than one-half that of his American counterpart, mainly because the former, being short in his caloric intake, would try to conserve energy for the more important need, i.e. the basal metabolism to maintain the life processes. There is a close correlation between adequacy of work calories and work productivity. If the work calories are below the required amount for the activity being undertaken, the body will first adapt somewhat to this lower food intake by avoiding effort (FAO, 1962; Keller and Kraut, 1962; Popkin and Lidman, 1972).

Improvement in mental performance is another important benefit of improved nutrition, although it is most effective in the early stages of brain growth. In children, improved nutrition can help prevent brain damage and improve cognitive development (Manocha, 1972). Hungry children cannot concentrate as well and hence learn less than the well nourished ones; they have poor judgment, are irritable, moody and unable to sustain mental application (Popkin and Lidman, 1972). Improved nutrition also reduces the chances of behavioral disorders which in malnourished children manifest themselves because of their loss in learning time and frustrations caused by expectations of their chronological age.

Not only the present, but the future generations also

benefit from improved nutrition standards of the population. Several studies have shown that the children of healthy parents are healthier and better motivated. Well nourished mothers produce healthier children and have an easier time raising them and, in turn, their children are better educated, and become more responsible citizens (Schultz, 1961; Weisbrod, 1962). These intergenerational financial gains have been estimated for the United States to be at least 14 percent of this generation's financial gains. When economic benefits from providing improved diets to the presently approximated 3.3 million children in the United States are estimated, the total gain in higher mental performance in lifetime earnings is up to 19.2 billion dollars, mainly due to higher achievement (Popkin and Lidman, 1972).

Environmental Quality

As we keep on increasing our usage of the natural resources year after year, in the name of progress, the biosphere of this planet gets progressively polluted with wastes. The carefully balanced ecological equilibrium begins to be disturbed, recoils itself and ultimately hurts man, for whose civilized progress the process was set into motion in the first place. In some respects the pollution is directly related to growing human population. Increased pollution is caused by increased agricultural activity and utilization of more and more fuel energy to increase agricultural productivity. But most of the pollution is caused by man's desire to create for himself material opulence. The industry and the technology must be pushed forward to utilize progressively larger quantities of resources. The thinking people who are sensitive to changes brought about by our industrialists are already beginning to worry about the increasing pollution. Hutchinson rightly believes that pollution is progressively decreasing the life of our biosphere, and its capability of sustaining healthy organisms and its ultimate life must be measured in decades rather than hundreds of millions of years. Our human species, although very ingenious, is systematically polluting this sphere in the most unintelligent manner.

What happens to the metals and fuels extracted from the earth after they have been used and discarded is a question that is most often asked by anyone interested in maintaining the ecological balance of our biosphere. In one sense they are never lost. They have served their industrial purpose or provided us with energy, or some other use, and are dispersed in the biosphere where their constituent atoms are rearranged and eventually dispersed in a diluted and unusable form into the air, into the soil, and into the waters of our planet. The natural ecological systems can no doubt absorb some of the by-products of human activity and reprocess them into substances that can again be used, but there are certain industrial products which can only partially be absorbed by our ecosystems.

If we release these wastes on a large enough scale, the natural processing or recycling mechanisms can become saturated. The wastes of human civilization can then build up in the environment until they become visible, annoying, and even harmful. Mercury in ocean fish, lead particles in city air, mountains of urban trash, and oil slicks on beaches are only some of the examples of human mishandling of the valuable resources in excessive quantities beyond the nature's ability to recycle. While we intend to pursue our energy hunger in our pursuit of material opulence, the substitution of fuels and natural gas by nuclear power may help to a great extent, but we are still unaware of the long term effects of radioactive by-products. In any case, we have to contend with pollution caused by industrial processes as well as agricultural practices because both of these activities are essential to maintain our large numbers. Whatever we do, we must realize that the cost of reducing pollution will keep on mounting if we let the environment deteriorate further. According to the estimate projected in the second annual report of the Council on Environmental Quality, the cost of reducing particulates by 22 percent from the aerial environment of a typical United States city is 50,000 dollars, but if we wish to reduce it by 66 percent, the cost jumps up to 7.5 million dollars. For an additional 3 percent reduction

(69%), the cost is 26 million dollars. A further delay in determined action to fight pollution could become prohibitively expensive, especially when we are aware that certain types of pollution such as thermal pollution, radioisotopes from nuclear power generation, fertilizer runoff, and asbestos particles are technically extremely difficult to control.

INFANT MORTALITY—A DISINCENTIVE TO VOLUNTARY POPULATION CONTROL

There is a strong relationship between the rate of infant mortality in a particular area or country and the people's attitude towards family planning practices. The infant mortality rate varies from 20 to 600 out of 1,000 live births all the way from Australia and New Zealand to parts of Africa. However, in most countries if a couple loses a child while they are still in the early reproductive age group (younger than forty years of age), they tend to replace him with another one. The same psychology operates in a wider sense in the people of those areas where the infant mortality rates have been traditionally very high. They tend to produce larger numbers of children in order to assure the survival of at least a few. In areas of high infant mortality, especially in Asia, Africa and Latin America, the population growth was not significant up to the early part of the 20th Century, because a heavy toll of life especially among the infants was taken by common epidemics such as cholera, malaria and common infections.

Starting from the Twenties, this pattern began to change in these areas. The level of nutrition and communications improved. Modern medical facilities came in slowly but surely, and the most vulnerable populations, i.e. infants, got a better chance of survival through the early difficult years. The rate of infant mortality came down in most of the overpopulated developing countries. India, for example, showed a remarkable decline in infant mortality rate from more than 250 to less than 100 per thousand live births within 3 to 4 decades. This is reflected in the average expectancy of an Indian from less than thirty years in the 1940's to more than

50 years in the 1970's. However, the social and cultural psychology which encouraged the large family pattern did not undergo any radical change. Since more children survived the early difficult period of infancy, large family size meant a rapid growth of populations.

There is a close relationship between voluntary restriction of family size and the rate of infant mortality, but it takes a long span of time to establish this relationship in the minds of people who for centuries have been conditioned to fight the high infant deaths with higher birth rates. In these countries, in spite of the lowering death rates, the message to simultaneously curtail the birth rate in order to stabilize population has not been effectively conveyed to the people. In the words of Dr. Chandrasekhra, even the vocabulary has not been developed to convey the message of restricting family size to those people who are culturally not conditioned to receive this message. For centuries they had accepted high death rates and larger numbers of births as normal and strictly in accordance with the will of God. It is hard to convince them that the lower infant mortality is no accident and that there is no need to have larger numbers of children to assure the survival of a few of them.

This is especially true in the tradition-bound Eastern societies where children are considered as their greatest assets and where they look to their children for sustenance in old age. For a Hindu in India, a son is a spiritual necessity who will perform his last rites when he departs from this world. In the presence of widespread infantile ailments, which take a toll of infant life, he is not going to be satisfied in having only one son, and in order to have at least two, he is likely to produce four children (assuming the statistical probability of two boys and two girls). It is not uncommon for a large number of people in India to produce up to six or more children in order to have a minimum of two sons, so that they can be certain that they would leave at least one son to look after their material and spiritual needs. There is in fact evidence from Bangledesh, showing a direct relationship between the death of a child and the probability of a birth in the family during the subsequent year (Brown and Wray, 1974). With minor modifications or objectives, this situation prevails in most of the tradition-bound societies of Asia, Africa and Latin America. According to Dr. Harold Taylor of the Population Council, "A basic dictum is that parents will not stop having children until they believe that those they already have are going to survive."

With a combination of better nutrition for infants (encouraging breast feeding, assuring comfortable supplies of animal's milk and availability of easily digestible infant foods), improved standards of sanitation and public health measures including compulsory innoculation or vaccination for the common ailments such as diphtheria, pertusis, tetanus, polio, measles, smallpox, cholera, etc., the infant mortality rate can be drastically reduced. Once the parents are convinced that their infant is healthy and is going to live longer and grow up to be a productive adult, it is likely that they will not contemplate producing another one. It appears that improved infant and child nutrition will provide in the long run one of the most effective means of lowering the birth rate in the developing countries. This will also give some relief to women who, through repeated pregnancies, get depleted of their own nutrient reserves and tend to succumb to minor infections (Chopra *et al.*, 1970). Old age insurance is another reason for having larger families. There is a natural urge to have a few living children who will be of some assistance to you in old age. This assistance may not necessarily be of a financial nature. The children give psychological comfort and a feeling of immortality to a person ready to depart from this world. Up to the early 20th Century, when the rate of infant mortality was high in both the technologically developed and undeveloped countries, men and women everywhere tended to have larger families for that reason.

Asians, Africans and Latin Americans are contributing heavily to the present population growth, but their fertility rate has never been extraordinarily high. Their numbers in the previous centuries were maintained by an equilibrium between birth and death. So was the case in Europe, Australia, America or other developed countries. The medical advances of these countries realized a few decades earlier than their counterparts on the Asian, African or Latin American continents that, since the chances of survival of their infants have vastly improved, they need not have a large family. The norm of the small family became the accepted pattern. In the developing countries, in spite of the significantly lowered infant mortality rate, this assurance has not penetrated the psychology of the vast majority of the mothers that their infant is going to survive and grow into adulthood and be of some help to parents in their old age. Once they get this assurance, there is less likelihood that they will have six or seven children. They are more likely to stop at two or three or, in Eastern societies, when they have satisfied the urge of fathering a son.

The large family size is directly related to the nutritional standard of all the members. A vast majority of the people in the developing countries lives on small fixed incomes, 90 percent of which is spent on getting food and shelter. When the number of children is large, not only is the level of food of all those sharing that fixed income likely to be low, but the standard of hygiene and sanitation of their shelter (dwelling or house) is likely to be correspondingly low. If a lesser number of children have to depend on the same income, they are likely to get better food, live in a more sanitary dwelling contract a lesser number of infections, and have brighter chances of survival. It has been established by a number of studies that the rate of infant mortality is much less in the first, second, or even third children than the subsequent ones. The rate of infant mortality is indeed high among those who are sixth in the arrivals. The rate of infant mortality is also lower among children who are spaced by two years or more than those who are born at closer intervals.

It is, therefore, essential that the planners of a country should not mourn the mistake of prematurely lowering the death rate by improved medical facilities without concomitantly decreasing the birth rate, thereby triggering population explosion because people will not decrease fertility until

they have security in terms of very low death rates, less malnutrition, and increase in per capita wealth or standard of
living. It is believed that in the developing countries it
is somewhat easier to "transmit the technology of health
and hygiene, pesticides and wonder drugs" than the technology of large-scale industrialization. By this approach, it
is hoped that a permanent long-term solution to the population problem will be found, rather than a short-term one.
While the population may still grow at a faster rate, a further
decline in the death rate will have a wholesome effect on the
cultural attitudes, which are ultimately going to determine
the outcome of this vexatious problem (Fredericksen, 1966).

> The basic assumption here is that demographic cause and effect is
> not a single plane phenomenon because several causes and effects are
> going on at various levels at the same time. An effective reduction
> of mortality need not wait till fertility is controlled. The increasing
> production of goods and services, at least food supply and health
> services, need not await the curtailing of rate of population growth,
> because small installments of all desirable processes will be in the
> nature of things happening simultaneously and not one at a time or
> one after another in some kind of preordained sequence . . . . such
> an unconventional and uneconomic approach will guarantee maximum
> dividends from investment on the development of human resources.
> Hitherto the approach has been a conventional one—spending more
> on birth control than on death control because of the common belief
> that even normal death control would lead to increasing investment
> in birth control. But while birth control is most essential, family
> planning ends will also be achieved by controlling the death rate,
> particularly the infant mortality rate (Chandrasekhra, 1972).

It may be reasonably concluded that the most effective method
of birth control is by lowering the infant mortality rates by
improving the nutritional level of the children.

POPULATION CONTROL MEASURES

Public Health Services

There are two main reasons for the high rate of population growth in a number of countries. The first one is the
ignorance about how to prevent the coming of new babies
year after year. Surveys indicate that parents with large

numbers of children realize that their poverty is a direct result of very large family size. A universal access to knowledge of contraception is a prerequisite to slowing down the rate of population growth. The second reason is the prevalent high rate of mortality among infants caused by a variety of pediatric ailments and, among the adults, caused by epidemics and natural disasters. This loss of life creates a psychological necessity to have a larger number of children to assure the survival of at least a few of them. In order to achieve a lower rate of population growth, it is most important that this psychology be reversed. This can be achieved by improving the public health services, maternal and child care services, and social services. This has been demonstrated by a recent study in India which shows that "families which have knowledge and have adopted good public health services as a way of life are the families which are more likely to have knowledge and practice family planning which over a period of time will be reflected in smaller families and lowered birth rates (Dutta, 1973). While it is true that the degree of knowledge about contraception as well as the improved public health services is essential to reverse a psychology of having large families, the period of transition could be one of great stress and strain. India is a classic example in this respect, as revealed by the following facts.

As a result of intensive well-organized public health programs, malaria was virtually eliminated as a public health problem. In 1947, there were recorded 75 million cases and 800,000 deaths from malaria; in 1964, the deaths were reduced to 56,000 (*Health Statistics of India,* 1970b). Smallpox has a similar story; in 1950, there were 150,000 attacks of smallpox which were reduced to 37,000 by 1964 (Samacher, 1965). Plague, which used to take a heavy toll of human life, is simply nonexistent because of the stringent public health measures (*Health Statistics of India,* 1970a; 1970b). The net result of all these improvements was that the average death rate of 27.4 in 1950 was reduced to 14.53 by 1971. This compares favorably with a large number of industrialized countries of the West. While the government was working on the health services of the country, the people did not take notice of the decreasing mortality rate as far as their psychology about family size was concerned. They kept on producing large numbers of children without giving any credit to the lives saved by the public health measures of the government. The net result was that in spite of all the democratic propaganda of the government about the need for family planning, the birth rate declined only from 39.2 in 1950 to 38.67 in 1971. The population grew at the rate of 2.4 percent, showing a net addition of about 13 million persons per year. In terms of figures, India increased its population from 439 million in 1961 to 547 million in 1971, a net increase of 108 million over a ten year period (Census of India, 1971). It might be recalled here that out of 147 countries, only seven countries in the world have a population of more than 100 million.

This raises many questions. Should India or other developing countries abandon the improvement in health services and let high death rates equalize the high birth rates? Nobody in his sane mind would recommend such a course because it involves a huge waste of human capital. The solution lies in a well organized, well planned system of population control measures while, at the same time, improving the health services all the more. While every effort should be made to save human lives and no one should have to die if the modern science and technology can help it, the uncontrolled growth in population could be equally catastrophic. If the people are not yet ready to reverse their psychological needs for larger families in order to assure the survival of a few children, the government may have to step in with its resources for voluntary family planning measures as well as legislative measures to control fertility.

Access to Commonly Used Methods of Family Planning

Birth control methods range from simple condoms to contraceptive steroids, intrauterine devices and sterilization (Contraceptive Technology, 1973–74). The condoms are relatively simple to use and are quite effective in preventing pregnancy as well as any contact with disease. Sexual intercourse among humans is also a very emotional phenomenon and the condom in a large number of situations takes the fun out of the process. They are widely used all over the world and their advantages lie in simplicity of use. They have made great contributions in preventing unnecessary fertility, especially in illicit relationships. The use of spermicidal agents (jellies and creams) deposited in the upper part of the vagina with special applicators and diaphragms are other methods which are equally simple. A well-fitted and properly used diaphragm is a highly effective contraceptive. Rhythm method or the periodic abstention is another method widely recommended. It involves avoiding sexual intercourse a few days before and after ovulation. However, none of these methods are popular because of the care needed in their implementation. Married couples, especially, tend to prefer other methods such as intrauterine devices, steroids or sterilization, which are almost foolproof solutions to unwanted pregnancy.

Intrauterine Devices

The intrauterine devices in order to prevent pregnancy have been used for centuries. The Hippocratic writings on "Diseases of Women" mention them quite frequently and the technique involved such as the insertion of all kinds of material ranging from lead, wool, ivory, wood, glass, silver, gold, ebony or platinum (Segal, *et al.*, 1965, Segal and Tietze, 1971). The medical literature of the 19th Century is filled with the merits and demerits of intrauterine devices. The question of infection, cancer and the formation of foreign bodies was reported in a number of cases. It was in the 1950's, however, that sterile, safe and effective intrauterine devices were developed.

Starting from the Pust intrauterine ring with a cervical extension, and the complete uterine ring of Grafenberg, a large number of devices have been made and tested. At the 1964 International Congress of Intrauterine Contraception, a large number of reports on the effectiveness of the intrauterine devices were reported from all over the world and at present the IUD is next only to the pill as a method of choice for the prevention of unnecessary pregnancy. About half a million births are prevented annually in India alone by the use of IUD's (Simmons, 1971). The rate of pregnancy among the two most popularly used IUD's (Large Lippes Loop and TCU 200) are 2.7 and 2.2 per 100 women per year of use respectively (Southam, 1973). The IUD's are available in a large number of shapes. They act by producing "an infiltration of polymorphonuclear leukocytes into the endo-metrius producing a normally sterile exudate which appears to be hostile to sperm and to blastocytes in experimental animals" (Southam, 1973). There is a small percentage (approximately 2 percent) of women who cannot tolerate the IUD's and tend to reject them or show side effects which may be as mild as pain and irregular bleeding during the early months of use or as serious as pelvic inflammation. The latter may even result in death and cases have been recorded to that effect. The IUD's are suspected to produce cervical and uterine cancer, but definite data are missing to prove or disprove it (*Report on Intrauterine Contraceptive Devices,* 1968; Segal and Tietze, 1971). The mortality rate from the use of intrauterine devices is 2 per 100,000 users. Based on the experience with the existing IUD's, new varieties are being produced as a result of extensive research. These are intended to decrease further the pregnancy rate, to lower the expulsion rate as well as to prevent pain and bleeding disturbances. The newly developed IUD's are either *inert* which are the new versions of the existing IUD's, or *medicated* (Johannisson, 1973). In the latter category, efforts are being made to develop IUD's which can deliver natural proges-terones directly to the target organ. One such IUD has been designed by Alza Corporation in California. It delivers a small quantity of progesterone daily and inhibits pregnancy by preventing implantation of the fertilized egg. Since the uterus lining destroys the natural progesterone, the side effects may be minimal. One IUD insertion may be good for as long as one year.

Steroids or Hormone Based Pills

The fundamental principal in the use of the pill as a method of contraception is the role of steroids in the suppression of ovulation. A number of steroids which are substitutes of progesterones and estrogens are available and are under active investigation. Most of the available pills contain a combination of one of several synthetic progestins and estrogens. In the United States alone, at least 20 brands are marketed and several million women are regular users. The 21 Pill Program is started from day five of the menstral cycle through the 25th or 26th day. When taken consistently over a long period of time, the oral contraceptives are associated with a very low failure rate. The rate of pregnancy by the use of combined type (progestin and estrogen) pills is only 0.7 per 100 women over a year's use.

However, the use of the pill as a method of contraception requires the constant drugging of the woman. Depending on the estrogen content, the pill is associated with the risk of thromboembolic disease. There have been many attempts, although inconclusive, to show the elevated risk of the woman on pills. Among the pill users, there is a three to seven times greater risk of uterine or breast cancer than among the nonusers. Also, among the users the mortality rate is 1.5 per 100,000 among the age group of 20 to 35 years, but jumps to 39 per 100,000 among women of 35 to 44 years of age.

The other complications resulting from long term use of the pills include nausea, vomiting, emotional changes, facial pigmentation and slight loss of hair. Some women who use pills as contraceptives complain of constant headaches and recently there is sufficient evidence to show that pills must not be prescribed to those women who have had migrane or similar vascular headaches (Man's Impact on the Global Environment, 1970; Weisbrod, 1972).

Since the pills act by suppressing ovulation, there are a lot of similarities between women who are taking pills and those who are actually pregnant. While a pregnant woman may add (exclusive of the fetus, membranes and amniotic fluid) approximately 10 pounds weight, the pill users add on the average 6 pounds weight. There is fluid retention and the enlargement of the breast in both conditions. Both pill users and pregnant women also show altered carbohydrate and lipid metabolism. (Goldzieber, 1970; Hodges, 1971).

Based on these facts a continuous effort is being made to improve on the pill, while at the same time getting the same benefits. One improvement is the *mini pill*. The *mini pill* contains only progestogen and in a daily dosage quantity almost one-third or less than that of the conventional pills used these days. "The low concentration of progestogen apparently prevents the sperm from reaching the oviducts, where fertilization occurs by maintaining the mucus at the opening to the uterus in a condition that hinders sperm migration" (Marx, 1973). The *mini pill* is designed to remove the biggest criticism that estrogen in the conventional pill is responsible for the often observed undesirable side effects. The Food and Drug Administration says, however, that progestogen in the *mini pill* is converted to an estrogen in the body. Secondly, the conventional pill has proven almost 100 percent effective. The trial use of the *mini pill* has shown a failure rate of 3 percent, which means that if 100 women use the *mini pill* over a one-year period, three of them may become pregnant. Further work on the *mini pill* needs to be done to improve upon its performance.

Sterilization

Sterilization of the male (vasectomy) and the female (tubal closure) are the most effective methods for the prevention of pregnancy. The ancient Egyptians, Chinese and Indians performed castration of the male and ovariectomy of the female for the purpose of preventing conception as well as other reasons. The castration of young male draft animals is still very common in India. In recent years, the procedure of sterilization has become very important in the drive to limit the human populations. India alone performs more than one million sterilization procedures annually. However, for the size of the Indian population and the high rate of population growth, this number is insignificant.

The vasectomy is a very simple procedure involving the bilateral interruption of the continuity of the vas deferens and does not require hospitalization. Since it is an almost irreversible procedure, there are several companies who freeze semen before vasectomy so that these men can still father children if the need arises. Several side effects such as pain, swelling, formation of hematomas, etc., have occasionally been reported, but there have been no deaths reported (Richter and Prager, 1972). Work is in progress at the Illinois Institute of Technology to develop a valve which will permit reversible sterilization of the male. This is likely to make this procedure more attractive.

Tubal ligation or closure is more complicated than vasectomy and requires several days of hospitalization. Newer methods have been developed by which tubal closure can be accomplished without hospitalization using local anesthesia. "The incidence of morbidity and mortality is much lower with the newer methods of culdoscopic visualization and closure of the tubes with clips or cautery" (Nortman, 1971).

Abortion

Abortion as a method of preventing unnecessary or extra additions to the family has been practiced world-wide, although in a large number of countries of the world it has been considered immoral or unwise. In countries like Japan, China and Russia, it is an accepted practice, whereas in others its availability is legally restricted. Despite legal restrictions, a large number of abortions are carried out in private clinics all over the world including the United States. Having realized the futility of unnecessary restrictions over the right of the mother to abort an unwanted fetus, several countries have loosened their laws. In a number of states in the United States, abortions can be legally performed in a well-equipped hospital. India passed an open abortion law in 1971 in order to strengthen the nation's family planning program.

The long term effects of abortion on the physiology and health of the female are still not clearly known. However, the data collected from countries where abortion has been legally practiced for several years show that repeated abortions may increase the frequency of premature births in future pregnancies (Brewer, 1972).

A hot controversy on the morality of abortion as a means of family planning or population control exists. The case can be argued endlessly. Especially controversial is the definition of what time the fetus becomes a human. Scientifically, one can say that as soon as the egg is fertilized, if given the opportunity, it will transform itself into a human. From this viewpoint, one can raise all kinds of arguments against induced abortion, based on social, humane or religious grounds. Cardinal Cook declared in 1972 that abortion is demeaning human life. Strong arguments can be given against the practice of abortion which, to some people, is nothing short of taking human life.

We have also to see the other side of the coin in the context of human existence in this world. Do we have to keep or do we need all the individuals that we are capable of producing? Like all animals, we also have the ability for prolific breeding. Do we have to force a woman to nurture an unwanted pregnancy and not give her the right to decide whether she needs to keep or wants that child? Can we worry all the time about the rights of the unborn and not the welfare of those who already have made their way into our world? In modern days of technology, we have to revise our attitude towards the rights of the unborn, especially when we know that it may not be long before babies may be produced by means of *in vitro* fertilization (Kass, 1971). We have to revise our legal standing to the effect that the infant is a being as soon as it is conceived (Diddle, 1973; *Mich Law Rev,* 1969). We should be concerned about the high rate of population growth and the ways and means by which to control our fertility in order to maintain a semblance of orderly society, which is extremely important from the point of view of the future of our species. Rouse believes that we may be forced into a situation where a couple may or may not be given the privilege by law to reproduce (Rouse, 1971).

Barnes lamented that "we are in a sense, a society of the walking wounded, collectively overcrowded and individually hurt, and the correction of this situation is the urgent task to which we should commit our thoughtful energy." Japan is a highly industrialized crowded society and has no legal, religious or medical restrictions concerning abortion. The individual couple should be given the choice of whether or not it would like to take care of an additional baby even if it has been conceived. Our medical knowledge is fairly advanced as to leaving no physical, physiological or emotional scar on the mother if she chooses to abort her fetus.

Illegitimacy is one of the biggest reasons in favor of making abortion legally available to those who wish to rid themselves of the unwanted pregnancy. In all countries of the world, where legal avenues are not available, the practice of illegal abortion by quacks and professionals alike is a flourishing business. It is the duty of the state to protect first the life of the would-be mother rather than the unborn individual for whom society is not yet ready. In the 25 years between 1940 and 1965, the percentage of illegitimate births increased from 3.8 to 7.7 percent of all live births. Out of the 291,200 out-of-wedlock live births in the United States, 44 percent were born to teenagers 19 years of age and under (Goldsmith, 1969). This is not to mention that 22 percent of all recent births in the United States to married couples were unwanted by at least one parent (Gold and Ballard, 1970). It is prudent to impart to our young generation useful instruction on sex, family life preparation, venereal disease prevention and knowledge of contraception. If they fail, as occasionally all do, the outlet of abortion should be available. It is better to abort a fetus who is unwanted than to bring him into the world.

Hormones

The recent discoveries of the secretion of hormones by the brain which regulate the reproductive processes have opened up new areas of research to regulate human fertility. One part of the brain—hypothalamus—directs the release of a certain category of hormones called luteinizing hormones by the pituitary gland which, in turn, triggers ovulation. The administration of a suitable preparation of this hormone may help a woman to control the time of her ovulation.

Prostaglandins, generally referred to as *miracle drugs,* are also being used to induce abortions in Europe. These drugs may either be given intravenously or injected through the vagina into the uterus.

Some important research work is also being pursued in the area of making an oral contraceptive for males. It will act by preventing sperm formation or by inhibiting sperm maturation. This approach has not been satisfactorily tested, although certain chemicals such as 'Danazol,' which is a synthetic analog of a male hormone, have been observed to decrease sperm counts.

Immunological Approaches to Birth Control

Immunological approaches have been successfully used over the last few decades to eliminate some diseases which take a heavy toll of human life. They may well be used to control human fertility as well. Antigens specific to sperm have been identified, isolated and used to immunize both males and females against the sperms that carry the antigen. These antibodies interfere with sperm production or viability. For example, Erwin Goldberg at Northwestern University in Chicago, Illinois, found that serum containing antibodies to the sperm-specific form of the enzyme lactate dehydrogenase suppressed the pregnancies of up to 60 percent of mice injected with the antiserum after copulation (Marx, 1973). The production of antibodies against female gonads is another approach. For example, it has been shown in mice that very early embryonic stages possess specific antigens on the membrane, which are not found at later developmental stages. Such an egg specific antigen might be used with a suitable immunization procedure so that a female would be sensitized to the antigen thus interfering with the implantation and further development of any early embryonic stages (Joshi, 1973). A lot of careful research is needed before a definitive statement can be made on the use of this method for birth control.

Family Planning Education

The biggest reason why family planning education should be imparted to our youth in an organized manner by the community is that more harm is done by misinformation rather than by accurate information. Many people have misgivings about family planning education. They believe that it will lead to rampant promiscuity and immoral practices. Recent sociological research has clearly shown that the knowledge or availability of contraceptives per se does not lead to increased sexual activity, whether it is premarital or in a married state. Pion pointed out that the adults opposing family planning education are those who in their youth based their own moral decision on a fear of pregnancy principle and who do not have any other moral argument when queried in depth by the youth of today (Pion, 1971). Pion also has some ideas about how to impart the family planning education to our youth on a formal and informal basis. On a formal basis, a young man should be aware of the problem of population in the context of its size, the cultural importance of family and the reproductive processes, while an attempt is being made to impart to him the awareness and availability of contraceptives. The involvement of the parents in such an education program is highly desirable because it has a positive moral influence on the mind of the young. He becomes more conscious about his role in the world at large and his community or family in particular. He realizes that the fast rate of population growth is the result of contributions of individual couples in their small way. Berelson (1973) emphasized that education in its nature is future oriented and hence makes planning more sensible, including family planning.

It is only natural for us to teach the innocent and young people who have not yet been misinformed by others, the truth about our reproductive processes. The stork stories do more harm than good. Living things, indeed, come from living things and the use of so-called *four letter words* is not *dirty* if they have been cleansed of *dirty* connotations. Since the processes of ovulation and spermatogenesis are indeed miraculous and awe-inspiring, they should be treated as such and open discussion should be invited. It is in this context that the young person should be initiated into the field of contraception or controlling fertility. Pion goes as far as to say that it is appropriate to discuss at some length to a 4, 5, or 6 year old the concept that human beings, unlike other species of living things, plan the creation of their offspring. Conception should not be an accident but a well designed, planned event. Young children can and should be taught that children are to be born into viable functional units so that ideal nurturing may occur. These facts are to be repeated and expanded in depth as the child nears reproductive capacity (Pion, 1971).

The community, by its own agencies, can impart the right information in the right spirit in a manner that is not likely to be misused. Newspapers and magazines ought to give space in a respectable place to population planning or family planning. The advertising world, who have proven their capabilities to persuade, motivate, suggest, decide and even stimulate, should rise to the task of educating our young men and women. "Family planning education is more than sex education, birth control devices and services or premarital examinations; it is the learning of a concept, a concept that would permit the system to respond to a priority need" (Pion, 1971).

Most adults in the developed countries have accepted family planning and are active participants in population control, but there is a great difference of opinion as to whether the birth control technology should be handed over to the teenager. Some fear that the measures that have led to a decline in fertility and an improvement in the quality of life may degenerate into a floodgate of immorality if they are handed over without restrictions to their growing teenagers. The free availability of contraceptives poses a moral issue. Most white Americans favor birth control education in high schools but are reticent about providing birth control services to teenage girls. They are afraid of the rising tide of premarital sex relations (Blake, 1973). This has caused a social problem of some magnitude, especially in view of the rising rate of unwanted pregnancies among single teenagers. Only an enlightened approach can solve this problem.

In the developing countries, the problems are of a different nature. Even today a major proportion of the births takes place outside the hospital without the help of an obstetrician. The midwives, trained and untrained, are still responsible for the prenatal care and the obstetrical service. In these circumstances, it is the midwife who can implement the family planning goals better than the physician. If midwives are trained and motivated properly, they will put a dent in the birth control program even without the necessary tools. In every village or clan, a midwife is almost omnipresent. She is a counselor and, in this capacity, she can be of useful service as a component of education. The rhythm method of contraception, which virtually failed in most developing countries, may have been due to a lack of knowledge or the motivation of the midwife. A proper education can go a long way. It may be surprising that Japan has the highest use of rhythm method of any other nation and the number of couples adopting the method exceeds that found in Catholic countries (Sai, 1973). Kohl *et al.* have outlined a training program for the midwife which they found extremely successful in Ghana within the 1½ years of its operation. If money and resources are utilized along with some enthusiasm, the practicing midwives in the developing countries can handle the family planning programs most effectively in the rural areas where 80 percent or more of their populations live. It may be worthwhile to quote here the outline of the course suggested by Kohl *et al.*

1. Comprehensive instruction in all phases of family planning.
2. Understanding of the basic concepts of the anatomy and physiology of the reproductive systems.
3. Complete indoctrination in the accepted methods of family planning and exposure to the experimental methods being investigated.

4. Attention to the development of proper methodology by each trainee.
5. Accurate record keeping and follow-up of patients.
6. Instruction in demography and the economics of family planning.
7. Orientation into social service problems of family planning.
8. Clinic planning and management.

At the outset of the course, our nurse-midwife staff evaluates each trainee's gynecological knowledge and skills. All trainees must become efficient in performing pelvic examinations. In order to properly care for patients medically, and in order to adequately prescribe family planning methods, the trainee must learn to:

1. Determine position, size and shape of the uterus and adnexa.
2. Determine the direction of the cervical canal.
3. Sound the uterus.
4. Recognize gross pelvic pathology.
5. Properly take vaginal and cervical smears for neoplasia detection.

The trainees are taught a minimum of laboratory techniques:

1. Hematocrit or hemoglobin determinations.
2. Trichomonas smears.
3. *Pap* smears.
4. Pregnancy test.

Each trainee is required to perform these tests whenever indicated on her patient. This is carried out under the direct supervision of her instructors. In addition to the clinical instruction, the trainees receive didactic instruction in:

Demography
Psychology of family planning
Ecology
Endocrinology of the ovulatory cycle and oral contraceptives
Disorders of menstruation.

After the third week of the course, the trainee begins to insert IUD's under very close supervision. After the sixth week, she is usually capable of doing this on her own. When she is ready to begin to work alone she has learned to perform as follows:

1. Secure and record an accurate history.
2. Perform a physical examination consisting of blood pressure determination, breast examination, thyroid palpation, and search for signs of circulatory problems, especially in the lower extremities and vulva.
3. Perform bimanual vaginal, recto-vaginal and speculum examinations, *Pap* smear and sounding of the uterus.

After carrying out the above, the patient and trainee are ready for a definitive selection of a method of family planning.

Encouraging Trends

Under the pressure of the high rate of population growth, a large number of countries all over the world have supported the family planning programs. It may be of some interest to the reader to have an idea of the countries who have active family planning programs. In Africa; Ghana, Kenya, Mauritius, Morocco, Nigeria, Tunisia and Egypt have an active family planning program. In Latin America; Barbados, the Dominican Republic, Guatemala, Jamaica, Puerto Rico, Trinidad and Tobago are quite actively working to control their populations. In Asia; Hong Kong, the Peoples' Republic of China, South Korea, Taiwan, India, Indonesia, Iran, Malaysia, Nepal, Pakistan, Philippines, Singapore, Thailand and Turkey have, over the last few years, pursued vigorously their family planning programs. However, there are some countries which, in spite of the need, do not have an active administrative policy of curbing their population growth. These are Algeria, Cameroon, Congo, Ethiopia, Madagascar, Sudan, Uganda, Brazil, Mexico, Peru, North Korea, Afghanistan, Burma, Cambodia, Iraq, Jordan, Laos, Lebanon, Saudi Arabia, Syria, North and South Vietnam and Yemen. It is hoped that in the coming years, these countries will also actively participate in stabilizing their populations.

India is a notable example among the developing countries to have an official family planning program, which shows the urgency and effort demanded by the situation. These include a wide publicity campaign with every available medium of communication emphasizing the desirability and benefits of a smaller family norm. Permanent and mobile clinics have been established throughout the length and breadth of the country which provide maternal health facilities, child care, immunizations against common infections as well as the education and material for family planning. Success in bringing down the rate of population growth would have been greater if some mandatory schemes were instituted, but a democratic India preferred the long, torturous road of persuasion, education and willing cooperation in order to achieve a long-term success. Many valid criticisms can be mentioned, but by and large this is one of the successful family planning programs in the world, considering the difficulties encountered in making useful contacts with a population steeped in ignorance, illiteracy, poverty, superstition and living in more than half a million villages not connected with one another by any modern means of communication.

India has done pioneering work in the distribution of 300 million condoms per year. The intrauterine devices have been tried on a large scale. Up to the end of 1972, India performed 12 million sterilizations. Impressive as this may seem, these efforts have only touched the periphery of the problem. Approximately 75 to 80 percent of the population has not been successfully contacted and has not been convinced of the need for restricting births. It is, however, believed that in the long run India will be successful in reducing its population growth to manageable levels, but it is the transition period of 10 to 20 years which is a matter of great concern to social scientists and agricultural experts.

Very little reliable information is available about the population figures and the family planning programs of the Peoples' Republic of China. Recent reports indicate that the Chinese are as active in the field of population control as any other overcrowded country. Late marriage with strict chastity before marriage is greatly reducing the birth rate. The ideal age for a man to marry is thirty; for a woman, twenty-five. The Chinese Peoples' Republic, according to the International Planned Parenthood News of June, 1972, has the best birth control program in the world, with 85 to 90 percent of Chinese couples participating. Female sterilization is the most popular method but vasectomies are also performed. Oral contraceptives rank second and condoms third (Faundes and Luukkainen, 1972; Southam, 1973). In some Chinese hospitals, abortions outnumber the live deliveries. A recent report indicates that the growth rate in urban areas is 1 percent or less. In China's most modern city, Shanghai, the crude birth rate is 12 per thousand, whereas the death rate is 5 per thousand, which yields a natural increase of 0.7 percent (*Scientific American*, 1973). It is stressed that it is no longer necessary to have children to guarantee security in old age and that planned birth is not something to be ashamed of; rather, it is something to be genuinely proud of.

It is also gratifying to note that in the United States there has been a family planning movement on a voluntary basis which is likely to make the proposition of zero population growth a reality. Starting from a birth rate of 24 live births per 1,000 population in 1960, the growth rate declined to 18 live births per 1,000 population in 1970, and has been declining steadily ever since. The greatest change that has happened is the awareness of family planning among the members of the lower and lower-middle classes. A Princeton University survey shows that fertility rates have significantly declined in recent years among the poor and near-poor women as compared to women above the poverty level. Three out of five couples using contraceptives employ the most effective methods such as pills, IUD's, or sterilization (Jafe, 1973).

REMEDIAL REMARKS

Reducing Population Growth

The *Homo sapiens* is a very intelligent species. He has gone through a series of adjustments, adaptations, setbacks and triumphs through his million year history in order to come to his present status as master of this planet. Now his own fertility and numbers if they are allowed to increase unchecked over the next century are becoming threats to his existence; it is more than probable that he will voluntarily go through other types of adjustments and adaptations before it is too late. The technologically developed countries of the west, as well as the east, have demonstrated that, given the social and economic impetus, the people will restrict their family size and their total numbers voluntarily.

There are some who feel so strongly about the catastrophic consequences of population explosion that they do not procreate at all to compensate for the extra baggage of someone else. Unfortunately, it is only the intelligent, thinking, concerned men and women who read the writing on the wall and act to protect the best interests of humanity. The ignorant or fanatics of the minority communities (who misread the message as some kind of an attempt to curtail their numbers and deprive them of their political powers) not only are not concerned about the growing human population, but want their numbers to increase as if on the doomsday, they want to proclaim that they died as a majority.

The unabated population growth has increased the density of population in areas which are the centers of industry, employment and material development. This, in turn, has raised problems of physical space, supply of food and water, and other resources. It has questioned the greatest moral issue of the "Quality of Human Life." Certain amenities, which have so far been taken for granted, may no longer be available if population keeps on increasing. In the industrially developed countries, the meaning of 'quality of human life' is interpreted in somewhat different terms than in the developing countries. In the former, overcrowding leads to excessive utilization of resources, which results in smog, pollution and unbearable pressure on social and natural environment. In the developing countries, the increasing density of population results in the denial of certain basic and fundamental needs of human existence. The scarcity of food results in a generation of people who are apathetic, lethargic and unable to understand or improve their conditions. The per capita income declines as more and more humans arrive with each passing year. The country finds itself unable to provide facilities for universal education, which is a prerequisite for decent citizenhood. The increasing population cuts down on savings and capital accumulation as substantial resources have to be spent on social services (Muller, 1973). In short, there is an overall deterioration of the quality of human life as the population increases at a rate much more than the replacement level.

The situation in the developing countries is the one that poses a threat as well as a challenge. Most of the populations of these countries are genuinely ignorant about the arith-

metic of one couple having 6 to 8 children in their reproductive period. All they can count is that their father had 8
children and he was able to feed them. Now they can have
6 to 8 children and they are going to feed them. No serious
catastrophe came in their father's time and nothing can be
expected now because all they have is a small number of six
children. These people do not have the intellectual background to understand the Malthusian growth of human populations and are therefore not equipped mentally to receive
the message of restricting their family size.

The means of communication in these countries is very
poor. In the absence of radio, television, good roads, rail-
roads and other communication channels, it is hard to impart the necessary education in this vital area of human welfare. It is this challenge that will determine the outcome of
any effort to curtail the human numbers on a voluntary basis.
Education and enlightenment are likely to have an impact
only over a very long period of time. By that time, we may
already be so overcrowded that the struggle for survival
may become a big burden. Because of the decreasing death
rates among the infants, the age structure of the developing
countries has drastically changed over the last two to three
decades. These overpopulated countries, especially in Asia,
have had a large population density to begin with, and even
a small percent increase caused by a stationary birth rate at
around 4 percent and a decreased death rate will add im-
pressively to their already large pool. This has resulted in
the preponderance of younger persons in their pre-reproduc-
tive age. When these persons marry and enter the pool of
those actively involved in the process of reproduction, the
numbers are bound to increase at levels higher than in the
past because of the significantly larger number of participants
in the game.

A successful family planning program needs a good management at the top and a missionary zeal on the part of its
workers. At the same time, it needs all the necessary legal
aids such as liberalization of abortion laws, raising the marriage age for boys and girls to more than 20 years, etc. The

communication media such as the press, radio, television, etc., can also play an important role in the creation of a favorable climate for couples to go through a sterilization procedure after 2 to 3 children without mental agony or uncertainty. It is only by a combination of a variety of family planning procedures, condoms, IUD's, pills, sterilization, etc., coupled with the prospects of economic betterment with a small family, that a dent can be made in the birth rate and the norm of a small happy family becomes a reality among all sections of the communities.

It is quite evident that at some point, we will have to put a ceiling on the family size in order to control the present rate of the world's population growth. Responsibility of restricting family size assumed voluntarily is much more effective than a regimented coercive approach from the top leadership downwards. The democratic system has much more resilience in this respect than an authoritarian regime that does not care to explain to the people the goals, in spite of their best intentions. However, in a democratic set-up, one may have to contemplate the infringement of one's private right to procreation. For the good of society, community and country, certain governments may be encouraged to seek from their legislators some measures of compulsory sterilization after two or three children before that catastrophic number reaches the point where the economy cannot sustain the demographic machine.

Reduction in the rate of population growth is desirable, not only for domestic reasons of improving the quality of life for one's citizens, but also from the point of view of worldwide stability. Our planet is no longer a big celestial body with inhabitants of one part not affecting the lives of those living in other parts. With faster and faster means of communication, growing international trade and interplanetary travel not far away, the people of this world have never been so interdependent before as they are today. Unabated population growth at a high rate in one country or region with the resulting deterioration of the quality of life for its inhabitants affects the social and political life of people in other regions or countries.

There is one more word of caution that may be needed here. The present writer has emphasized in great detail the need of the overcrowded developing countries to curtail their populations or at least stabilize them at their present figures. This should not be taken that, since the industrially advanced countries have the economic resources, they should indulge in the luxury of procreating at will. On the contrary, the rich face a bigger responsibility. It is well known that the rich consume a larger share of energy and food per capita, as well as other resources of the earth. The rich people occupy much more space, consume more of each natural resource, disturb the ecology more, and create more land, air, water, chemical, thermal and radioactive pollution than poor people. So it can be argued that from many viewpoints, it is even more urgent to control the numbers of the rich than it is to control the numbers of the poor (Mayer, 1972).

Our axiom here is to restrict the human numbers to a level where the mother earth can provide its resources without disturbing its ecological balance. The exploration of space is giving evidence that the earth is one of the most beautiful planets. We must be lucky to have taken possession of it. Let us not pollute it and make it unlivable. Let us keep it beautiful and let us prove that the ingenious human species, when challenged, always rises to the occasion. The conclusions arrived at by Ehrlich and Ehrlich are quite pertinent in this context.

1. Considering present technology and patterns of behavior our planet is grossly overpopulated now.
2. The large absolute number of people and the rate of population growth are major hindrances to solving human problems.
3. The limits of human capability to produce food by conventional means have very nearly been reached. Problems of supply and distribution already have resulted in roughly half of humanity being undernourished or malnourished. Some 10 to 20 million people are starving to death annually now.
4. Attempts to increase food production further will tend to accelerate

the deterioration of our environment, which in turn will eventually *reduce* the capacity of the Earth to produce food. It is not clear whether environmental decay has now gone so far as to be essentially irreversible; it is possible that the capacity of the planet to support human life has been permanently impaired. Such technological *successes,* as automobiles, pesticides, and inorganic nitrogen fertilizers are major causes of environmental deterioration.

5. There is reason to believe that population growth increases the probability of a lethal worldwide plague and of a thermonuclear war. Either could provide an undesirable *death rate solution* to the population problem; each is potentially capable of destroying civilization and even of driving *Homo sapiens* to extinction.

6. There is no technological panacea for the complex of problems composing the population-food-environment crisis, although technology, properly applied in such areas as pollution abatement, communications, and fertility control can provide massive assistance. The basic solutions involve dramatic and rapid changes in human *attitudes,* especially those relating to reproductive behavior, economic growth, technology, the environment, and conflict resolution (Ehrlich and Ehrlich, 1970).

Reducing Food Wastes and Encouraging Economical Food Consumption Patterns

Reducing food waste is as important as the effort to increase food output. The developing countries, where food needs are the greatest, are the ones that lack the technology as well as resources to store extra food and avoid wastage at different stages of food production. A large quantity of food is eaten in the fields by pests and an equally large quantity is wasted in storage. According to the estimates of FAO, the world food losses are as high as 50 billion dollars, most of it in the developing countries. It is estimated that in Latin America, the annual losses are as high as 40 percent of the total crop, and in tropical Africa, they are over 30 percent of their produce. It is believed that even if half of the world's storage losses were prevented, enough calories would be saved to satisfy the diets of half a billion people. Disinfecting cereal grain alone would net an estimated extra 9 million tons of protein a year, equivalent to the protein needs of 375 million people. In many countries, especially the needy ones, the combined losses due to rodents, insects and fungi are double or triple the food deficits (Berg, 1973a). The developing countries need to develop and implement a comprehensive system of avoiding such heavy food losses. Surveillance should start in the fields and must continue to the time when the food is actually consumed.

Food consumption patterns is another area which needs attention. In general, consumers know little about the nutritional value of foods. A typical consumer depends greatly on the honesty of the food advertiser and feels cheated when he learns to the contrary. For example, in a number of survey studies, consumers were asked to describe a nutritionally balanced meal; only about 50 percent came reasonably close. The primary concern of a typical housewife, entrusted with the job of guarding the health of the family, is to please the tastes and food preferences of the members of her family (Bauman, 1973).

Independent organizations, such as the Nutrition Foundation, can do a good job of educating the people in nutrition and encouraging economical food consumption patterns through the sophisticated techniques of mass media. The government, educators, and especially the food industry have failed to get the message of good nutrition across to the people. Good nutrition perhaps necessitates certain important changes in food habits, and the consumers should know that it is not how much you spend but what you select to eat that matters to the body from the point of view of nutrition. Dr. Pearson, the former President of the Nutrition Foundation, rightly pointed out that:

> food manufacturers, sensing a good selling point in nutrition, rush to advertise how nutritious their products are. The consumer movement has unwittingly encouraged food faddists by raising public alarm over the chemicals and additives in processed foods. Nutritionists themselves have failed to agree, causing confusion in the minds of the public, and further aiding food faddists by failing to help the public to choose the most economical and nutritious foods.

A most important need is the promotion of understanding of nutriton, not just by teaching the nutritional alphabet or nutritional biochemistry but an applied knowledge of the

available foods and how they can be most economically consumed to promote the maximum nutritional welfare (Darby,
1972).

The American concept of food based on substantial
quantities of meat, poultry and dairy products, along with
bread or cereals, is the ideal nutritive standard for proper
health and well-being of human beings. In order to obtain
the superior animal products, an average American utilizes
one ton of food grains. This is in sharp contrast to 450 pounds
used by an average Asian. More than 2 billion, or ⅔ of the
human population, comes in the latter category. It is simply
inconceivable that food can be produced in such large quantities that the American concept of diet and nutrition can
be provided for all human beings. It is, therefore, essential
that consumption patterns be modified to provide adequate
nutrition but also eliminate the wasteful method of utilizing
food grains to convert them to meat, especially when it is
becoming increasingly clear that excessive consumption of
meat increases susceptibility to cholesterol and fat problems
(Holden, 1974).

Recent research has shown that vegetable proteins used
in a sagacious combination are as good as animal proteins
in promoting growth and maintaining perfect health. If the
wealthier countries simplify their diet only to some extent,
enough food could be saved for those who cannot afford the
bare necessities of survival. In certain respects, vegetable
sources of food may be superior to those of animal sources.
Vegetable oils are one example in that category. The widespread use of polyunsaturated vegetable fats has led to a
decrease in cardiovascular problems. Modern technology
has produced meat substitutes out of soy based products
that possess the taste, texture and cooking qualities of meat,
but do not contain its harmful saturated fat. One of the greatest benefits of modern technology is the utilization of vegetable proteins to augment meat proteins in ground meat.
"Soya protein *extenders* as they are known, are being added
to a variety of processed and ground meat products, frequently improving flavor, cooking qualities, and nutrition

as well as reducing prices" (Brown, 1973). The affluent communities of the developing countries can greatly help utilize the scarce animal proteins for the good of larger numbers of people by increasing the use of vegetable sources of food.

Learning to Live and Grow Within the Resources of our Planet

It is futile as well as dangerous to continue to use the earth's resources at the rate at which the United States is using them at present. If the presently underdeveloped and developing countries start using the earth's resources at the level of the United States, or develop a standard of living equivalent to that of the United States, all the known resources of earth will disappear within 50 years (Lebowitz, 1973a). Even without that happening, the limit to the earth's resources could come within a few decades, which could lead to a collapse of the whole system (Forrester, 1971; Meadows, 1972). Technology could support a population three to ten times its present size, but the standard of living of that larger population would be at much lower levels. The study of Meadows *et al.* is very interesting in this respect. They have shown the extent of our vulnerability if the population is not stabilized in the near future. Figure 3 represents a world model, which assumes no major changes in the physical, economic or social relationships that have historically governed the development of the world system. The variables (resources, food per capita, population, per capita industrial output and pollution) follow the pattern shown during 1900 to 1970.

The natural resources in such an uncontrolled system diminish so rapidly that it forces a slowdown in industrial growth with the result that food per capita will be drastically reduced and so will the population. Meadows *et al.* concluded that for a state of global equilibrium, population number and capital investment must be in an equilibrium state. By various computations, the emphasis from the factory produced goods should be shifted to health and educa-

tion facilities. Figure 4 shows the world model which supposes that, by 1975, the population is stabilized by setting
the birth rate equal to the death rate. The industrial capital
is allowed to increase naturally until 1990, after which it,
too, is stabilized by setting the investment rate equal to the
depreciations. In that ideal stabilized world model, the pollution level is low, the per capita industrial output as well
as per capita food output will be high and the resources of
the earth will be deleted at a gradual rate. In this system it
is supposed that 100 percent of the human population practices birth control and the average family size consists of two
children. The birth, deaths, investment and depreciation
are kept to a minimum level.

The undertaking of such a supreme effort is "a challenge
for our generation. It cannot be passed on to the next. The
effort must be resolutely undertaken without delay, and
significant redirection must be achieved during this decade."
If we do not heed the warnings at this stage and continue the
population growth as well as the rate of investment, Meadows
et al. concluded that "population and industrial growth will
certainly stop within the next century at the latest," under
its own weight. "The crux of the matter is not only whether
the human species will survive, but even more whether it
can survive without falling into a state of worthless existence." Technology has been extremely helpful to man's
survival as well as progress, but to rely upon it blindly may
not be so wise, although Boyd (1972) would have us believe
that irrespective of growth, technology could ultimately be
depended upon for continuous survival as well as prosperity.

In the past, Boyd's philosophy has worked successfully.
Technology always helped ease the natural pressures released by growth processes to such an extent that we have
now evolved a whole culture around the principle of fighting
against limits rather than learning to live within them. This
culture has been reinforced by the apparent immunity of the
earth and its resources and by the relative smallness of man
and his activities (Meadows *et al.*, 1972). This is indeed a
very optimistic way of believing that technology, whose

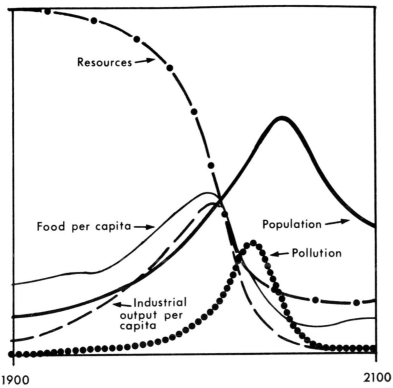

1900   2100

Figure 3. A world model which assumes no major changes in the physical, economic or social relationships that have historically governed the development of the world system. The variables (resources, food per capita, population, per capita industrial output and pollution) follow the pattern shown during 1900 to 1970. The natural resources in such an uncontrolled system diminish so rapidly that it forces a slowdown in industrial growth, with the result that food per capita will be drastically reduced and so will the population.

abundance can be continuously increased with human effort, will also greatly determine the world's future (Starr and Rudman, 1973). Meadows *et al.*, however, warned that

> the relationship between the earth's limits and man's activities is changing. The exponential growth curves are adding millions of people and billions of tons of pollutants to the ecosystem each year. Even the ocean, which once appeared virtually inexhaustible, is losing species after species of its commercially useful animals. Yet man does

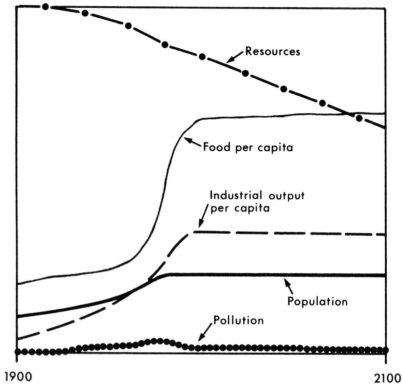

Figure 4. A world model which supposes that by 1975 the population is stabilized by setting the birth rate equal to the death rate. The industrial capital is allowed to increase rapidly until 1990, after which it, too, is stabilized by setting the investment rate equal to the depreciation. In that ideal stabilized world model, the pollution level is low, the per capita industrial output as well as food output is high and the resources of the earth will be depleted at a gradual rate.

not seem to learn by running into earth's obvious limits. Is it better to try to live within that limit by accepting a self-imposed restriction on growth? Or is it preferable to go on growing until some other natural limit arises, in the hope that at that time another technological leap will allow growth to continue still larger? For the last several hundred years, human society has followed the second course so consistently and successfully that the first choice has been all but forgotten.

There may be much disagreement with the statement that population and capital growth must stop soon. But virtually no one will argue that material growth on this planet can go on forever. At this point in man's history, the choice posed above is still available in almost every sphere of human activity. Man can still choose his limits and stop when he pleases by weakening some of the strong pressures that cause capital and population growth, or by instituting counter-pressures, or both. Such counter-pressures will probably not be entirely pleasant. They will certainly involve profound changes in the social and economic structures that have been deeply impressed into human culture by centuries of growth. The alternative is to wait until the price of technology becomes more than society can pay, or until the side effects of technology suppress growth themselves, or until problems arise that have no technical solution. At any of those points the choice of limits will be gone. Growth will be stopped by pressures that are not of human choosing.

Such a situation may be worse than those which the human society might choose for itself.

Meadows *et al.* took pains to explain that, in recommending a restriction in growth of capital as well as population, they do not foresee any limitation on the growth of technology.

Technological advance would be both necessary and welcome in the equilibrium state. A few obvious examples of the kinds of practical discoveries that would enhance the workings of a steady state society include:

1. new methods of waste collection, to decrease pollution and make discarded material available for recycling;
2. more efficient techniques of recycling, to reduce rates of resource depletion;
3. better product design to increase product lifetime and promote easy repair, so that the capital depreciation rate would be minimized;
4. harnessing of incident solar energy, the most pollution-free power source;
5. methods of natural pest control, based on more complete understanding of ecological interrelationships;
6. medical advances that would decrease the death rate;
7. contraceptive advances that would facilitate the equalization of the birth rate with the decreasing death rate.

As for the incentive that would encourage men to produce such technological advances, what better incentive could there be than the knowledge that a new idea would be translated into a visible improvement in the quality of life? Historically mankind's long record of new inventions has resulted in crowding, deterioration of the environment, and greater social inequality because greater productivity has been absorbed by population and capital growth. There is no reason why higher productivity could not be translated into higher standard of living or more leisure or more pleasant surroundings for everyone, if these goals replace growth as the primary value of society.

Similar conclusions have been arrived at by Forrester (1973), Behrens and Meadows (1973) and Randers and Meadows (1973), although some others tend to dispute their thesis on counterintuitive behavior of social systems, determinants of long-term resource availability and the carrying capacity of our global environment. Some of the counter arguments to the Meadows predictions may be in order. The Science Policy Research Unit of The Sussex University severely criticized the Meadows team and projected that the living systems are not passive victims of entropy and that population as well as capital could grow beyond the year 2100 without any catastrophic effects (Streatfield, 1973). Rothkopf (1973) stressed that the world model would not work simply because it would reflect the thinking of basically pessimistic and basically optimistic specialists. Fyodorov (1973) also voiced criticism against the conclusions of the limits to growth, believing that the continuous creation of new scientific and technological possibilities enables man to satisfy his increasing needs faster than his rate of population growth. Boyle (1973) believed that affluence without restrictive policies is attainable, provided corrective measures such as exploration of resources, new sources of energy, recycling, pollution control, agricultural technology and family planning are instituted simultaneously. Ridker (1973), however, posed the most pertinent question that the choice is not between grow or not to grow, but the inequities in the distribution of resources. Meadows and co-workers agreed that their model may have some flaws created by typographical and other errors, but warned that the physical planet has its limits to growth and significant delays in the feedback processes that act to contain population and capital within the global carrying capacity are likely to deteriorate the quality of life. The crux of the matter is "not only whether the human species will survive, but even more whether it can survive without falling into a state of worthless existence" (Meadows *et al.,* 1972). In light of the above discussions, it may be pertinent to add that, whatever the merits and demerits of the world model created by Meadows' team may be, we cannot afford to ignore the writing on the wall and we cannot permit population growth and resource consumption to continue at the present rate without serious consequences.

Cooperation Among Nations

Global poverty, with its ramifications such as technological backwardness manifesting itself in ancient agriculture and primitive health services, is mainly responsible for a losing battle between the food supply and the explosive population growth. It is time that the spirit of internationalism takes over the parochial interests. The developed countries ought to come forward, not to dole away food to the needy, but to reduce the technological and economic gap between themselves and the poor countries. By doing so all will benefit in the long run. Education and social improvement are the key to a realization of one's responsibilities towards himself and the human race. Ultimately education is the best way of implementing the goal of lowered birth rates along with improved quality of life for those who have chosen to stay on this planet. It is only by international cooperation that some worthwhile objectives can be achieved. The overcrowded developing countries are too poor to afford the huge capital demands necessary for massive literacy programs along with adequate social services, public health and nutritional measures.

The cooperation among the developed and developing countries can lead to a proper exploitation of the potential of the poor countries to the benefit of all mankind. It is the developing countries that have the greatest reservoir of unexploited food potential which they have not been able to utilize for lack of resources and resourcefulness. Given the appropriate economic incentive, fertilizers, water, capital input and the proper seeds, the per acre yield of the developing countries is likely to jump up significantly.

Readiness for Emergencies

Preparedness for emergencies is important because a vast majority of the human race lives in impoverished, underdeveloped, overpopulated countries in a perpetual state of undernourishment. A natural disaster such as drought, flood, or an earthquake, would drive many millions of such people to hunger, starvation and an extreme degree of malnutrition. The recent tragedies in West Africa and acute food shortages in Asia caused by droughts and floods or mass migration of populations of Bangladesh in 1971 remind us that we are not found ready to face the challenges on an emergency basis. The world has been steadily moving to a situation of chronic scarcity of agricultural products as the population keeps growing. Some of the thinking men have suggested various ways and means to combat crisis situations. The feasibility of such proposals must be seriously considered. The Director General of the Food and Agriculture Organization of the United Nations, Mr. A. H. Boerma, suggested in early 1973 the adoption of the concept of *minimum world food security*. This scheme would ask member nations of the United Nations to hold certain minimum levels of food stocks to take care of international emergencies. The food situation with respect to these buffer stocks would be reviewed periodically so that in the event of a crisis a machinery could be cranked up within the shortest possible time. The world community must have a basic humanitarian interest to ensure that unnecessary hardships are not borne by individuals hit by drought, famine, earthquake or other natural disasters. A world food bank is a natural corollary to any suggestion of international cooperation. Such a bank could be internationally managed and could be a great asset as well as have a stabilizing influence on the world food economy. A bank could build up reserves of food at the time of abundance, which could be utilized at the time of scarcity. It is indeed a complex undertaking, which requires great dedication and determination if we have to ensure adequate food supplies to countries who have the misfortune of being in the grip of crop failures or natural disasters.

REFERENCES

Allison, A. C.: *Proc R Soc Med, 66:* 110, 1973.

Asian Student, December 9, 1972.

Barnes, A. C.: *The Social Responsibility of Gynecology and Obstetrics.* Baltimore, Johns Hopkins, 1965.

Bauman, H. E.: *JAMA, 225:* 61, 1973.

Behrens, W. W. and Meadows, D. L.: In *Toward Global Equilibrium,* D. L. Meadows and D. H. Meadows (eds.) Cambridge, Wright Allen Press, 1973.

Bennett, I. L.: *World Rev Nutr Diet, 2:* 1–16, 1969.

Berelson, B.: *Persp Biol Med, 16:* 446, 1973.

Berg, A.: *The Nutrition Factor: Its Role in National Development.* Washington, Brookings, 1973.

Berg, A.: *Population Bulletin, 29:* 13, 1973.

Berg, A., and Muscat, R.: *Am J Clin Nutr, 25:* 939, 1972.

Blake, J.: *Science, 180:* 708, 1973.

Bogue, D. J.: *Principles of Demography.* New York, John Worley & Sons, 1969.

Boyd, R.: *Science, 177:* 516, 1972.

Boyle, T. J.: *Nature, 245:* 127, 1973.

Brewer, M. F. (Ed.) : *Population Bulletin, 28:* 4, 8, 1972,

Brown, L. R.: *Population Bulletin, 29:* 2, 1973.

Brown, R. E. and Wray, J. D.: *Nat History,* January, 1974.

Census of India in 1971, Series 1, Part I of 1971. Government of India.

Chandrasekhra, S.: *Infant Mortality, Population Growth and Family Planning in India.* Chapel Hill, U of NC Pr, 1972.

Cheney, E. C.: *Am Scientist, 62:* 14, 1974.

Chopra, J. G., Camancho, R., Kevary, J., and Thomson, A. M.: *Am J Clin Nutr, 23:* 1043, 1970.

Christian, C. S.: In Junk, Mudd (Ed.) : *The Population Crisis and the Use of World Resources.* The Hague, 1964.

Clark, C.: In *Food Supplies and Population Growth.* Edinburgh, Oliver and Boyd, 1963.

Cloud, Wallace: *The Sciences, 13:* 836, 1973.

Commission on Population and American Future. Findings, 1972.

Contraceptive Technology, Emory Uni. Family Planning Program, 1973–74.

Cooke, T.: *U.S. News and World Report, 72:* 50, 1972.

Dalrymple, G.: *A Survey of Multiple Cropping in Less Developed Nations.* FEDR-12, USDA, Washington, D.C., 1971.

Darby, W. J.: *Nutr Rev, 30:* 27, 1972.

Davis, K.: *The Population of India and Pakistan.* Princeton, Princeton U Pr, 1959.

Desai, P. B.: *India News,* Indian, Washington, D.C., June 8, 1973.

Diddle, A. W.: *Obstet Gynecol, 41:* 782, 1973.

Dutta, R.: *Am J Public Health, 63:* 158, 1973.

Ehrlich, P. R., and Ehrlich, A. H.: *Population, Resources, Environment.* San Francisco, Freeman, 1970.

FAO: Nutrition and Working Efficiency. In *Freedom from Hunger Campaign Basic Study 1,* Rome, FAO, 1962.

FAO: *U.N. Main Conclusions and Policy Implications of Provisional Indicative Plan, 3,* Rome, FAO, 1969.

FAO: *Provisional Indicative World Plan for Agricultural Development, 1,* 41 Rome, FAO, 1970.

Faundes, A., and Luukkainen, T.: *Studies in Family Planning, 3,* Suppl. 7, 1972.

First Annual Report of the Council of Environmental Quality. Washington, Government Printing Press, 1970.

Forrester, J. W.: *World Dynamics.* Cambridge, Wright-Allen, 1971.

Forrester, J. W.: In *Toward Global Equilibrium,* D. L. Meadows and D. H. Meadows (eds.) Cambridge: Wright Allen Press, 1973.

Fredericksen, H.: *Public Health Reports, 81:* 1008, 1966.

Fyodorov, Y.: *New Scientist, 22:* 431, 1973.

Gold, E. M., and Ballard, W. M.: *Clin Obstet Gynecol, 13:* 145, 1970.

Goldsmith, S.: *Fam Plann Perspect, 1:* 23, 1969.

Goldzieber, J. W.: *Fed Proc, 29:* 1220, 1970.

Hammonds, T. M., and Wunderle, R. E.: *Am J Clin Nutr, 25:* 419, 1972.

Hardin, G.: *Science, 162:* 1243, 1968.

Hawley, A. H.: *Science, 179:* 1196, 1973.

Health Statistics of India. Ministry of Health, Family Planning and Urban Development, Table 23, pp. 124–125, 1970.

Health Statistics of India. Ministry of Health, Family Planning and Urban Development, Table 24, pp. 128–129, 1970.

Hodges, R. E.: *J Am Diet Assoc, 59:* 212, 1971.

Holden, C.: *Science, 186:* 548, 1974.

Hutchinson, G. E.: The biosphere. *Sci Am,* p. 53, Sept., 1970.

Jafe, F. S.: *Sci Am, 229:* 17, 1973.

Johannisson, E.: *Contraception, 8:* 99, 1973.

Joshi, S. H.: *Am J Phar, 145:* 22, 1973.

Kass, L. R.: *New Engl J Med, 285:* 1174, 1971.

Keller, W. D., and Kraut, H. A.: Work and nutrition. *World Rev Nutr Diet, 3:* 75, 1962.

Kohl, S. C., Majzlin, G., Burnhill, M., Jones, J., Solish, G., Okrent, S., and Pendleton, E.: *Am J Public Health, 62:* 1448, 1972.

Lebowitz, M. D.: *Perspect Biol Med, 16:* 599, 1973a.

Lebowitz, M. D.: *Soc Biol, 20:* 89, 1973b.

Luce, H. R.: In Farber, Wilson and Wilson (Eds.) : *Food and Civilization.* Springfield, Thomas, 1966.

Manocha, S. L.: *Malnutrition and Retarded Human Development.* Springfield, Thomas, 1972.

Man's Impact on the Global Environment. *Report of the Study of Critical Environmental Problems.* Cambridge, MIT Press, 1970.

Marx, J. L.: *Science, 179:* 1222, 1973.

Mayer, J.: *Human Nutrition.* Springfield, Thomas, 1972.

Meadows, D. H., Meadows, D. L., Randers, J., and Behrens, W. W.: *The Limits to Growth.* New York, Universe Books, 1972.

Meadows, D. H. and Meadows, D. L.: *Nature, 247:* 97, 1974.

Michanek, E.: *UNICEF News,* Issue #71, March, 1972.

Mich Law Rev, 63: 579, 1969.

Moreland, W. H.: *India at the Death of Akbar.* London, McMillan, 1920.

Muller, C.: *Am J Public Health, 63:* 519, 1973.

Nath, P.: *A Study in the Economic Conditions of Ancient India.* London, Royal Asiatic Society, 1929.

Norman, D.: Population and Family Planning Program: A Fact Book. *Reports on Population/Family Planning,* No. 3, June, 1971.

Paarlberg, D.: *World Rev Nutr Diet, 16:* 1973.

Pearson, P. B.: *Nutr Rev, 30:* 31, 1972.

Pilon, R. J.: *Clin Obstet Gynecol, 14:* 409, 1971.

Pollack, H., and Sheldon, D. R.: *JAMA, 212:* 598, 1970.

Popkin, B., and Lidman, R.: *Am J Clin Nutr, 25:* 331, 1972.

Pyke, M.: *Food and Society.* London, John Murray Publ., 1968.

Ramsey, P.: *JAMA, 220:* 1346, 1972.

Randers, J. and Meadows, D. H.: In *Toward Global Equilibrium,* D. L. Meadows and D. H. Meadows (eds.) Cambridge: Wright Allen Press, 1973.

Report on Intrauterine Contraceptive Devices. Advisory Comm on Obstet Gynecol, Washington, FDA, 1968.

Richter, R. M., and Prager, D. J. (Eds.) : *Human Sterilization.* Springfield, Thomas, 1972.

Ridker, R. G.: *Science, 182:* 1315, 1973.

Rothkopf, M.: *New Scientist,* March 22, 1973.

Rouse, H.: *Spectator, 5:* 4, 1971.

Sai, F. T.: *Proc R Soc Med, 66:* 123, 1973.

Samachar, Swastha: Ministry of Health, Government of India, October, 1965.

Sanyal, S.: Indian Broadcaster and News Commentator. Writing about Chandrasekhra, 1972.

Schultz, T. W.: In *Social Forces Influencing American Education.* Chicago, Chicago University Press, 1961.

Scientific American, November, 1973.

Scrimshaw, N. S.: In Brock, J. C. (Ed.) : *Recent Advances in Human Nutrition.* Boston, Little, 1961.

Segal, S. J., Southam, A. L., and Shafer, K. D. (Eds.) : Proc 2nd Inter Cong. on Intrauterine Contraceptives, New York, 1964. *Excerpta Medica Foundation Int. Cong Series No. 86, 1965.*

Segal, S. J., and Tietze, C.: Contraceptive technology: current and prospective methods. *Rep Popul Fam Plann, No. 1,* July, 1971.

Shaffer, P., and Coleman, W.: *Arch Intern Med, 4:* 538, 1909.

Simmons, G. B.: *Population Council,* New York, 1971.

Slater, E.: In Cox, P. R. and Peel, J. (Eds.) : *Population and Pollution.* New York, Acad Pr, 1972.

Sokolov, I. P.: *New Scientist,* Feb. 22, 1973.

Somerset, N. J.: *Metal Statistics.* American Metal Market Company, 1970.

Southam, A. L.: *Contraception, 8:* 1, 1973.

Spengler, J. J.: *Values and Fertility Analysis Demography, 3:* 109, 1966.

Starr, C., and Rudman, R.: *Science, 182:* 358, 1973.

Streatfield, G.: *New Scientist,* March 8, 1973.

Taylor, C. E., and Deseweemer, C.: *World Rev Nutr Diet, 16,* 1973.

Thant, U.: Speech of the Secretary General in the United Nations, 1969.

Tuncer, B.: *The Impact of Population Growth on the Turkish Economy,* 31, Ankara, Hacettepe University, 1968.

U. S. Bureau of Mines, Minerals Year Book. Washington, Government Printing Office, 1967.

U.S. Bureau of Mines, Minerals, Facts and Problems. Washington, Government Printing Office, 1970.

U.S.D.A. World Food Population Levels. Report to the President, Washington, 1970.

U.S. News and World Report, March 20, 1972.

Wade, N.: *Science, 181:* 634, 1973.

Weisbrod, B. A.: *J Polit Econ, 19:* 117, 1962.

Westoff, C. F.: *Family Planning Perspectives, 4:* 9, 1972.

White, C. L.: In Mudd, Junk (Ed.) : *Population Crisis and the Use of World Resources.* The Hague, 1964.

Willett, J. W.: *The Impact of New Grain Varieties in Asia.* ERS-For. 275, p. 15, Washington, USDA, 1969.

Williams, R. M.: In Farber, Wilson and Wilson, (Eds.) : *Food and Civilization.* Springfield, Thomas, 1966.

Woodham, A. A.: *World Rev Nutr Diet, 13:* 1, 1971.

World Bank Atlas. Washington, International Bank for Reconstruction and Development, 1970.

CHAPTER II

FEEDING THE TEEMING BILLIONS

THERE ARE VERY FEW socio-economic or political tangles that face the human race which match the gravity and enormity of the problems involved in feeding the human population at an acceptable and adequate level of nutrition. The problem is two-fold. First, the existing population has to catch up from their low plane of existence and join the standards of living that the 20th Century man has set before himself. Secondly, we have to face up to the needs of approximately 70 million new arrivals every year, knowing well that these are the most vulnerable members of our society in terms of nutritional needs. The net result is that we have to produce extra food, not only to improve the nutritional standard of our existing population, but also for the 2 percent per year increase in its numbers. This makes it essential that we increase our food production every year by a margin of at least 5 percent. Our experience in this respect in the Sixties has not been encouraging enough to bring out optimism in the Seventies. Food and Agriculture Organization reported that in 1965–1967, food production failed to increase in the world as a whole, and declined in the developing areas. In 1966, in both Africa and Latin America, food production decreased. According to FAO, the decreased food production during 1965 to 1967 wiped out what little progress in per capita food production had been achieved in the developing countries in the previous decade (Bender, 1969; FAO, 1967). Vast areas of Asia and Africa faced near starvation conditions. Although not many starved to death, there are millions who are left chronically undernourished and malnourished as a result of unsatisfactory performance in producing food.

The success of the 'Green Revolution' in Asia and South America in 1969 to 1971 brought back some optimism and demonstrated that we do have the will and the ability to apply our technical knowledge to the benefit of all mankind and provide adequate food for our runaway populations. No sooner had this optimism taken roots than cracks began to appear in our strategy of using mass scale technology to produce ample food for all. The new technology increased tremendously the requirements for agro-industrial products such as machinery, fertilizers, pesticides and seeds. At the same time, it sharpened the socio-economic problems between the rich and poor farmers and threatened to blow up the very foundations of the coherence that binds the old traditional societies. Some of these implications have been discussed in the next section. It is progressively more difficult to bring additional land under cultivation because of the overcrowded conditions in the developing countries and land needs for socio-industrial use. Intensive cultivation of the existing land is the only answer. The net result is that pessimism again came into vogue in 1972 to 1973. In that context, we are still wondering whether we can tackle, along with the food problem, the overriding socio-economic and environmental problems of the modern society if proper physical, mental and cultural development are ever to be achieved for all human beings.

There is a distinct relationship between nutrition and a number of social problems (Mayer, 1972). We cannot lose any more time in our planning to solve the urgent problems facing us. We must develop new strategies of increasing the food output, while at the same time striving to reduce the population growth rate and bring about certain social changes favoring a change in attitude. It is quite probable that we may have to change radically our thinking about food. We may be faced with making the maximum use of plant sources to provide us with the bulk, whereas we may depend on our technology to produce proteins from petroleum, microorganisms, ocean food, etc. Even the human wastes can be converted into edible proteins. For bulk and energy, we may have to utilize to the maximum our land resources, which means conservation of arable land and conversion of land not now cultivated into food producing acres. The land which is now used for pastures will be put to use to produce more food.

It is well known that much more efficient use of solar energy to provide energy for man is possible through plant life than through the intermediate step of raising animals suitable for food. In that context, the amount of land now used for nonfood plant life may have to be reduced. Man may have to consider using only foods of high nutrient density and forget about eating for pleasure (White, 1970).

Dr. Darby, the President of the Nutrition Foundation, rightly stressed that the hope for the future lies in the production of nutrient enriched unconventional foodstuffs, such as unicellular proteins, through the application of the knowledge of biosynthetic chemistry. We cannot stick forever to our traditional diets, without feeling the pinch of scarcity and hunger. There are other unconventional sources of food which must be tapped. Professor Bigwood, Director of the Food Land Research Center, Institute of European Studies in Brussels, pointed out that "if one does not find other methods and new sources of proteins, which would have the same high biological value as animal protein, and could be produced in sufficiently short time, on an individual basis, the situation might become desperate in ten or twenty years time. Some of the prospects of increasing protein production lie in the area of developing on a large scale the capacity to produce yeast protein, microorganisms and plankton of the sea. Protein from microorganisms which are the by-products of petroleum refineries, is of extremely high biological value. Considering the amount of petroleum utilized, if factories are set up to tap this source of edible protein, the shortage of the latter could disappear in a short period of time. It is about 2,500 times quicker to produce a given amount of protein in that form than to produce meat protein" (*World Health,* 1969).

By the use of different methods that our technology has put at our disposal, it is highly probable that significant contributions to the world protein pool can be made and the spread of protein deficiency among millions can be halted, until world-wide population regulation is a reality (Gray, 1966). We must not forget, however, that technology can only buy us some time to help prevent the further deterioration of the quality of human life, but if we close our eyes to the urgent problem of stabilizing our numbers and let it double every quarter of a century as it threatens to do, all the technology and resourcefulness at our command may not prevent the catastrophe that will be the fate of the human race in the 21st or 22nd Century (Ehrlich and Ehrlich, 1970).

GREEN REVOLUTION—THE STRATEGY OF MODERN AGRICULTURE

Cereals

Cereals provide more than 60 percent of the energy needs of the human population all over the world. The production of cereals has played a great historical role in ancient times in transforming human existence from an unsettled nomadic style to permanent settlements. The principal cereals are rice, wheat, corn, millet, oats and rye. Rice and wheat, together, are the staple foods of more than two thirds of the human population. Rice is predominant among the crops of damp tropical climates and, because of its large water needs, grows best in the deltas of the great rivers. China grows about 35 percent of the world's total rice, India and Pakistan 27 percent, Japan 7 percent, Indonesia 6 percent and some countries of Southeast Asia and Latin America about 25 percent.

Wheat is the predominant cereal of people living in temperate or dry climates and is mainly grown in the United States, U.S.S.R., Canada, France, Australia, Europe, India, Pakistan, Argentina, Egypt and Turkey. The United States produces about 15 percent of the world's wheat, the Soviet Union 24 percent, Canada, France and India 5 percent and Italy 4 percent, Turkey 3 percent, Argentine and Australia

2.5 percent, and the rest of the world 34 percent. Corn is grown extensively in the United States, Italy, Yugoslavia and parts of India and Africa. More than half of the world's supply is grown in the United States, Russia and Brazil 5 percent each, Yugoslavia, Mexico, Argentina, Rumania, South Africa combined 13 percent, and the rest of the world 25 percent. Millet grows in hot climates and can be cultivated even if the water supply is poor. Oats are a hardy crop. Rye is a cousin of wheat and can grow on poor soils in cold climates. It is sown in Scandinavia, Russia and Poland (Davidson *et al.*, 1972).

Most of the cereals are a good source of energy in the form of carbohydrates. In addition, they have significant quantities of protein, although the latter are somewhat deficient in one or two of the essential amino acids and need to be supplemented with proteins from other sources. They also contain calcium, iron and a useful amount of water soluble complex vitamins. However, when the cereal grains are milled and the outer portion of the seed discarded, there is a serious loss of B vitamins. It is essential that the cereals be lightly milled in order to get the maximum nutritive value out of them.

In addition to cereals, there are some starchy roots which are in some countries as popular as cereals as a source of energy. Potato, cassava, yams, sweet potato and taro are the most important of them, which are rich in starches. Potato is the native of the New World and was introduced to Europe by the early explorers. It is, indeed, a cheap alternative crop to cereals and yields more energy per acre than any cereal crop. In Ireland, the potato flourished so well and became so complete a food staple that it ousted the other cereal crops that were grown before its introduction. Potatoes contain 70 to 90 k cals of calories per 100 gms weight; 7.6 percent of the calories being derived from protein and the rest from starch. They have some B group vitamins, a small amount of vitamin C and good quantities of potassium. They are easily digested and can support life when fed as a sole article of diet. Cassava, known variously as manioca, yuca, tapioca, etc., is the native of South America, but is widely grown in Africa and parts of Asia. Cassava is very poor in protein (approximately 1%) and consists mostly of starch. Cassava is a staple food in many African communities and, because of its very low protein content, is responsible for protein malnutrition in those areas. It is essential that the persons using cassava as a source of energy must consume, along with it, foods which are rich in proteins. Yams are rich in starch, but also contain significant amounts of protein. Sweet potatoes and taro are similar to yams and potatoes in their nutritive property. They are rich in starch and are good sources of calories.

Sugars are, of course, sheer energy and do not have other nutrients. It is extremely agreeable to the palate and is extremely popular as a sweetener for all kinds of dishes. Crystalline sugar is almost 100 percent sucrose, with 4 k cals in every gram. Honey is 20 to 25 percent water and 75 percent sugar, mostly fructose and glucose, which are readily absorbed in the digestive tract.

Cereals and Green Revolution

As the population grows unchecked, large quantities of extra food will be needed in the coming years. In general, there are two recognized ways of expanding the food output: expansion of area and increasing the yield of food grain per acre. The prospects of continuous increase of area under cultivation are not bright, indeed. The growing population increases the demand for more roads, residential and commercial areas, industries, schools, hospitals, etc., in addition to the farm land. Until recently in most countries of the world, the food output was increased by enlarging the size of the farmland. However, this policy of extending the areas under cultivation had its own disastrous effects. Once the forests were cleared to use the land for cultivation, the soil deteriorated for lack of protective cover of the forests. In India, much of the precious land under cultivation has been deteriorating because of soil erosion. In the developing countries, with the exception of some areas in Africa and

South America, much of the once potentially cultivatable land has already been converted into farmland, leaving little room for further expansion.

At present, it appears that the only way to increase the food production is to try to increase the yield per acre. The developed countries produced food over the last three decades with matchless efficiency by raising the yield per acre significantly. Japan is a notable example of a country with limited farmland and a heavy pressure of population. With intensive farming they increased their rice production from a 2,000 lbs/acre to about 4,500 lbs/acre. The countries of northern Europe and North America achieved similar successes in increasing the production; but the greatest success story has probably come from the United States, which could not only increase the per acre yield but also bring a lot of additional land under cultivation. As an example, corn yields per acre have doubled to more than three tons in recent years.

The developing countries remained backward in the use of technological methods for intensive farming due to a number of reasons; their status as colonies under the rule of colonial powers was one of them. However, in the early 1960's, the food production in the developing countries began to fall behind the population growth, bringing a shortage of crisis proportions. Serious attention was then paid to investing energy and capital in the improvement of agricultural practices (Scrimshaw, 1972). Money was invested in developing new technologies of developing high yielding new grain varieties, as well as production of fertilizers and development of irrigation facilities. Drs. Mertz and Nelson and their co-workers at Purdue University took the lead in this area. By the use of gene mutations and selective breedings, these scientists have changed the composition of the endosperm proteins in corn, wheat and sorghums (Mertz, 1966; Nelson, 1966).

Numerous other studies have been done in other research institutions, notably at the Agricultural Institutes of India and International Rice Research Institute in the Philippines.

As a result of these studies, the protein content of the commonly used cereals (wheat and rice) has been improved by as much as 60 percent. Recently Drs. Singh and Axtell of Purdue University discovered a high lysine gene in two strains of sorghum, which is likely to improve significantly the biological quality of sorghum protein. In addition to manipulating the genes, mutant hybrid varieties of cereals have also been developed. Special mention may be made of a hybrid between durum wheat (triticum) and rye (secalis) generally referred to as triticale. It is a new man-made cereal produced after lots of research work and contains 18 to 20 percent protein compared to 10 to 16 percent protein in wheat. It also contains more of the limiting amino acid of wheat, i.e. lysine, which is an essential amino acid for good nutrition and growth. As a commercial crop, triticale has certain additional advantages over wheat because it resists dry weather and could, therefore, prove an ideal high protein crop in the semi-arid areas of the world. Recent studies using the improved quality cereals in the diets of pregnant animals have shown their superiority over traditional cereals in terms of growth and development of the young (Jansen, 1973).

In the area of wheat research, it has been noted that the newly evolved varieties differ in their genetic make-up and yield per acre ability depending on the local climatic conditions, quality of soil as well as availability of essential ingredients such as water, fertilizer and pesticides. The most successful varieties are "Mexipak,"® evolved in Mexico and Pakistan, and several varieties in India such as "Kalyan sona,"® "Sonora 63,"® "64,"® "Lerma Rojo,"® etc. These new varieties have raised the per acre yield to four times India's national average.

Rice is the staple food of about $1\frac{1}{2}$ billion people and is probably the most important and most widely used cereal in the world. A number of new rice varieties have been developed during the last few years, which have the promise to raise the yields of this cereal in a spectacular manner. By selective breeding, the quality of rice protein has been greatly improved and compares well with that of wheat proteins.

More than any other cereal, breeders have produced many hybrid varieties of corn which have greatly increased its per acre yield as well as improved on its protein quality. The protein quality of some of the recently evolved varieties is as good as milk protein. In areas where corn is the staple diet, this could make a significant contribution in improving the diets of millions of people who are fighting desperately to eliminate the prevalent malnutrition in their midst.

The strategy has proved a great success so far. As a result, Mexico got rid of its chronic shortages of food. The Philippines achieved self-sufficiency in rice after half a century of dependence on imported rice. Pakistan not only was able to feed adequately but became a net exporter of grain. India has greatly improved its food supply, although still short of its goals of providing adequate diets for its huge population. Brown states that "during the seven year span from 1965 to 1972, India expanded its wheat production from 11 million tons to 27 million tons, an increase in a major crop unmatched by any other country in history.

The 'Green Revolution,' as it is called, has great potential. Only a fraction of the potential benefits has been reaped so far. A series of spectacular advances in agricultural technology lie ahead that will vastly improve the availability of food for the teeming billions of humans inhabiting this planet. For example, most of the plant's dry bulk consists of carbon products, produced by fixing atmospheric carbon during photosynthesis. In this respect, much higher yielding varieties can be evolved by making photosynthesis more efficient (Tudge, 1973). However, in our enthusiasm, we must not forget that the 'Green Revolution' has its limitations and if the human population keeps on growing at the present high rate of 2 percent, the technology at our disposal may not be able to save us for an indefinite period of time. Dr. Normal Borlang, who was awarded the Nobel Prize for his contribution to the 'Green Revolution,' strongly stressed that the new technologies do not represent a solution to the food problem of the world. Probably we have bought from nature a few extra years in which to apply brakes to our runaway population growth. The ultimate solution of the food problem is curbing the world population growth.

Socio-economic Implications of Green Revolution

The 'Green Revolution' has resulted in a substantial increase in the total output of food with the result that it has been instrumental in averting famine and crisis caused by chronic food shortages in the countries who do not have the resources to buy food from rich countries. A closer examination of the socio-economic implications of the 'Green Revolution,' clearly reveals that it is not enough to say that the 'Green Revolution' is doubling yields (*UNICEF News*). The 'Green Revolution' has brought in its trail those complications which led in the first place to the division of this world into rich countries and poor countries. The benefits of the 'Green Revolution' have been reaped greatly by the rich and resourceful among the poor countries who have the water and fertilizers to nourish the new crops and the acreage to make full use of the technology, and this has led to social, economic and political tensions. If these *side effects* of a desirable phenomenon (a technical solution to food shortages by the use of new high yielding seed varieties, fertilizers, irrigation and pesticides) are not properly handled, the resulting tensions may adversely affect the lives of millions of people.

The rich farmers who have gotten the taste of quick and large returns, are likely to exploit the small farmers who do not have the necessary economic capability for the kinds of inputs required by the modern agricultural technology. The rich farmer, on the other hand, will invest his earnings in mechanization and resort to multiple cropping by a method of quick harvesting and replanting. The poor farmer, with small holdings, is out-maneuvered, because of his dependence on traditional tools and his bullock as a source of energy. Seu, in his first volume dealing with modernizing Indian agriculture, has described this phenomenon in various states of India, how the process of mechanization in the management of large farms has created unemployment among the landless. In Indonesia, tensions between the land owners and the landless had become so great in 1964 that violent confrontations were frequently reported from the countryside (Franke, 1974).

The big farmers have generated enough money within a short period of time to be able to buy land from the smaller farmers, driving them to cities to look for jobs in the industrial sectors which can't absorb any more men, either. This has resulted in economic disparities, social tensions, economic misery, agricultural unemployment, increased migration to urban areas in search of employment and perhaps a greater degree of malnutrition, since the poor and unemployed do not have the resources to buy the newly produced food. The very possibility of technological success is creating a human disaster. Richard Critchfield described that it is a revolution all right, but this revolution has also created glaring socio-economic disparities. "A landless laborer's income in West Pakistan today is still just about what it was five years ago, less than 100 dollars a year. In contrast, one landlord with a 1,500 acre wheat farm told me when I was in Pakistan this winter that he had cleared a net profit of more than 100,000 dollars on his last harvest." Similar reports have come from India, Southeast Asia and Mexico. In the latter, for example, there has been a steady 5 percent increase of agricultural production from 1940 to 1961. However, in the latter decade, the landless laborer had fewer working days (100 as compared to 194) and his real income decreased from 68 to 56 dollars. Eighty percent of the increased agricultural production came from 3 percent of the farmers (Meadows, 1972).

In order that maximum benefit can be obtained from the technological advances of the 'Green Revolution,' some timely measures must be adopted which should assure not only greater production, but should distribute their benefits almost equitably among all sections of the society. The governments of these countries must decide now how best to spread the benefits of the 'Green Revolution' as widely as possible to make certain that they reach the lowest income level of the agricultural population (*UNICEF NEWS*). The 'Green Revolution' should help create jobs and not unemployment. In the rural areas, where the bulk of the populations of the developing countries live, the problem of unemployment looms as far more intractable than that of food supply. With it comes not only human misery but social unrest and political instability (Wade, 1973).

If, however, the benefits of modern technology are shared by the vast majority, it could not only provide enough food for everybody, but the infant institutions of self-rule and democracy might take deeper roots. This may create an impetus for faster economic development. Wade rightly commented that if the Asian 'Green Revolution' continues to operate successfully, it could well become the most significant world economic development since the economic rebirth of Europe following World War II. It is extremely important that this strategy of modern agriculture succeeds. In that case, it could have a salutary effect on the psychology of masses as well as the national leaders, whose faith in modern technology can go a long way in improving the well-being of the downtrodden in their countries (Wade, 1973). It may give them the needed impetus to pursue the policies which should assure that the 'Green Revolution' provides maximum participation of maximum numbers of people and that it does not become an instrument of the rich to become richer.

Future Prospects

'Green Revolution' has produced many optimistic estimates of our ability to feed the projected 4 billion population by 1975. Because of the wholesale use of 'Green Revolution' techniques, India expects this year (1973–1974) a crop of 120 million tons, which may suffice to feed her vast population of approximately 570 million people. So far, so good, but we must be careful not to project an overoptimistic picture of our ability to feed adequately the ever-growing population. In the developing countries, there are a number of factors which were historically operative two decades back, that cannot be applied to the present day. Some of them may be mentioned here.

1. Heavy load of populations, agrarian subsistence economies and almost stagnant or very slow growing industrialization do not leave the nations with enough savings to make the investments needed to modernize agriculture.

2. Modern agriculture needs not only investments in the land and in irrigation projects, but also investment in industry to produce tractors, agricultural machinery, fertilizers and, above everything else, it needs the energy (petroleum) to sustain the mechanized agriculture.

3. More than 80 percent of the populations in the developing countries are employed in agriculture. If food is to be produced efficiently, economically and in larger quantities, it will necessarily mean having good management, which may throw lots of unskilled persons out of work. In the absence of a flourishing economy, which could create additional jobs for these displaced agriculturists, the country may end up in political chaos.

Modern methods of agriculture necessitate high inputs of energy, especially in fuel in the forms of fertilizers, pesticides, hybrid seeds and irrigation. The latter requires huge capital input that could greatly strain the investment capacity of developing countries like India (Wharton, 1969). The energy shortages are fast becoming a world-wide phenomenon and the finite reserves of fossil fuels are getting depleted at a very fast rate. Since the continued success of the 'Green Revolution' depends greatly on the progressively increasing availability of fuels, the energy crisis is expected to have a significant impact on food production technology (Pimentral, *et al.*, 1973). The analysis of Pimentral *et al.* reveals that in 1970 energy equivalent to 80 gallons of gasoline was used to raise an acre of corn. If this is taken as a yardstick, the energy for raising food for 4 billion people is indeed colossal and if the population keeps on growing, our ability to produce enough food for everybody may be in great jeopardy merely because of the shortage of energy.

Let us give some figures from the U.S. agriculture in order

to bring home the point that familiar methods cannot be used in the overcrowded developing countries whose resources are indeed limited. Within a period of three decades during 1920 and 1950, the number of tractor horsepower increased from 5 million to 92 million and is over 200 million today. The consumption of energy similarly went up (Steinhart and Steinhart, 1974). The tractors alone consume about 8 billion gallons of gasoline a year, and the total energy consumed in farming runs to a figure equal to more than 30 billion gallons of gasoline per year. This kind of mechanization was possible in response to labor shortage. At the same time, the nonagricultural economy of the country grew at a rate that enabled it to absorb profitably the people displaced from agriculture. The number of small farms have been shrinking steadily and today only 223,000 farms (7.6 percent of the total number) produce slightly over 50 percent of the agricultural produce. "Farmers have been going out of business at a rate of 2,000 a week since the 1930's. During World War II, we had over six million farms; today there are less than 2.7 million. This process is expected to continue. Secretary of Agriculture Earl Butz says there may be only 1.8 million farms by 1980" (Cloud, 1973). If this trend continues, it is very probable that within 2 or 3 decades, 70 to 80 percent of the total agricultural produce will come from about 100,000 farms (Cloud, 1973).

This kind of mechanization of agriculture cannot be adopted by the developing countries (Pimentral *et al.*, 1973). Black has strongly urged us to take stock of benefits, cost and risks of high energy demand of 'Green Revolution' agriculture in order to make sure that what is considered a remedy today may not aggravate the already serious world food situation.

> To gain some idea about what the energy needs would be for different diets if U.S. agricultural technology were employed, an estimate is made of how long it would take to deplete the known and potential world reserves of petroleum. The known reserves have been estimated to be 546 billion barrels. If we assume that 76 percent of raw petroleum can be converted into fuel, this would equal a usable re-

serve of 415 billion barrels. *If petroleum* were the only source of energy and if we used *all* petroleum reserves solely to feed the world population, the 415-billion-barrel reserve would last a mere 29 years. The estimate would be 107 years if all potential reserves (2000 billion barrels) of petroleum were used for food production. However, if the world population were willing to eat nothing but corn grain, potential petroleum reserves could feed a projected 10 billion humans for 448 years (Pimentral *et al.,* 1973).

There are some inherent dangers in total dependence upon technology. The availability of energy is one aspect. If energy sources are heavily imported, it leaves a country open to economic and political blackmail by those who provide the sources of energy. It is also not completely safe to depend entirely on the genetically manipulated varieties, even if their yields are much higher than the wall-adapted but lower yielding, traditional crops. The pattern of disease resistance by the genetically mutated varieties of food crops is another area which must be carefully looked into. Current estimates show that in India (a representative of a developing country), approximately 20 percent of the food grain crop is from the new high-yielding wheat varieties, and a desperate attempt is being made to increase it to 80 percent or more, not only in wheat, but rice, sorghum, millet, legumes and peanuts as well. Were a new rust strain or other pestilence to strike these recently introduced varieties, India could suddenly lose a major portion of its food supply. That this is no idle gossip is demonstrated by the recent devastating corn blight in the United States, the roots of which lay in the *genetic engineering* procedures of the corn hybrid (Paarlberg, 1973).

Legumes, Oilseeds and Nuts

For the populations depending heavily on cereals for intake of energy, the legumes, oilseeds and nuts truly serve the purpose of meat in their diets. Legumes are the seeds of different kinds of plants belonging to the family *leguminosae* and including different varieties of peas, beans and lentils (see Appendix II for the nutritive value of these seeds).

Legumes were domesticated by man along with cereals as early as six millenium B.C., long before the initiation of agriculture. Whereas the cereals (grass kernels rich in starch) provided a rich source of energy, the leguminous seeds proved rich in protein and together they supplied a balanced diet to the prehistoric man (Zohary and Hopf, 1973). There are a number of varieties of peas and, according to English terminology, they are widely referred to as pulses. The pulses have a high protein content as compared to cereals; as much as 20 gm protein/100 gm dry weight. The biological quality of pulse protein is not high by itself, but since they are generally eaten in combination with cereals, they supplement the cereal protein.

For example, cereals are deficient in an amino acid, lysine, whereas the pulses are rich. The sulfur containing amino acids are deficient in pulses, but are well supplied in cereals. A combination of cereal and pulse protein may have a nutritive value quite close to that of animal protein. Pulses, in addition to their high protein content, are also rich in B complex vitamins. Sprouted pulses also contain significant amounts of vitamin C. The best known of the pulses are Bengal gram, black gram, green gram, red gram and the garden peas. The latter have become popular all over the world, and they are cultivated on a very large scale. They are available in dry form as well as in canned and frozen states. Lentils are closely allied to pulses and are also rich in proteins. They are extensively cultivated in India and are popular in Europe as well. However, the pulses are not as important in the diets of European and North American populations as in India, China and Southeast Asia.

In the category of oilseeds, certain varieties of beans and nuts are the most important, although corn is also a good source of oil. Soybeans and peanuts are the major items for oil production, as well as rich sources of protein. In addition, there are other kinds of beans which are mainly used as pulses, described above. These are kidney beans, broad beans, lima beans, etc. Peas and beans are two of the outstanding sources of vegetable proteins. Just to clear a distinction between the two, peas bear round seeds and have small leaflets on their plants, while beans have rather flat seeds and the leaves are large. India and Pakistan together produce about 90 percent of the world's production of chick peas, whereas 60 percent of the world's crop of sweet peas comes from China, with India the next largest producer. China is also the main producer of broad beans and India is the major producer of lentils. These legume plants can provide valuable supplementary proteins to those obtained from cereals, which are staple diets of the developing countries. Cereals and legumes together may contribute 70 to 90 percent of the calories in the daily diet and an almost similar proportion of dietary protein in these areas.

Soybeans and ground nuts are popular all over the world for their high protein contents, and a hundred and one different kinds of food items are prepared from them besides oil, which is used as a cooking oil. The reader is referred to a recent "Symposium on soybeans," sponsored by the American Oil Chemists' Society for details. The dry soybeans contain as much as 40 percent protein and 20 percent fat. During recent years, when animal proteins are getting scarcer, the soya proteins have become extremely important (Dovring, 1974). Simulated meats, milk and other products which are of high nutritive value are made out of soya. The pragmatic methods developed centuries ago by the people of Southeast Asia to process soybeans into a great variety of foods are widely known. One can list the tofu (soybean curd) of China and Japan and the *tempeh* of Indonesia and the large variety of fermented products derived from it (Milner, 1966). Some details have been given in the section on processed foods.

The United States and China are main producers of soybeans, but because of its nutritive value, many other countries, notably Indonesia, Central Europe, India and Pakistan, have started cultivating this bean. A good deal of research work is being done on improving soybean with respect to its antitrypsin, or hemaglutamin factors, as well as its yield per acre. The 'Green Revolution' is being extended to soybeans. Already the soybean processing industry is coming out with processes which may assume great importance in human nutrition in the future. Soybean protein concentrate containing 70 percent protein content is being used, along with cereals or meat products, to form new and fancy foods. Peanuts are rich in protein as well as fat, more so the latter. The whole seeds contain about 20 percent fat, twice the amount in soybeans, and that is why peanuts are cultivated mainly for their fat value. India is one of the largest producers of peanuts and more than 80 percent of the crop is simply used to crush oil and the residue, which incidently is very rich in protein, used as animal feed or fertilizers.

Informed sources suggest that 80 percent of India press cake, which contains up to about 40 percent protein (not to mention residual oil of 10 percent) is used mainly as manure. This is indeed tragic and unfortunate to note that the largely vegetarian Indian society has not made an effective or rational use for this valuable protein source. (Milner, 1966). During recent years, India has done some research work in order to find several other uses of peanuts besides oil and a number of products such as peanut-based milk and peanut flour are being made. Some details have been given in the next section on processed foods. Sunflower seeds also come in the same category as soybeans and peanuts because of their high fat and protein content. They are widely cultivated in Russia and during recent years are becoming quite popular with food faddists.

Among the nuts, almonds, Brazil nuts, cashew nuts, Spanish chestnuts, walnuts, pecans and pistachios are the most prominent. They are not produced in large quantities and are mainly used as snacks or as a pleasant adjunct to the main food. Because of their production in small quantities, they are relatively expensive. They are rich in proteins as well as fats. Most of the nuts grown on trees are either large trees such as those of Brazil nuts which grow in tropical forests, or large sized shrubs such as those of almonds or cashew nuts. The latter predominantly come from India.

Walnuts grow on large trees, as do pecans. The latter are grown mostly in the United States. Pistachios are nuts with green kernels, covered with purple skins. They are mostly grown in Turkey, Italy and some parts of Afghanistan, Pakistan and India.

Vegetables and Fruits

There are hundreds of common vegetables eaten in different parts of the world. A large number of varieties like okra, cauliflower, cabbage, turnips, carrots, etc., are grown almost everywhere. They range from leaves and roots to fruits of small sized shrubs. Davidson *et al.* described that in spite of the fact that everyone knows what *vegetables* are, they are not easy to describe and they defy exact classification. Only to give a few examples, some vegetables like spinach, cabbage and lettuce are leaves; others such as onions, turnips and radishes are roots. Egg plants (brinjals), gourds and marrows are fruits, whereas celery is a stalk and cauliflower and artichokes are flowers. (Davidson *et al.*, 1972). Most of the vegetables are not rich in calories or proteins. They provide roughage to the diet and are a source of satiety. However, depending upon the vegetable, they are good sources of vitamins and minerals. Some are rich in calcium, others in iron, still others have significant quantities of vitamin A or B group of vitamins (see Appendix II) (Altman and Dittmer, 1968). They also contain valuable amounts of vitamin C, but since most vegetables are eaten after cooking, the vitamin C may be lost to some extent, but still enough is present to prevent scurvy if the vegetables are eaten regularly. Because of their vitamin and mineral content, the vegetables should occupy a respectable place in our menus. This is especially true in the developing countries, where a large number of people do not get a variety of foodstuffs.

Like vegetables, fruits also present a great variety. Fruits are not only rich in energy, but are good sources of vitamins and minerals. Fruits are eaten fresh. They are preserved in the form of jellies and jams, and some of the delicious wines are made from them. There is an endless variety of pleasant and attractive flavors in the many kinds of fruits familiar to us. Apples and oranges can be produced on as much of a mass scale as the cereals. The oranges and other members of the citrus family are especially rich in vitamin C. Most fruits also contain vitamin B complex as well as carotene (precursor or vitamin A). Some countries specialize in the production of certain categories of fruits, probably because their climate is most suitable for their growth. For example, mangoes are the major fruit of India while oranges and apples are produced in large quantities in the United States. Bananas are grown in East Africa and several countries in South America. Grapes are grown almost universally. In smaller quantities, most countries produce pears, apricots, plums, peaches or strawberries. Most of the fruits are rich in sugars, but bananas probably contain much larger amounts of carbohydrates than most other fruits and therefore have caloric value of about 80 k cals/100 gms. Green bananas, before they ripen, are also cooked and eaten as a vegetable. When ripe, the starch in the fruits is converted into sugars, such as sucrose, fructose or glucose. Coconut, strictly speaking, is not a fruit but may be mentioned here. They are enclosed in a tough, stone-hard cocoon. The white fruit which is called copra, has a high oil content. Dried coconut is also used as a fruit in confectionary, but most of the coconut production is used for oil and the residue is fed to animals. In the fresh state, the sap of the fruit is a pleasant drink. Sweet toddy is readily fermented by yeasts and this product has been the chief alcoholic drink in many parts of the tropics (Davidson *et al.*, 1972).

PROCESSED FOODS BASED ON CEREALS AND OILSEEDS

Need and Basis for Formulating Processed Foods

In the developing countries where protein deficiencies are endemic and where animal proteins are not available in adequate quantities, a well-planned vegetarian diet, based on the concept of mutual supplementation, seems to be a logical solution to the protein problem (Narayana and Swaminathan, 1969). The desirability of using vegetarian sources of food for the good of a maximum number is also evident from the economic viewpoint. Even though the meats, milk and eggs contain proteins of high biological value, their production is less economical than that of vegetable proteins. Slade and his coworkers estimated that 3 to 6 times the amount of land space is needed to produce animal proteins as compared to the same quantity of vegetable proteins. The amount of protein (lbs/acre/year) that could be derived from land varies with its use: under grass it is 600, under beans 370, and under wheat 269, but only 90 if the land is used for milk production and 54 if the land is used for meat production (Slade *et al.*, 1945). The available acreage in the overpopulated developing countries can be better utilized if the land is put to use for the production of vegetable proteins. The situation in some countries in Southeast Asia, Bangladesh and India is especially critical from this point of view. Unused land hardly exists and arable land cannot be used to produce milk and animal protein to feed their ever-increasing populations. The biggest drawback in the use of vegetable proteins is their deficiency in one or two of the eight essential amino acids which the body cannot manufacture and must be supplied from an external dietary source. The nutritional deficiency status in populations of the developing countries is not quantitative because even a low protein cereal such as rice, eaten in sufficient quantity, would provide the recommended daily needs of protein, but it is of a qualitative nature because of amino acid imbalance of proteins of cereal origin.

The processed foods are formulated on the basis of amino acid patterns of various foods of vegetable origin. A combination of two or more vegetable proteins could make up an amino acid pattern of the final product which is similar to that of egg or milk, believed to have a perfect combination for promoting body building processes and maintaining a satisfactory growth pattern in children. This highlights the significance of mutual supplementary relationships between vegetable proteins (Dean, 1953; Oliviera and De Souza, 1967). The world supplies of animal proteins are grossly inadequate, and it is becoming evident with each passing day that feeding conventional foods to infants (animal milk and other dairy products) will be more difficult in the future despite efforts to increase dairying and stock raising. It is important, therefore, to look for vegetable foods which are protein rich, palatable, digestible and of good biological value. As an example, the high methionine content of sesame flour can be used to balance the low content of sulfur containing amino acids in soy flour. The amino acids of sesame and soy then become mutually supplementary when each supplies 50 percent of the protein of a diet. Similarly, a mixture consisting of 60 percent sesame flour and 40 percent fish meal is found to be equal to casein with respect to its protein quality (Howe *et al.*, 1965). Certain combinations of barley, wheat and soy proteins or corn and soy mixtures are nearly perfect and complete substitutes for milk in the diet of children. In the same way, proteins of chick peas *(Cicer arietinum)*, which are deficient in methionine and rich in lysine, and those of sesame, which are rich in methionine and deficient in lysine, mutually supplement each other. There is indeed a remarkable supplementing effect of proteins of legumes, oilseeds and leafy vegetables to those of cereals (Narayana and Swaminathan, 1969).

During recent years, a considerable amount of research work has been carried out in the preparation of processed protein foods suitable for supplementing diets of those children and adults whose traditional diets are qualitatively imbalanced. These foods are being prepared in a number of developing countries at a medium scale. It is hoped that after feeding, distribution, marketing and other related problems are solved, large scale production of these foods will begin in the near future. Broadly speaking, the processed foods can be grouped into three categories: protein foods based on blends of oilseed meals and legumes and fortified with vitamins and minerals; precooked roller dried foods based on cereals, oilseed meals and legumes and fortified with vitamins and minerals; and spray dried milk substitutes based on blends of oilseeds, protein isolates from oilseeds and skim milk powder (Tasker *et al.*, 1966). Table II lists some of the important new food products. Most of these foods have a long shelf life and studies have shown that the products keep well at 37° C in sealed containers for 9 months without any appreciable loss of nutrients. At the end of a 9 month storage period, the processed foods are well accepted by the consumers. The foods that have been prepared for the weaning infants are reconstituted in 10 times the weight of boiling water and sugar added to improve the taste. The resulting paste is suitable for feeding infants.

The FAO/WHO expert committee on nutrition suggested that in the planning of new food mixtures, the following criteria must be taken into consideration:

(1) the amino acid content of the individual ingredients and the final product; (2) the possible presence of toxic or interfering factors; (3) the need for obtaining exact specifications for each of the components; (4) the necessity of avoiding processes that may damage protein quality; (5) the desirability of using products of local origin; (6) the low cost and good-keeping quality of products; (7) suitability of the product for feeding weaned infants; and (8) the acceptability of the product to the consumers. At the same time, the processed protein foods should possess high nutritive value and should have a significant supplementary value to the diets normally consumed by the people in the region. Although the primary objective should be to provide a supplementary source of protein of good quality, it is desirable that a vegetable protein food should also contain or be fortified with adequate quantities of vitamins and minerals that are likely to be lacking in the diets (FAO/WHO, 1955; Subrahmanyan, *et al.*, 1961).

The manufacturing processes should satisfy most of these criteria; for example, optimal heat processing eliminates partially or wholly the nonnutritional or toxic factors present in the vegetable proteins and improves their nutritional value. Their suitability in weaning infants has been proven by numerous feeding experiments, and if made available in larger quantities at moderate prices, the consumers have shown a definite preference for them. In this manner, the

TABLE II

LIST OF IMPORTANT NEW FOOD PRODUCTS

	Product	Country	Composition	Protein content (%)
1.	IncaParina	1.1 Guatemala	Maize, cotton seed flour, vitamin A lysine, $CaCO_3$	27.5
		1.2 Colombia	Same plus defatted soya flour	27.5
2.	Fortifex	Brazil	Maize, defatted soya flour, vitamins A, B_1 and B_2, DL-methionine, $CaCO_3$	30.0
3.	Pro-Nutro	South Africa	Maize, skim milk powder, peanut, soya, FPC, yeast, wheat germ, vitamins A, B_1 and B_2, niacin, sugar, iodized salt	22.0
4.	Saridele	Indonesia	Extract of dry soya, sugar, $CaCO_3$, vitamins B_1, B_{12} and C	26.0–30.0
5.	Protone	UK, Congo	Maize, skim milk powder, yeast, vitamins, minerals	24.40
6.	Arlac	Nigeria	Peanut flour, skim milk salts, vitamins B_1, B_2, B_{12} and D	42.0
7.	Indian MPF	India	Peanut flour, chick-pea flour, vitamins A, B_1 and B_2	40.0
8.	Prolo	UK	Soya flour, DL-methionine, minerals, vitamins A, B_1, B_2 and PP	49.0
9.	Alpine MPC	USA	Marine protein concentrate	80.0
10.	FAP	Morocco	Fish protein concentrate (FPC)	80.0
11.	Superamine	Algeria	Wheat, chick-peas, lentils, skim milk powder, sugar, vitamin D	20.0
12.	SM	Ethiopia	Teff, peas, chick-peas, lentils and skim milk powder	15.0
13.	Bal Ahar	India	Mixed wheat flour, vegetables & defatted oil seed flour, vitamins, Ca	22.0–26.0
14.	Lactone	India	Vegetable protein-toned milk, ground nut protein isolate, glucose, syrup, minerals, vitamins, water blended with buffalo milk	12.0
15.	Aliment DE Sevrage	Senegal	Millet flour, peanut flour, skim milk powder, sugar, vitamins A and D; Ca	20.0
16.	CSM	USA	Maize (precooked), defatted soya flour, skim milk powder, $CaCO_3$, vitamins	20.0
17.	Supro	East Africa	Maize or barley flour, torula yeast, skim milk powder, salt, condiments	24.0

From: D. B. Jelliffe, *Infant Nutrition in the Subtropics and Tropics* (Geneva, WHO, 1968). S. L. Manocha, *Malnutrition and Retarded Human Development* (Springfield, Thomas, 1972).

scarcity of animal protein experienced lately all over the world can be overcome. The available quantities of animal products could then be used to supplement the vegetable mixtures, which could go a long way to improve their biological quality and protein efficiency ratio. As the human population grows and the demand for more food increases, the animal proteins are likely to become more and more scarce. Brown rightly remarked that in the years to come, "the supply of animal protein will lag behind growth in demand for some time to come, resulting in significantly higher prices for livestock products during the remainder of the 1970's than prevailed during the 1960's. The world protein market may be transformed from a buyer's market to a seller's market, much as the world energy market has been transformed over the past few years (Brown, 1973).

Special mention may be made here of the unique position of peanuts in an overpopulated country like India, where prevalent undernutrition is of a great magnitude. India produces 40 percent of the world's production of peanuts, which properly utilized, could provide significant quantities of good quality protein when incorporated at 20 percent level in the average poor vegetarian diets of this country. Feeding trials on school children, given 1 ounce of peanut flour besides their regular diets, have shown significant increases in height, weight and hemoglobin content over control groups not receiving additional supplements (Lal, 1952; Sundaravall: and Narayana Rao, 1969). In India, the common cereals, particularly wheat and maize and barley, are eaten in the form of flat-pan cakes, *chapatis* (unleavened bread). It is most convenient to mix peanut flour in the cereal flours. A number of mixed flours are available in India but not in quantities needed by the population. For example, Mysore flour is a blend of 75:25 tapioca flour and peanut flour. Paushtik flour is a blend of wheat flour, peanut flour and tapioca flour in the ratio of 75:8:17. The essence of the problem is to provide 40 to 50 gm of protein from these protein mixtures which will adequately supplement the 10 to 15 gm of protein derived from the traditional foods (Subrahmanyan *et al.,* 1961). It is now well recognized that peanut proteins supplement wheat, oat, corn, rice and coconut proteins to a significant extent.

Milk occupies a unique place in the nutrition of infants, preschool children and other vulnerable groups because of its nutritive value, flavor and the ease with which it can be fed. In many developing countries of South and Southeast Asia, Africa and Central America, it is in short supply or not at all available. Attempts are being made in most of these countries to enhance the production of milk, but at best the task is unequal to the problem of bridging the gap between the available and the required (Chandrasekhara, 1972). A number of methods have been evolved to solve the problem of short supply of milk by either supplementing the available milk by other means, e.g. toned milk produced by combining skim milk powder and milk fat, or by producing milk-like substitutes using vegetable protein mixtures. One such example is the production of Miltone® by the Central Food Technological Institute of India, in which half of the total protein comes from peanuts and the other half from milk. Half of the carbohydrate is lactose, while the other half is sucrose. The composition of Miltone resembles that of cow's milk in the gross constituents, vitamins and minerals. In a similar manner, soy milks with improved flavor have been prepared and recommended as a solution to countries with nutritional deficiencies (Mustakas *et al.,* 1967).

It is evident that the production of milk substitutes based on soybeans and sesame possesses a high nutritive value comparable to milk proteins. These milks provide a possible solution to the shortage of milk in the developing countries, provided the vegetable protein resources are properly utilized for human feeding. Throughout Southeast Asia soy milk is suddenly a popular drink. In Hong Kong, it is called Vitasoy; in Bangkok, Vitamilk; in Singapore, vegetable milk. It is bottled as any other soft drink and is sold mainly on its taste appeal in addition, of course, to its nutritive value. In some countries, it has been such a tremendous success that it sells in quantity next only to Coca Cola® (Streeter, 1969).

It is most desirable that the sources of vegetable protein for the preparation of processed foods be procured from local sources. It is only then that long term success can be achieved in the manufacture and acceptance of these food products in areas or countries where malnutrition exists. A climate can then be created for the human consumption of some of the raw materials such as the oilseed press cakes, which are now used for animal feeds and fertilizers. It generates a lot of optimism to note that most of the developing countries do have ample vegetable sources, which can provide raw materials for the mass scale production of nutritionally balanced processed foods. For example, India is the major producer of wheat and rice in the cereal category and of oilseeds and beans in the legume category. India is the largest producer of peanuts and sesame. It also has substantial quantities of cottonseed and coconut. China is next only to the United States in the production of soybeans and is a major producer of wheat as well. Having all the raw materials needed, the effort at the production of nutritional well-balanced processed foods is only a matter of investment in technology, determination in eradicating undernutrition and imaginative marketing, so that these foods do not directly conflict with the established eating patterns of the people. There is no doubt that by applying modern science and technology to farming practices, increasing use of fertilizers and preventing infestation, the availability of these food supplies for the production of processed foods can be increased substantially (Parpia, 1966). Already there is a drive to maximize the output of cereal grains. A number of new varieties of rice, wheat, sorghum, corn, millet, etc., have been evolved. A similar research effort needs to be put into evolving high yielding varieties of legumes (beans, lentils, grains, etc.) and peanuts. A combination of cereals and legumes is ideal for the purpose of balancing the amino acid pattern in the manufacture of processed foods. These foods have a great potential in removing the undernutrition caused by the qualitative deficits of proteins, in the diets of more than half of the human population.

A note on the fermentation of various edible products may be in order. It is widely believed that the processes of fermentation greatly improve the nutritive value of the product. This may be somewhat of an exaggeration, but the fermentation process often facilitates the use of a product, which otherwise might have been considered inedible or indigestible. The use of soybeans in the preindustrial societies is a classic example. Soybeans are very rich in their protein content, but at the same time, they are not easy to eat. They are difficult to digest as well as taking a long time to cook. The Indonesians have solved both of these problems by fermenting the soybeans with a mold after soaking and partially cooking them. The mold, they believe, makes the soybeans more digestible. The well-known preparation, *Tempeh*, is prepared by a fermentation process involving a mold, *Rhizopus oryzae*. This mold grows rapidly at temperatures of 37° to 45° C. Incubated at 37° C, the beans are covered with mold in 24 hours. The higher temperatures inhibit the development of the mold, which is highly proteolytic and will produce enough ammonia in unbuffered substrates to kill itself (Steinkraus, 1961). Besides Tempeh in Idonesia, old Japanese produced another product, *Natto, or Kojbean,* by a process of fermentation. This product is very rich in proteins of good quality and it is believed that the nutritive value and flavor of soybeans are modified favorably by the process of fermentation (Sakurai and Nakano, 1961).

Fermented foods are also prepared from other cereals, pulses or legumes, fruit, milk or fish. In Burma, fermented fish (*Nappi*) is used as a supplement to a staple rice diet, which greatly balances the rice diet with respect to its protein quality. In India a mixture of black grain and rice is allowed to ferment by air-borne microorganisms in the preparation of *Idli* and *Dosa*. Similarly, Bengal grain is used in the preparation of a fermented product, *Dokhla*. Feeding the fermented product, *Idli,* to the experimental rats at 50 percent replacement of dietary casein lowered the fat percentage of the liver. This was quite significant as compared with the feeding of the same preparation before fermentation.

Chemical and microbiological studies on the fermented and unfermented preparations have shown that, as a result of fermentation, there is an increase in choline, methionine and folic acid values. Fermentation, however, does not influence the B_{12} content of the mixture of black grain and rice. On the other hand, the fermented food preparation, *Idli*, possesses a better regenerating capacity for red blood corpuscles as compared with the unfermented preparations (Ramakrishna Rao, 1961).

Nutritive Value of Processed Foods

A number of studies and field trials on the nutritive value of these products have been carried out and have shown that vegetable proteins of moderately high nutritive value can promote adequate growth when fed at somewhat higher levels (Gordon and Scrimshaw, 1972; Narayana Rao and Swaminathan, 1969). As supplements to the traditional foods based on cereals, the blends of vegetable proteins have proven to be extremely useful. A 4:4:2 blended mixture of peanut, soybean and sesame flour alone or as a supplement to a predominantly rice diet increased significantly the growth rate of experimental rats as compared to those which were maintained on traditional cereal levels of the developing countries (Dreyer, 1968; Srinivas, *et al.,* 1966; Tasker *et al.,* 1967).

Studies on the regeneration of plasma proteins with vegetable proteins, as compared to milk proteins, indicate that the rate of regeneration is somewhat slower with vegetable protein mixtures in the early stages, given sufficient time, the rate returns to normal values with vegetable proteins alone (Tasker *et al.,* 1962), but when small quantities of skim milk powder are added to predominantly vegetable protein mixtures, the rate of regeneration of plasma albumin is distinctly improved. A 2:1 blend of peanut protein isolate and skim milk, in which the latter provides only 15 percent of the total protein, is as effective as skim milk powder itself in the regeneration of serum albumin in kwashiorkor children (Bhagavan *et al.,* 1962).

In feeding experiments with children, the Indian multipurpose food (a mixture of peanut flour and chick-pea flour with added vitamins and minerals) produces highly significant improvements in height, weight, RBC counts, hemoglobin, and nutritional status compared to the control group receiving regular vegetarian foods. When this formula is supplemented with 20 percent skim milk powder, it results in a marked improvement in kwashiorkor patients within eight to ten days.

Here it may be important to define the chemical evaluation of the quality of protein, which is responsible for the difference in metabolic absorption of protein from one source of food as compared to another.

> The chemical evaluation of the quality of a protein rests on the comparison of its amino acid pattern with the patterns found in proteins of high biological value. From a practical point of view the most useful basis for comparison is the hypothetical FAO *reference protein*, the essential amino acid requirements of man as far as these are known. This protein is theoretically 100 percent utilizable and a rough indication of the biological value of a protein can be obtained by calculating its *protein score,* i.e. by expressing concentration of its most *limiting* amino acid as a percentage of the concentration prescribed in the reference pattern (Editorial, 1968) .

In order to compare the biological quality of protein in the commonly used blends of vegetable mixtures with those of animal proteins, a number of studies have been conducted to test the efficiency of vegetable mixtures. Prasana *et al.* undertook a detailed study of the relative efficacy of the microatomized protein foods based on blends of low fat peanuts, soy and sesame flours and skim milk powder, fortified with vitamins, calcium salts and limiting amino acids, on twenty children suffering from kwashiorkor. Besides routine clinical observations, nitrogen balance and serum constituents studies were undertaken in detail. They concluded that the blends of oilseed meals and skim milk powder are readily acceptable and are quite effective in initiating a cure, and the food was well absorbed by the patients. The nutritive values of protein-enriched cereal foods based on wheat, soybean and peanut flours containing varying amounts of proteins (22.6, 19.2 and 15.6%) have also been thoroughly investigated (Narayana-swamy, 1973). It was concluded that not only are these vegetable blends efficient in promoting satisfactory growth, but a protein content of about 22 percent may be optimal for a protein-enriched cereal food meant for feeding preschool children.

A vegetable protein mixture prepared from the foods available in the Middle Eastern countries has been evaluated in the experimental animals and children. The mixture consists of 47 percent autoclaved chick-peas, 35 percent defatted sesame flour and 18 percent heat processed, low fat soybean flour, and the final product contained 37.8 percent protein content. These investigations have shown that children receiving this mixture compared favorably with respect to metabolic studies, as well as nitrogen retention and weight gain with those in a control group receiving a whole milk diet or another vegetable protein food mixture, Incaparina, which has been produced in the Institute of Nutrition of Central America and Panama (Matoth *et al.*, 1968).

Pretorius made a thorough assessment in South Africa of the nutritive value of multipurpose food (mixture based on vegetable sources of protein) in the treatment of convalescent kwashiorkor patients. Based on clinical investigations, balance studies, analytical methods and statistical methods, they concluded that there was no indication that the efficacy of the vegetable mixture differed in any way from that of skim milk in the treatment of kwashiorkor patients. The vegetable mixture has an advantage over skimmed milk in that it contains added vitamins and minerals. Ballarin estimated that the protein-rich food mixtures should supply in the diets of preschool children at least 350 calories a day as a compliment to their regular diet. The mixtures should contain at least 30 percent protein and have a nutritive value of at least 80 percent of that of milk protein (Ballarin, 1963). At the same time, for the children to eat the food to their benefit, it is essential that the vegetable mixtures should have the flavor and texture compatible with general eating habits.

TRADITIONAL FOODS OF ANIMAL ORIGIN
Dairy Products

Dairy products are excellent sources of high quality protein and calcium as well as a number of other vitamins and minerals. Milk is in many respects a complete food and the human infant during its first few months thrives on it. Milk can play a very important role in human nutrition, but the unfortunate fact is that three fourths of all the milk in the world is produced in the developed countries, which contain not more than one fourth of the human population (Josephson, 1966). The developing countries produce only one fourth of the quantity of milk in spite of the huge cattle numbers that they possess. India alone has a cattle population of 250 million. Technology again makes all the difference. In India, an average cow produces about 600 pounds of milk per year. This is in contrast to about 10,000 pounds of milk produced in the United States. Many well-managed cows average 15 to 16,000 pounds of milk per year. A Maryland cow, *Rheihart's Ballad,* holds the world record of producing as much as 42,000 pounds of milk in a year (Cloud, 1973).

No wonder in North America we consume about a quart of milk (in all forms) per capita per day, while the average Asian is limited to one quart equivalent every 14 days (Josephson, 1966). It is in these countries that intensive efforts need to be made to improve the supply of milk and raise the milk production per cow per year by genetic improvement in the quality of the cattle. While this may take some time, the scanty resources of milk may to a great extent be stretched by using them in combination with constituted milks produced out of vegetable sources. These are the milk substitutes produced in various countries out of soy protein (soy milk) or peanuts (peanut milk). The vegetable proteins singly are not of high biological value but a combination of several sources of vegetable proteins supplemented by cow's milk produces a milk-like commodity which contains all the essential amino acids, vitamins and minerals and can promote satisfactory growth in children.

While milk, as such, is a very nutritious and well-liked commodity, the various products of milk are equally nutritious and pleasing in flavor, and are very much liked all over the world. The most commonly used milk products are yoghurt, different varieties of cheese, cream, butter, buttermilk or whey. Milk is converted into yoghurt by curdling it with the help of various bacteria such as *Lactobacillus acidophilus*. These bacteria break down the lactose in the milk to form lactic acid. The yoghurt formed by the action of these bacteria has all the protein, fat, calcium and vitamins of the original milk. It is indeed a safe preparation in those countries where standards of dairy hygiene are low, because the original milk is sterilized by boiling and the subsequent profuse growth of *L. acidophilus* will overgrow any chance of pathogenic contaminant (Davidson *et al.*, 1972). Yoghurt in its thick form or after diluting it with water is quite popular in a number of eastern countries, especially India, Pakistan, Iran and Afghanistan. Yoghurt is also popular in Greece, Rumania, Hungary, Bulgaria and Turkey.

Whey is the fluid which separates from the milk when the latter is clotted with some weak acid solution. It contains most of the lactose, a little lactalbumin, but almost no casein or fat. Its nutritive value is not very high. On the other hand, the cream contains all the fat and from one third to one half of the protein. But when the fat has been removed from the milk to make either butter or cream, the remaining part is called skimmed milk. Since this can be readily dried, it can be easily converted into powdered milk. Except for its very low fat content, the skimmed milk is as nutritious as the original milk. It contains most of the protein, nearly all the calcium of the whole milk and the B complex vitamins.

Cheese is the most common form in which the dairy products are consumed. When in the summer months, milk is in surplus, the ideal way of preserving it along with all the nutrition, is to either convert it into powdered milk after separating the butter or to convert it into cheese. The latter use has been so popular that at present there are more than 400 varieties of cheese. Most of the commonly used varieties contain 25 to 35 percent protein of very high biological value. They are also rich in calories, and their fat content varies from 16 to 40 percent. Cheeses are a good source of calcium, vitamin A and vitamin B. The procedures used at present in milk processing to make products like yoghurt, cheese, dried milk, concentrated milk, etc., are generally conservative and the losses of nutritive quality are very small (Rolls and Porter, 1973).

Nutritious, tasty and popular as the different varieties of cheese are, it may be important to warn some susceptible individuals about the reaction of cheese.

> Many cheeses contain tyramine, the amine of the amino acid tryosine. The amounts vary greatly, but a portion of cheddar may contain 20 mg. Tyramine stimulates the sympathetic system and, in particular, may cause a big rise in blood pressure. The tyramine naturally present in foods is normally destroyed in the tissues by Mono-amine-oxidases (MAO). Cheese, therefore, does not contribute to the causation of high blood pressure. However, a group of drugs which are used for the treatment of depression, inhibit MAO. If patients on these drugs eat a large portion of cheese, the tyramine present is not destroyed and may produce alarming reactions. Headache, severe nausea and dizziness frequently occur, to be followed by confusion and occasionally a fatal cerebral haemorrhage or cardiac failure. In practice it is not necessary to forbid patients on these drugs to eat cheese, but they must be warned to take only small portions (Davidson, *et al.,* 1972).

Milk and its products contain exceptional food values and supply more of the essential nutrients in significant amounts than any other single food with the exception of eggs. Because of the high cholesterol content of the eggs, one cannot use too many eggs but one can consume large quantities of milk without any fear of excessive intake of any particular nutrient. Whereas milk contains 12 mg/100 gms of cholesterol, the whole egg contains 500 mg of this nutrient. Milk can be rightly considered as a single natural food, excellent for promoting growth, muscle building, sound teeth, strong bones, normal vision, physical vigor and good health (Rusoff, 1971).

Milk fats rate high for their pleasing flavor, which improves not only the palatability of other foods but is easily digested and increases the satiety value of meals. About two thirds of the milk fats are saturated and one third unsaturated. The latter contain essential fatty acids such as linoleic and arachidonic which are necessary for good nutrition. Milk contains biologically high quality protein and one quart contains 50 percent of the daily allowance for an adult. The main carbohydrate in milk is lactose whose presence in the gastro-intestinal tract stimulates the growth of harmful bacteria but also helps in the increased absorption of calcium, phosphorus and magnesium. Milk is a good buffering agent when there is pain caused by peptic ulcers or by simple hyperacidity. Lactic acid, a product of lactose fermentation present in fermented milk products such as sour cream, buttermilk, yoghurt, etc., has a favorable influence on intestinal micro-organisms during the oral administration of antibiotics and helps re-establish normal intestinal microflora.

All of the 14 essential minerals (calcium, phosphorus, potassium, magnesium, sulfur, sodium, chlorine, iron, copper, cobalt, manganese, iodine, zinc and fluorine) known to be needed for good nutrition are present in milk (see Appendix III). Milk is especially rich in calcium and phosphorus, the two major tooth and bone building elements, and a quart of milk contains more of these minerals than is recommended for daily consumption by average-sized adults. Since approximately 20 percent of the calcium in the skelton is replaced every year, the importance of milk in the diet is greatly enhanced in order to maintain vitality and vigor. Milk is also rich in a number of vitamins, especially riboflavin and a number of other B vitamins. Some of the vitamins are present in large quantities but there are others such as ascorbic acid which are present only in small amounts. However, milk can be considered a whole food in terms of its vitamin content because all the fat soluble vitamins (A, D, E, K) and water soluble vitamins (ascorbic acid and the B family—thiamine, riboflavin, niacin, pantothenic acid, pyridoxine, folacin, biotin, choline, inositol and vitamin B_{12}) essential for good nutrition are present in milk. During these days, most of the commercial milk is fortified with vitamin D. Because of its high nutritive value, nonfatted milk (fat being the main source of calories) can be an ideal diet for reducing weight. Buttermilk, skim milk, cottage cheese and nonfat milk solids are ideal reducing diet foods, since they are low in calories and high in health promoting essentials (Rusoff, 1971).

Meats, Poultry and Eggs

Animals represent a useful source of high quality protein, because they provide all the essential amino acids in amounts which are desirable for body building purposes. Man started his life as a hunter and has a natural appetite for flesh. The modern technology has brought to his dining table meat from a hundred or more species of animals. The modern man cultivates animal farms and maintains them with the same economic incentive as an agriculturist maintains and harvests his crops. These animal farms are in the strict sense of the word, crops. The animals breed in captivity, eat, fatten themselves and pass through a slaughter house and are then passed on to the kitchen of the consumer, in the same manner as a package of cereal made out of wheat.

Almost every part of the animal body is eaten. The lean muscle is the most popular, but liver, kidney, heart, tongue are well-liked. In addition, in some areas organs like pancreas, thymus, brains, testicles, etc., are considered delicacies.

The preference and prices of different organs are generally not based on their nutritive value, but their socio-cultural preference in a certain area. Brain, for example, is not rich in protein and contains large amounts of lipids, especially phospholipids, but may be sold as a delicacy at a very high price if it is locally preferred. A lean cut of muscle generally contains 20 percent protein, 5 percent fat, 1 percent mineral ash and the rest water. Most meats are rich in fat content unless lean muscle is especially selected. Sausages contain a lot of fat content, which may provide a satiety value to the food because a fat meal is known to cause delay in emptying the stomach. The variable amounts of fat in the meat make great differences in its energy value. In addition to protein and fat, meats contain fibrous connective tissue which is hard to digest. Actually, the degree of connective tissue determines the quality of meat. Muscle mass from younger animals has more lean meat and less fibrous tissues, whereas the older animals contain more fibrous connective tissue. The latter is tougher to chew and sells cheaper than the meat from younger animals.

Meat is superior to cereal not only for its protein of high biological value, but also because it is relatively richer in iron, phosphorus, calcium, nicotinic acid, riboflavin, thiamine, etc. If liver is eaten, it is rich in vitamin A. Liver contains more vitamins and iron than muscle and is highly recommended in certain conditions such as anemia.

Mention may also be made of the nutritive value of white and red meats. "Many textbooks of medicine have insisted until quite recently on the superior quality of white meats (poultry and game) in contrast to red meats (beef and mutton) especially for invalids and convalescents. The superiority of white meats has never been satisfactorily demonstrated. It is a myth" (Davidson *et al.*, 1972). However, the large quantity of highly saturated fats in the red meats may make some difference to the health and welfare of an obese person or the one prone to cardiovascular disorders. For him, the white meats may prove superior for providing biologically high quality proteins without the necessity of taking in large quantities of saturated fats. Whereas the poultry contains minimal fat, 100 gm of sausage may contain 12 gms protein, 20 gms fat, 12 gms carbohydrates and 280 k cals. (Davidson *et al.*, 1972).

The developed countries of the world take adequate quantities of meat in their diet. In North America more than 60 gms out of a total of 90 gms protein in an adult diet comes from animal sources. This is in contrast to almost 5 gms animal protein out of a total of 50 gms taken by an average adult in India. The conditions in China, Africa, Pakistan, Bangladesh and Southeast Asia are no different. There is an acute dearth of meat products for human nutrition in these countries. It is argued that animals are not efficient converters of feed to food and it may be better strategy to supply to the

vast human populations adequate diets from plant sources
(Wilcke, 1966). However, it must not be overlooked that
in spite of the overpopulation, the developing countries have
considerable sources of foodstuffs not fit for human consumption. With better management, these sources can be developed to augment animal sources of food.

From the point of nutrition, some of the insects can be
extremely useful. In various parts of the world, there are
religio-cultural taboos against their use as articles of food,
but wherever they are eaten, they have contributed significantly to the nutrition of the human population. In Indochina and Thailand, besides the full-grown insects, the larvae
are considered delicious and are eaten by the wealthy and
poor alike. An impressive list of insects is eaten by man after
properly cooking or roasting them. "Properly cooked and
served, locusts can be an attractive and nourishing food.
Flying ants cooked in butter are considered to be a delicacy
in certain parts of Africa" (Davidson, *et al.,* 1972).

Eggs are in all respects a complete food. The biological
quality of other sources of proteins is always measured in
terms of the proportion of essential amino acids and other
nutrients found in the egg because an egg, by itself, sustains
the growth of the embryo into a full-fledged animal. All kinds
of bird eggs are eaten by humans but the hen's eggs are by
far the most popular. No longer does the hen have to sit on
the eggs to provide the body's warmth, essential for the
growth of the embryo. Eggs in thousands can be incubated
in automatic machines and chicks hatched with an extremely
low rate of mortality. The modern genetical selection has led
to the development of species which give a large number of
eggs per year. Whereas an average hen in a developing country like India lays about 65 eggs per year, a genetically selected breed in the United States produces 227 eggs per year.
Recently a Japanese farmer produced a hen which layed 365
eggs in 365 days. It could mean that eggs could become an
important source of food for millions. An average hen's egg
weighing about 2 oz or 60 gms, contains 6 to 8 gms of protein, 6 gms of fat and contains about 80 k cals. In addition,

an egg contains 30 mg calcium, 1.5 mg iron and significant quantities of vitamin A, thiamine, nicotinic acid and ribo-flavin (Davidson *et al.*, 1972).

Fish and Other Foods from the Ocean

Fish is another source of animal protein, which is of bio-logically high quality as well as low in fat, which is most dreaded by the opulent, well-fed, overweight modern man. Lean fish contains 30 percent proteins with approximately 50 to 80 k cals per 100 gms. In this category, the common fishes are cod, haddock, pollack, saithe, brill, ling, whiting, John Dory, lemon sole, etc. The fat fish contain 8 to 15 per-cent fats, and has an energy value of 80 to 160 k cals per 100 gms. These include herring, salmon, white bait, eel and sar-dines. The intermediate species of fish, i.e. containing 2 to 7 percent fat are hake, halibut, mullet and trout (Davidson *et al.*, 1972).

Besides fish, the crustaceans such as lobsters, crayfish, crabs and shrimps form an important item of diet and a source of good nutrition. They are low in fat and rich in proteins. Due to their lesser catch as compared to the fish, they are valued more and are expensive enough to take the place of delicacies and prestigious foods. The other edible varieties of marine animals are the mullusks such as oysters, cockles, mussels, clams, scallops, whelks, winkles, etc. The mollusks contain 15 percent protein, 5 percent carbohydrate and very little fat. Oysters are prized as delicious foods in a number of countries.

The rate at which the demand for more food is increasing year after year indicates that the future existence of mankind may very well depend on the seas and oceans that cover 70 percent of the globe. The oceans contain a great variety of living organisms, from microscopic single-celled plants to the giant whales. At present, our major catch from the oceans belongs to the category of fish, which provide approximately 1 percent of the world's total food production. If the sea's resources were used in a rational manner with due respect for its ecological environment, an acre of its surface could produce twice as much protein-rich food as an acre of high class pasture. Not only is fish a valuable food for man, but its waste products and unmarketable varieties can be transformed into products for feeding animals and poultry. Moreover, the sea contains several times as many shellfish, crabs, lobsters and other valuable sources of food as it does fish. (Bogorov and Stepanov, 1969). This is indeed a very optimistic way of putting things, but as the realities stand, it becomes evident that the oceans are not a veritable storehouse; that all we have to do is to take to our fishing fleets and we have solved our food problem. On the contrary, by doing so we are hurting our vital interests. As Ehrlich pointed out, in spite of the vast quantities of food that can be obtained from the ocean, it would be quite foolish to assume that the food crisis facing the human species as a result of unthoughtful proliferation can be solved by harvesting the *immeasurable riches* of the ocean. The notion that we can extract vastly greater amounts of food from the sea than our present catches is just an illusion, promoted by the uninformed. We should have learned our lessons from the whale hunting and overfishing for anchovy in Peru. We must strictly regulate an International Code of Fishing which would allow the stocks of edible species of marine animals to build up their numbers again. The entire ocean is not as rich in marine life as it may seem (Ehrlich and Ehrlich, 1970).

During recent years, the commercial fishing has been greatly expanded, with Japan and Russia in the forefront, in utilizing the protein capacity of the oceans to its limits. The search for high quality animal food is bringing into the news clashes among the nations which can be rightly described as fish wars. If it were only for human consumption, probably the oceans covering the $2/3$ of this planet could sustain the needs of 3.9 billion aspirants, but a large quantity of the catch is fed in the form of fish meal to livestock in order to get still better quality animal protein. This has put a tremendous strain on the fish resources of the oceans. Lester Brown, a Senior Fellow of the Overseas Development Council, recently remarked that world fisheries are in serious trouble, largely because of overfishing. Many marine biologists now feel that the global catch of the table-grade fish is at or near the maximum sustainable level. A large number of the 30 or so leading species of commercial grade fish may currently be overfished, i.e. stocks will not sustain the current level of catch.

We must recognize that all the surface of the oceans is not equally productive and rich in life. Ryther pointed out that "the open sea—90 percent of the ocean and nearly three fourths of the earth's surface—is essentially a biological desert. It produces a negligible fraction of the world's fish catch at present and has little or no potential for yielding more in the future" (Ryther, 1969). The main reason cited for this pessimistic estimate is that the upper layer of the open sea, where there is enough light for photosynthesis, lacks the nutrients necessary for high productivity. The photosynthetic producing organisms that live in this layer are extremely small in size. In certain offshore or coastal areas where powerful currents bring nutrients to the surface, the level of productivity is 2 to 6 times. Ryther estimated that 90 percent of the ocean, which is equivalent to 326 million square kilometers, is likely to produce annually 160,000 metric tons of fish. The coastal zones which comprise 9.9 percent of the ocean (approximately 36 million square kilometers) will produce annually as much as 120 million metric tons of fish. The coastal up-welling regions which are approximately 0.1 percent of the ocean's area (approximately 36,000 square kilometers) are likely to produce another 120 million metric tons. According to this estimate, the total annual production of the ocean is in the neighborhood of 240 million tons, out of which not more than 100 million tons are available for harvesting and this, too, would require sustained effort and a high level of economic input.

The oceans are, however, ideal for regular farming. As new technology develops and economic inputs are made in the same manner as for agricultural production on land, the coastal areas could become quite profitable farming lands with great potential for food production. At this time marine fish culture is not popular due probably to man's concentration on tapping other sources of food production (e.g. improving the yields of traditional staples such as cereals), but as need for more food is felt, the ocean farming will take its rightful place. At present, Japan and France cultivate on a small scale certain kinds of fish, crustaceans and seaweeds in the shallow water. It is estimated that the shallow water ideally suited for farming may be as much as the whole of Europe. In these areas, just like developing new lands, the unwanted weeds and forms of life can be removed and replaced by plants and animals which will serve as food for man and beast. This could provide a huge quantity of extra food. At least the quantities, in which the food is deficient at the present time, can be easily produced with minor investments and hard work.

There are optimists who go too far in depending on marine farming as a source of food for our growing populations. Some of them argue that 80 percent of the solar energy is absorbed by the marine plants as compared to 20 percent by the land plants. If that part of the solar energy which is at present absorbed by the natural vegetation in coastal waters is applied to marine plants suitable for transformation into human or animal foods, it could produce a harvest sufficient to feed 58,000 million people. If the total resources of the oceans could be used in the same way, it would be possible to produce four to five times as much, or sufficient food for 290,000 million people (Bogorov and Stepanov, 1969). Professor L. Zenkevitch, an oceanographer of the Soviet Academy of Sciences, is all the more optimistic in the ability of the oceans to produce fantastic quantities of food for the humans to flourish on this planet. He believes that the productive capacity of the sea is more than a thousand times that of the arable land area. As an example, he states that

> 15 tons of underwater plants can be collected from an area which, on land, could scarcely produce four tons. It must also be remembered that marine vegetation contains four or five times as much organic matter as land plants. It has been calculated that five million tons of vegetable products could be harvested each year in the Baltic, the

Black Sea, and the Far Eastern coastal waters of the Soviet Union (*World Health,* 1969).

These kinds of estimates are grossly optimistic and, to some extent, misleading into a belief that we need not be serious about stabilizing our numbers. It is an overstatement of the fact that human ingenuity would always produce ample food, irrespective of the numbers. We must point out that, in spite of the great potential of both fresh and salt water fish culture, farming the sea is not as easy as it may seem. It could present an array of formidable problems, especially of fertilizing and harvesting and, despite the large capital investment, the actual food production may be only a small fraction of the potential. About the only planting and harvesting of marine plant crops done today is some seaweed culture in Japan, and this is really an extension of land agriculture into shallow water (Ehrlich and Ehrlich, 1970).

The other big obstacle in realizing our food potential from the oceans is the ever-increasing pollution of the sea due to our industrial activity. As population grows, the industrial activity is likely to increase and, along with it, the pollution of waters. The present level of pollution is threatening to have a negative effect on our present production. If some urgent steps are not taken to minimize the water pollution, there is a real possibility that our total catch from the oceans may even decline from our present level.

TECHNOLOGICALLY PRODUCED UNCONVENTIONAL FOOD PRODUCTS

Synthetic Amino Acids and Proteins

It is evident that a vast majority of the human population gets its food predominantly from a few cereal staples. These staples such as rice, wheat, corn, millet, sorghum, etc., are good sources of calories and, to some extent, proteins, but are deficient in one or two amino acids which are essential for the proper utilization of their protein content. These are called limiting amino acids. The widespread and predominant use of cereals in the diet has resulted in varying degrees of undernutrition, and, according to an estimate, more than 50 percent of the world population is undernourished (Howe *et al.*, 1965). Either additional varieties of foodstuffs that contain extra amounts of the limiting amino acids should be eaten along with these staples, or these staples should be fortified with the limiting amino acids by means of synthetic preparations.

A combination of cereals and legumes in the same diet serves to a great extent the former proposition, but it is not always possible due to the overwhelming poverty of certain communities that cannot afford to buy any other variety of foodstuffs. In such cases, the cure lies in the supplementation of cereals. The synthesis of some amino acids is already established on a commercial basis. The manufacture of lysine and methionine in large quantities is technically and economically feasible (Woodham, 1969a). By fermentation methods amino acids can be prepared from low-grade materials which are not suitable for human consumption. Such a measure could be extremely useful not only in the prevention of kwashiorkor but also to improve the diets of the undernourished populations (Scrimshaw *et al.*, 1968). A South African group of nutritionists has made an important contribution by showing a definite improvement in kwashiorkor symptoms by the use of vitamin-free casein or a mixture of synthetic amino acids. In most cases not only has there been a distinct improvement in anorexia, apathy, cutaneous lesions and edema, but the amino acid mixture has provided a satisfactory *initiation of cure* (Trustwell and Brock, 1959).

Laboratory investigations have shown that wheat proteins are improved by supplementation with lysine (Hutchinson *et al.*, 1959); maize proteins by lysine, tryptophan and threonine (Sauberlich *et al.*, 1953); and rice, ragi, sorghum and millet proteins by lysine and threonine (Leela *et al.*, 1965). Supplementation with these amino acids leads to a marked increase in nitrogen retention in children fed these cereals supplemented by appropriate amino acids. Lysine, tryptophan and isoleucine supplementation of maize diets, supplying children and adults with 0.5 to 1.0 gm protein/kg/ day, results in significant increase in the retention of nitrogen in all subjects.

Supplementing oilseed proteins (with much higher protein content than the cereals) with the deficient amino acid is another method of providing additional high-quality protein to the human population. Supplementation of soybean protein with methionine raises its protein efficiency ratio (PER) to a level almost equal to that of milk proteins (Joseph *et al.*, 1960). Howe *et al.* showed that supplementation with lysine, threonine and methionine, singly or in combination, raised the PER of oilseed proteins to the level of animal protein, casein. Similarly, supplementation of sesame with lysine; peanut with lysine, methionine, tryptophan and threonine; cotton seed with lysine and methionine; and chick-pea proteins with methionine will have the same effect.

It is, therefore, technically possible as well as desirable to supplement the cereals and oilseed protein with synthetically produced amino acids. Such a procedure will also cost much less than other foods which have the same quality protein content. Since it is not possible to produce the oilseeds in quantities as large as those of cereals, more emphasis must be placed on improving the quality of cereal proteins.

It is because of the high per acre yields of cereals that a vast majority of the human population depends on them as a staple food. These people are almost certain to benefit from the judicious supplementation of these foods with lysine, lysine and tryptophan, or lysine and threonine. In addition, there is no other method at present by which the protein quality of the foods of many of these poor and undernourished people can be improved without a concurrent sacrifice of available energy-yielding foods, which hungry people can ill afford (Howe *et al.*, 1965).

Fish Meal and Fish Protein Concentrate

With the increasing populations, almost all the countries of the world are looking towards the vast oceans in a manner which would indicate that the final battle for human survival is going to be fought at the high seas. The high quality animal protein is the scarcest commodity. The land animals use vegetables very inefficiently to convert into meat and, as time passes, there may not be extra pasture land left. In addition to the traditional methods of exploiting fish stocks by hunting, it may be profitable to husband marine animals just like farm animals. If this is done, fish farming on a major scale can provide significant amounts of food for the human populations.

There are only a few varieties of fishes that are at present liked and eaten. A number of other varieties are available in the oceans, which are equally nutritious but are not fit to be eaten in the conventional way due to a variety of reasons. Preparing fish meals or fish protein concentrates out of these varieties is the ideal solution. These fish products can be used in combination with other types of food to provide the needed nutrients, especially biologically high quality protein. With a little imagination and management, we can easily multiply ten times our present catch of fish, estimated at 65 million tons per year. Catches that are not palatable, such as menhaden, or those which are surplus to immediate needs, can be converted into fish protein concentrate (FPC) which contains 70 percent protein of high biological value if it is properly dried and stored. The FPC

has been incorporated in breads and infant foods in South Africa, corn products in Guatemala, hard bread in Sweden, baby foods in Ethiopia and Chile, pasta in Chile, biscuits in Brazil, flavored beverage tablets in Pakistan, and a variety of wheat products in Peru. It is, however, expensive, running about 22 cents a pound, more than twice the cost of most oilseed flours. Without significant technological advances to lower the cost, it is unlikely that fish protein concentrate will have much impact on the nutrition problem in the near future (Berg, 1973).

Fish meals have been used to great advantage in the animal feeds, but so far they have not been considered ideal for human consumption. The main problem is the rancid fat content of these meals, which could not only be toxic in the long run but may also precipitate a deficiency of fat soluble vitamins. For this reason, some 40 percent or more of the world fish catch is presently converted directly into fish meal to be used as animal feed. The production of fish meal is also simpler as well as more inexpensive, because of the relatively simple process of cooking, pressing out most of the oil and about half the water, and drying the press cake.

This product, however, is not a stable one and cannot be used by humans. It is important that a stable preparation such as fish protein concentrate be prepared from the fish meal. FPC is quite suitable for human consumption and should become a major industry in the developing countries, which are short of animal protein. As things stand today, coal is being transported to New Castle. The developing countries catch fish, prepare fish meal and export it to the developed countries as animal feeds in return for hard cash. Peru has been exporting to the United States 100 percent of the fish meals prepared from an oily fish, anchovy.

FPC, prepared under satisfactory conditions, is an acceptable human food and is considered tasty in many areas of the world. It is indeed a wise use of this valuable source of protein, since in most cases it is prepared from species that would be of little commercial value for human consumption. In Malaya, dry FPC is eaten straight from the can with delight because of its taste, like small dried salted fish, already familiar in their diet. It has been found acceptable when added to cooked rice or vegetable soup (Lovern, 1966). It has been suggested that at about 70 percent protein content, approximately 20 gms of FPC should be added to the regular diet, which would provide 15 gms of good quality protein. Even if this contains 10 percent residual oil, it may contribute not more than 2 gms of rancid fat. It is most unlikely that this quantity involves any significant risk (Lovern, 1969). It is estimated that 10 gms of FPC daily can support the minimal animal protein needs of an average adult human being. Five generations of mice were kept on FPC prepared from whole red hake and it was found that growth, reproduction and lactation in 5 succeeding generations from conception to death were satisfactorily favorable to those maintained on casein and laboratory chow. These observations are a strong argument in favor of extensive utilization of FPC to aid in the alleviation of protein deficiency in the overcrowded developing world.

There are some practical difficulties which have to be surmounted before FPC takes its rightful place in the eradication of prevalent protein deficiency. The preparation of a fat-free, odorless and tasteless fish protein concentrate, not easily detected if mixed with some cereal-based food, is not an easy matter. In the first place, fish is a poor starting material for the preparation of a permanently tasteless and odorless dry powder. It is poor in antioxidants, and its lipids are very highly unsaturated. Even after multiple extraction with a lower aliphatic alcohol, up to 0.2 percent lipids remain. Apart from the constant presence of a disagreeable odor, FPC has a gritty texture that is detectable in the mouth even after very fine grinding. Used in a milk shake, FPC leaves the impression of a mouthful of chalk. It is essential that for use with other foods, FPC must be finely ground, which could increase its cost terribly (Lovern, 1969).

Simulated Foods

We are so accustomed to eating the traditional foods that the new food products which simulate them in appearance, texture, color and taste are more likely to be readily accepted than those which are presented to us in a different form. A number of staple foods have been prepared by using mixtures of foodstuffs that provide a nutritionally balanced product. Rice is the staple food of the areas where protein deficiency is most evident. The production of simulated rice grains is a major technological breakthrough which could have a desirable impact on the problem of chronic undernutrition among vast sections of the human race. The simulated rice grains are prepared from a mixture of tapioca, peanuts and wheat flour (Parpia, 1968). Similarly, milk and other dairy products have been prepared from nondairy ingredients. Soybeans, peanuts, coconuts, almonds and other oilseeds have been used to produce milk of high nutritive value. These products not only resemble milk, but also have comparable nutritional value. The promotion of such products is likely to be successful because they do not interfere with the traditionally established food habits. It is fervently hoped that such products are produced on a large scale in the developing countries.

The production of simulated foods was prompted to provide high quality protein from a mixture of vegetable sources to those populations whose intake of these body building materials is qualitatively and quantitatively inferior. Recently the emphasis has shifted to the production of highly sophisticated foods by processes which make them quite expensive. Much effort is spent in providing the same flavor and texture as the original food. Because of their expense and the small quantity in which they are produced, they are becoming a source of adding variety to the diets of western menus. As an example, Woodham described the menu given to the delegates of the International Symposium on New Sources of Protein, held in Amsterdam in 1968.

> This included *chicken* soup made with artificial chicken flavouring and containing soybean protein, and a *game pie* was made from the soybean meat analogues. Hamburgers contained one-third vegetable protein, and biscuits, cassava, soya flour and fish protein concentrate. It was claimed that the retail price was 10 percent of a normal meal, and 25 percent of that of milk and cheese (Woodham, 1971).

Protein Isolates from Vegetable Sources

The protein deficiency of the present day world and even the future needs can be easily met, if the vegetable leaves not consumed at present by humans are used for the isolation of protein. This extra source of protein is especially important because the raw material for its manufacture can be produced indigenously in the areas which have the most need. The populations at present which are in most need of extra food live in the rural areas of the wet tropics, which abound in vegetation. First of all, the use of leafy vegetables can be encouraged in these areas so as to obtain the protein from them. In large areas of India, the leaves of mustard, turnip, radish and other leafy vegetables are routinely cooked and eaten, but the human physiology puts a limitation on the consumption of amounts which may be desirable to get a certain quantity of protein. It is here that technology can help. The fiber can be separated and leaf protein could be used for human consumption. In tropical areas with regular rainfall, the leaf proteins can be a great extra source of food for the people. In Britain, 1.4 tons of protein were extracted from a hectare in a year, whereas in a tropical region such as Mysore in India, as much as 3 tons per hectare were reached. This is quite comparable to protein yields from soya or peanuts.

Leaf proteins have another advantage over other sources. Leaf proteins could be the by-product of some other crop; tops from early potatoes, sugar beets, radishes, carrots and sweet potatoes. Even the jute, cotton, ground nut, sugar cane, etc., have good potentials. Green cereal leaves have been shown to yield protein concentrates of high nutritive value (Woodham, 1965). Not only can protein for human production be extracted, but the residue can still be used for feeding livestocks. The extracted protein makes up approximately one fifth of the total and the residue is still satisfactory feeding stuff for ruminants (Woodham, 1969b). Extensive research work in this area is badly needed.

At this time, we do not know the yields of extractable protein from a number of different crops growing in different climates and how much yields will differ after given quantities of fertilizer are used. Answering this will give us a better idea of the economic feasibility. Only to outline briefly the method of preparation of leaf protein in the laboratory, protein is usually precipitated by adding salt or acid to the juice pressed out of the pulp; in large scale work it is more convenient to use heat (70° C) because the curd is then easier to filter off. The curd is then washed at about pH 4 to remove flavor and alkaloids, should any be present in leaves used, and also to promote easy filtration and to yield a product that has, in the moist state, the keeping qualities of cheese or sauerkraut. The press cake is dark green and contains 40 percent of dry matter. The dry matter is 60 to 70 percent protein (Pirie, 1969).

Regarding the nutritive value of the leaf proteins, a good deal of analysis has been done in a number of laboratories and, based on the nutritive value, it is suggested that leaf protein is a better supplement in a protein deficient diet than the seed proteins. As a matter of fact, the leaf protein compares very well with the animal protein, apart from those in eggs or milk. Feeding experiments showed that 6 to 12 year old children grow better on a diet supplemented with leaf protein than on one supplemented with oilseed protein such as sesame protein (Doraiswamy *et al.*, 1969). The leaf proteins have high levels of lysine and other essential amino acids. A combination of cereal seeds and leaf proteins would provide a balanced protein to the diet. Waterlow showed that a mixture of leaf protein concentrate and milk was a satisfactory diet for malnourished children. However, the vitamin losses during preparation are quite significant, which have to be made good by supplementation (Woodham, 1973).

In countries where vegetarianism is well accepted and widely practiced, leaf protein cannot only be easily or readily accepted, but can go a long way in overcoming the protein deficits. In India, parts of Asia and Africa, vast populations already eat large quantities of leaves after cooking and spicing them. In New Guinea, children and adults are accustomed to eating powdered dry leaves. It should not be difficult for them to accept leaf protein concentrate.

Unicellular Protein and Microorganisms

One of the most exciting developments of recent years has been the interest in unicellular proteins, to ameliorate the protein hunger of human populations. No longer are yeasts looked down upon as cheap sources of some vitamins. They are now acclaimed as the potential suppliers of large quantities of edible protein. The potentialities of yeast as a source of protein in the diet of poor people of the developing countries is well recognized. Yeast is capable of synthesizing proteins from inorganic nitrogen in the shortest time. The efficiency of conversion of carbohydrate to protein by yeast is stated to be on the order of 16 to 33 percent. Yeast thus provides us with an excellent means of utilizing industrial carbohydrates for producing protein (Parpia, 1964). "While a 10 cwt bullock produces rather less than 1 lb of protein daily, 10 cwts of yeast may produce over 50 tons of protein in the same time" (Woodham, 1969b). The yeasts produced by fermentation of either pure n-paraffin or heavy gas oil grow fast and efficiently on cheap substrates.

> When the substrate is something which is of no commercial value and when the value of a primary product is enhanced by its removal, the use of single-cell protein is peculiarly attractive. Such a situation obtains in the crude petroleum refining industry and it has been satisfactorily demonstrated that not only can deleterious waxes be removed from the gas oil, thus facilitating the refining process, but good yields of protein may at the same time be collected (Woodham, 1969b).

Regarding palatability, Shacklady fed a ration with 65 percent gas oil grown yeast to a pig for 11 weeks without any trouble. After slaughter, he submitted hams from this pig and those from a control pig to testing by 250 people. Both were equally acceptable. This is indeed a most favorable condition because petroleum is always available in large quantities. The sterilization of the medium may be somewhat expensive, but the final protein may still be economically competitive with other sources. Besides petroleum, cane sugar may be another attractive alternative. Willcox calculated that an acre of land could produce approximately 45,000 lbs sugar cane from which 20,000 lbs dry yeast could be prepared which, in turn, can give as much as 10,000 lbs of protein (Willcox, 1959). Experimental evidence indicates that yeast protein incorporated at 5 to 10 percent level in human diets is quite safe. In Germany, a level of 5 percent has been fixed as the legal limit although experiments suggest that 10 percent is equally safe (Woodham, 1969b). Unicellular protein can thus provide the badly needed protein. However, despite its tremendous advantages, the future of single cell protein for human consumption is not very clear. It requires a substantial production facility as well as a ready market. "A 50,000 to 100,000 ton plant is necessary for economic production, since the unit costs are 40 percent greater in a 10,000 ton plant than in a 100,000 ton plant. Even at that volume, single cell proteins, although cheaper than milk, may not be competitive with oilseeds (Berg, 1973).

It has been the experience of social workers that the poorer the communities, the more rigid or conservative are their food habits and preferences. Will it be easy to convince an average American to eat snakes or grasshoppers? In some parts of the world, they are considered delicious. We may face a problem of the same magnitude, trying to convince some of the poor nations that single cell proteins are edible and will satisfy their deficits of protein. It has been estimated that three million tons of dried yeast can meet the protein requirements of 100 million needy children (Parpia, 1964).

Proteins from unicellular algae, bacteria and fungi are also quite promising in their scope. Much has been written recently about algae culture. Under optimum conditions, an algae (chlorella) attains a protein content of 50 to 60 percent. Feeding trials carried out on humans have shown that consumption of 100 gms of powdered algae daily is well tolerated. At levels of 250 gms per day, algae proteins cause cramps and diarrhea and may result in nausea, vomiting and abdominal distension. Similarly, the bacterial protein preparations are well tolerated in smaller quantities. Certain categories of fungi can also make large contributions to the world protein supply because they are rapidly growing organisms and can synthesize their amino acids directly from carbohydrates and inorganic nitrogen compounds. As sources of carbohydrates for the production of proteins, the commonly used cereals and sugars can be profitably used (Gray, 1966).

The unicellular proteins, like the cereals, have the drawback of having one or two limiting amino acids. These protein sources are generally deficient in methionine and, to some extent, tryptophan. They are, however, good sources of lysine. Since methionine as well as tryptophan can be commercially synthesized, their supplementation should not pose any major problems. There is a lot of scope in unicellular proteins, as has been the case with corn and other cereals, for the manipulation of genes to modify their protein composition in a favorable sense.

FOOD PROCESSING AND FOOD ADDITIVES

Man, for several hundred years, has been concerned with the problems of the storage of food so that he could use it at a later date when his needs would be greater. Food processing fundamentally involves handling the food in a manner that would serve the above purpose. Early man used the processes of smoking, curing, drying or dehydrating. Man's adventures into oceans involving long-term voyages were made possible by the availability of food in the processed form and, in recent times, space travel for as long as three months has been achieved because we have the ability to process and preserve foods to last long periods of time. However, the general question remains: do we preserve all the nutrition of the food during the course of processing for preservation for future use? No definitive statement can be made to answer this question because the preservation of food can affect the nutritional quality favorably as well as adversely.

> Processing destroys thiaminase in fishes and fishery products, anti-trypsin factors in cereal grains, and biotin and iron binding factors in egg white. In heat processing of cereal grains the digestibility may be markedly increased, thus making both the proteins and carbohydrates of these products more available . . . Generally, however, processing of food materials by fermentation, drying, freezing, thermal processing, or dehydration tends to decrease the supply of nutrients, particularly vitamins and minerals. Thermal processing or long storage times may significantly reduce the protein availability of foods while dehydration, accompanied or unaccompanied by smoking, may reduce the stability of the lipid components. Since there is an interaction between the carbohydrates, proteins and lipids, carbohydrate availability may also be affected by thermal processing (Chichester, 1973).

Food processing for the purpose of long-term storage is not as destructive as it may seem. The curing of meat results in only a small reduction in nutritive value (Burger and Walters, 1973). The process of cooking, which is essential before consuming the food, may hurt the nutritive value more than losses which may occur during processing and storage. In this respect, vitamins are especially sensitive. During the normal process of cooking, the loss of vitamins may be as high as 75 percent, whereas during the course of food processing for storage, the vitamin losses may never exceed 25 percent (Hein and Hutchings, 1971). The vitamins most sensitive to heat and cooking are the water soluble thiamine, riboflavin, niacin and ascorbic acid. Riboflavin, is also lost in the presence of light in addition to heat. Heat processing is in many respects more destructive, but is a better method of protection against microbiological deterioration and, because of its superiority, high-temperature short-time sterilization is receiving more attention during recent years.

The processes of dehydration or freezing do not destroy the vitamins or minerals. The freezing below —18°C results in excellent retention of vitamins, even an easily labile vitamin C. Temperatures above —9°C result in losses of easily oxidizable vitamins over a period of time. With respect to proteins, tryptophan, methionine and lysine are heat labile essential amino acids and must be given attention during the course of food processing. Short-term baking of wheat during bread preparation does not result in any loss of lysine but after 50 minutes of cooking at 232°C, as much as 30 percent lysine is lost (Benden, 1966). When peanuts are processed, they lose part of their lysine content but if after cooking the ground nut flour is mixed with powdered milk, the amount of lysine available biologically to the consumer is considerably greater (Carpenter and March, 1961). The lysine content of meat is not affected by heat treatment or during the course of normal cooking. Heller *et al.* studied the effect of heat treatment on lysine in meat and found that 74 to 92 percent is available after standard cooking procedures. It is only when meat is subject to 16 hours of autoclaving that the amount of available lysine is significanctly reduced (Heller *et al.*, 1961). During canning of common fruits and vegetables, however, an average of 15–50% of the nutrients are lost. For example, about 40% of nutrients are wasted in canning apples, beans, beef roots, potatoes, spinach, etc. (Henshall, 1973). Freeze drying or irradiation are other standard methods of preservation which have been considered harmless by some, but hazardous by others. In general it may be safely said that modern methods of food processing succeed to a very great extent in preserving the nutritive value of the foods and are generally safe. It is difficult to do justice to this vital subject in a limited space. The reader is therefore referred to some excellent reviews to get an insight into this subject (Bender, 1966; Chichester, 1973; Harris and Loesecke, 1960; Hollingsworth and Martin, 1972; Sabry, 1969; Tape, 1969).

Food preservation may not only involve processing by thermal treatment, freezing or other methods briefly mentioned above, it may require the addition of certain harmless chemical reagents. Strictly speaking, a food additive is defined as a "non-nutritive substance added intentionally to food, generally in small quantities to improve its appearance, flavour, texture or storage properties" (FAO/WHO, 1956). These additives are added in minute quantities and very seldom are ingested in quantities larger than 1 gm per day. The food additives may be categorized as flavoring agents (such as spices, synthetic imitation flavors, sweetening agents, sucrose, salt, salt substitutes or mineral hydrocarbons), food colors (e.g. synthetic dyes and naturally occurring substances), consistency improving agents (emulsifiers and stabilizers and anticaking agents), and preservatives (antioxidants, antimicrobial agents, nitrates and nitrites, nicotinic acid and sodium nicotinate, antibiotics, animal feeds, etc.). The food additives may be in the form of nutritional supplements as well, such as iodine compounds, vitamins and amino acids which may be used for the fortification of flours.

While our list of food additives is increasing year after

year, we need to be extremely careful about their use in terms of their safety.

> They must be studied not only away from food but also from the point of view of what happens to them during the processing of food and whether this alters any effect they may have after being consumed; we need to know more about the interaction of additives and food and metabolites of food additives. Special consideration is required in the case of food additives that have a slow or cumulative effect. Tests in animals are of limited value because of species differences and technical or other considerations, so that positive or negative results that are observed are not necessarily transferable to man (Sapeika, 1973).

A ready example is that of the widely used monosodium glutamate. Very large quantities of this chemical have been used over the years in baby foods and other products. During recent years, a number of discomforting reports have appeared regarding its effect on the physiology as well as nervous system. A report in *Nutrition Review* dealt with the effects of monosodium glutamate on the nervous system (*Nutrition Reviews* 1970), and described the brain lesion in mice and infant monkeys when this chemical is administered subcutaneously, the infants being more susceptible than the adults. Kuher also observed lesions and has explained a possible mechanism for the pathogenic action of monosodium glutamate (MSG) (Kuher, 1971). Used in large quantities to improve the taste, as has been done in Chinese restaurants, MSG is responsible for a burning sensation at the back of the neck, which later spreads into the arms and chest. Face muscles are especially affected, accompanied by lacrimation and palpitation (Kwok, 1968). These are indeed serious effects reported for an additive that has been in use for a long time. This calls for extra caution in using additives for the purpose of flavoring or preserving.

Due to increasing incidence of obesity and greater awareness of the desirability of weight loss among large numbers of people, saccharin became quite popular as a substitute for sugar. "The continuous use of small amounts of saccharin appears to be harmless but large doses daily may produce hyperacidity and enormous doses (5–25 gm daily) or a single dose of 100 g may cause anorexia, nausea, vomitting, diarrhea, abdominal pain, spasm of muscles, convulsions, and stupor. In hypersensitive persons it may even in small doses produce vomitting, diarrhea and skin eruptions" (Sapeika, 1973). Sugar is not an additive. It is a food in its own right, however, it must be eaten with restraint. Not only is sugar known to cause dental caries, but taken in large quantities, it increases the chances of developing myocardial infarction (Yudkin and Watson, 1969).

We take common salt (sodium chloride) regularly every day in order to make our foods tasty and palatable. In small quantities it is desirable as well as essential but when eaten in large amounts it could result in poisoning. This is especially true of the babies whose salt intake must be carefully monitored. A mistake such as putting 2 teaspoons full of salt instead of sugar could be very dangerous. The symptoms may range from vomitting, fever, respiratory distress to such serious conditions as cyanosis, convulsions or death (Calvin *et al.*, 1964; Finberg *et al.*, 1963).

It is in the area of food preservatives that special attention must be given with respect to their desirability and possible effects on the human physiology. A number of antioxidants, antimicrobial agents, antibiotics, nitrates and nitrites have been used to make the meat attractive, through interaction with haem pigments; nitrites also have antimicrobial action and retard the spoilage of meat, but a number of deaths have also been attributed to them (Steyn, 1973). Sapeika has rightly emphasized that "all food additives both new and old need to be studied for the possibility that they may prove to be harmful. An extensive literature is available dealing with the thousands of food additives currently in use; there are many technological, legislative, as well as toxicological problems that need to be solved."

FOOD SAFETY AND TOXICITY OF COMMON FOODS

It may not be wrong to state that there are very few

foods which are completely safe and harmless. Whether it is potato or wheat, the staple foods of millions, or the cabbage which goes into our tasty cole slaw, or the onions, straw-berries or peanuts, there is some problem or the other re-garding their toxicity and safety of consumption. The prob-lem of the nutritionist concerned with food safety is quite subtle and precarious. Humans, since ancient times, have suffered from food-borne diseases, and experience and study have revealed a long list of foods which should be avoided and a much longer list of foods which can be used if care is taken to eliminate their toxicity. Much of our daily foods come in this category. In addition to the natural toxicity of common foods, there are certain other causal agents such as bacterial, parasitic, viral, chemical agents and substances of still unknown etiology. During recent years, because of the everincreasing use of new food products, there have been in-creased incidences of food-borne diseases, especially in the advanced countries such as the United States, the United Kingdom, Japan and Western Europe. Bacterial and viral food poisoning represent the most common types. Viral poisoning is hard to determine as compared to the bacterial. In the United States, bacterial food poisoning represents 63 percent of all reported outbreaks and 83.5 percent of all reported cases; in Japan, 96 percent of all outbreaks and 87.5 percent of all cases; and in the United Kingdom, 69 per-cent of all outbreaks and 73.2 percent of all cases (Center for Disease Control, 1970; Vernon, 1967). This may be due either to changes in eating habits from home prepared meals to communal meals in restaurants, schools and other mass-feeding establishments, or may be a result of mass production of processed foods and their nationwide or inter-national distribution exposing large segments of the popula-tion to potential dangers. It may also be due to increased consumption of slightly heated products of animal origin because of ignorance or undue faith in the protective effect of food sanitation (Genigeorgis and Reimann, 1973).

There is a great need for tightening the procedures of food inspection not only at the level of production, but also through processing, preservation and distribution. In terms of potential carrying ability of food-borne diseases, meat is at the top and yet there are no elaborate methods except visual inspection, of ensuring safety. In addition to being the carriers of infections, the food could carry certain toxic material, which may be the result of metabolic products formed by microorganisms while they multiply in foods. Some poisonous substances may be incidentally added to foods during the course of production, processing, transport or storage. For details the reader is referred to an excellent review by Genigeorgis and Riemann.

Let us briefly discuss the toxicity of the foods which are used by a vast number of people almost daily. It is not intended to scare anybody from these foods, but only to provide a few illustrative examples of how the common articles of food carry with them certain amounts of toxic material. Starting with our staple foods, potatoes are known to contain a poisonous substance, solanine, in a quantity as high as 90 parts of solanine per million. This figure could go to 400 parts per million if the freshly dug potatoes are exposed for a long time to the sun. At this level of toxicity, it could be poisonous. The greatest redeeming factor in potato toxicity is that solanine is mainly concentrated in the green sprouts and in the process of boiling most of this toxic substance is extracted out (Bamford, 1961; Pyke, 1968). Wheat is not toxic in any sense of the word. But there are a large number of individuals who are sensitive to the gluten fraction of the wheat and celiac disease has been associated with it. During the last world war, there was a marked increase in celiac disease among the Dutch infants when in periods of stress wheat became the primary dietary staple (*Nutrition Reviews*, 1963).

A brief mention may be made of the commonly used vegetables. A harmful and toxic substance, 1-5-vinyl-2-thiooxazolidene, is present in a large number of highly recommended wholesome vegetables. It has been isolated from kale, brussels sprouts, broccoli, rape, kohlrabi and cabbage (Nordfelt *et al.*, 1954). Eaten in large amounts in the raw form, this could lead to very undesirable symptoms related to goitre. Oxazolidene acts by preventing the accumulation of iodine. Under normal circumstances, when iodized salt is eaten, some of these vegetables may not interfere with the functioning of the thyroid. In parts of the world where the local foodstuffs do not contain iodine, eating cabbage in large quantities can have a strong toxic effect. Onions are not free of blame. Although no direct influence on human physiology has been verified, Sebrell discovered that feeding raw or cooked onions to dogs can lead to severe anemia. Spinach is a valued food in our daily diet and often is recommended wholeheartedly to children. The spinach leaves are known to contain insoluble calcium oxalate crystals which may make up to 10 percent of their dry weight. It is believed that the insoluble oxalates prevent the absorption of calcium from spinach and other green vegetables, such as Swiss chard, beet tops, marigolds, halogeton (goosefood plant), sorrel, purslane and rhubarb. In halogeton, it approaches 37 percent of the dry weight of the leaves (Mickelsen 1967; Mickelsen and Yang, 1968).

Beans of different kinds generally referred to as legumes are regarded as the meat of the poor people. In combination with cereals, they can provide a balanced mixture of essential amino acids so necessary for proper growth and maintenance. However, before we recommend their large-scale use, it may not be inappropriate to warn of some of the toxic substances present in them. In view of our present knowledge, it will be only prudent to suggest that a major scientific effort should be made to look deeper into their toxicity. The commonly used varieties of peas (*Lathyrus sativus, L. cicera, L. cylmenum*) cause a neurologic disease called lathyrism, which in extreme cases manifests itself as spastic paralysis. After the ingestion of these peas, a feeling of heaviness of the legs appears accompanied by great weakness, so much so that while standing the leg muscles become tremulous and when the individual starts to walk, he may drag his feet. The young ones are especially susceptible and are permanently deprived of the use of limbs below the waist. It is associated with lesions of the spinal cord. In periods of drought it has been observed in India that these peas survive and their consumption by the local population increases and, according to some reports, as much as 7 percent of the population may be affected (Liener, 1966; *Nutrition Reviews*, 1967).

Toxic substances in soybeans have been studied extensively. It is now well-known that, whereas the ruminants are not affected by the toxic substances present in soybeans, human beings are quite sensitive. Liener and his group isolated from raw soybeans a protein which has the property of causing red blood cells to agglutinate (Liener, 1952). This hemagglutinating factor, which could result in inhibition of growth, must be eliminated before consumption. Soybeans also have some goiterogenic agents which produce a marked enlargement of the thyroid gland. This factor can be eliminated by heat treatment or the extra supplementation of diet with iodine. Raw soybeans may also produce a systemic disturbance in methionine metabolism (*Nutrition Reviews*, 1965). Luckily, all the toxic elements of soybeans can be eliminated by proper heating and processing. Due to their high level of biologically superior quality protein, soybeans are indeed indispensible for eliminating widespread undernutrition in the world.

In the raw state, some other beans, such as kidney, navy, lima and pinto beans, also contain toxic substances which can be removed by heat treatment. According to a report, navy beans when fed uncooked to rats not only inhibit growth, but produce acinar atrophy of the pancreas, fatty degeneration of the liver, and atrophy of the thyroid (Mickelsen, 1967). The eating of a broad bean *(Vicia tabor)* causes a disease commonly known as tavism. This condition is not common at all and afflicts only certain individuals who are hereditarily susceptible to it. The attack can be precipitated by a simple exposure to the pollen of the blossoms of this legume (Liener and Pallansek, 1952). Peanuts were for a long time suspected to have some kind of toxicity. Before the real reason was discovered, a large number of poultry, pigs and other animals were either killed or poisoned by the feeds which contained peanuts. It was later found that a fungus identified as *Aspergillus flavus* was responsible for the contamination which could take place in any warm and humid environment during the process of harvesting, drying or storage of the valuable peanuts. It is now know that the fungus contaminated peanuts may not only be toxic, but also carcinogenic (Pyke, 1968). Molds such as *Claviceps purpurae* growing on wheat when eaten along with flour made from even 1 percent contaminated wheat results in a disease called ergotism. This could lead to symptoms as severe as lameness and necrosis of the extremities due to contraction of the peripheral vascular bed (*Nutrition Reviews,* 1962). There are other molds which contaminate peanuts, cottonseed meal, yams and corn. They are generally termed aflatoxins (*Nutrition Reviews,* 1964).

Most of the fruits that we consume are relatively safe but we may mention some of the substances that interfere with nutrient utilization. The orange peel contains *citral,* which produces changes in eyes similar to those created by vitamin A deficiency. Based on certain studies it is assumed that citral is probably an antagonist of vitamin A. A person ingesting the peel, while eating oranges, may get sufficient quantities of citral as to create vitamin A deficiency. There are some other fruits, especially the wonderful juicy strawberries, which contain a toxic aromatic organic compound, *coumarin.* This compound interferes with the clotting of blood, which in case of an injury, may result in uncontrollable bleeding.

That one man's food may be poison for another is literally true of some groups of individuals who during the course of a treatment for depression or other conditions are on drugs which inhibit the activity of monoamine oxidase. Isoniazid is one such drug which is widely used. If these individuals eat cheddar cheese, they might be asking for real trouble in the form of hypertension, severe headaches, palpitation, etc. It appears that during the process of making cheddar cheese, the bacterial culture used to curdle the milk may contain a mixture of organisms which produce tyramine, which is a potent vasopressor substance. Under ordinary circumstances, a body would metabolize it through the action of monoamine oxidase, but among these individuals who are on drugs inhibiting the monoamine oxidase, a severe reaction will result with quite unpleasant consequences.

A number of animals also contain toxins produced as a result of their normal metabolic processes. These animals are not fit for human consumption and may be categorized as poisonous species. A large number of fishes have been reported to be poisonous. A number of poisoning cases as a result of eating fish have been reported from Japan, which produce neurologic symptoms for which there are no palliative measures. The puffer fish may be illustrated as an example of a poisonous species. The toxin is especially concentrated in the viscera and special skill is required to remove it before consuming the rest of the fish. Mickelsen and Yang described an episode recorded by Mosher *et al.,* that "four soldiers came upon a bonfire where native fishermen had roasted some of these fish. They had left the livers of the fish on shells. Despite the dire warnings of a native, the soldiers ate a little of the liver—some of them only chewing one bite without swallowing any. The first soldier who ate a little of the liver died in half an hour, the others at varying intervals during the next 24 hours."

It is believed that all over the world, the poisonous animals produce a greater degree of morbidity and mortality than do the poisonous plants. At least 500 species of marine animals are known to be poisonous to man. Among the common mammals, the dogs, seals, sea lions and polar bears are the ones who could be poisonous, especially if their livers and kidneys are eaten. This is probably due to a high concentration of vitamin A in their organs. It is apparent that extremely high levels of vitamin A could be very toxic and dangerous. One does not have to eat the livers of seals or polar bears, three fourths of a pound of which may contain as much as 7,500,000 I.U. of vitamin A. There are people who indiscriminately swallow lots of vitamin pills which may contain high levels of vitamin A. Infants younger than 6 months of age may develop symptoms of toxicity with doses of 18,000 to 60,000 I.U. of vitamin A per day. Vitamin D in larger quantities is no less toxic. The primary symptoms are anorexia, vomitting, constipation, failure to gain weight, fever, systolic murmurs, hypertension or even mental retardation in extreme cases (Stapleton *et al.*, 1957).

In order to protect ourselves from eating the toxic animals, it is essential that the meat processor as well as the public be educated in their identification and their use as food, especially in regard to the avoidance of certain organs and tissues. A food inspection service may also help eliminate dangerous products from the market (Genigeorgis and Reimann, 1973).

Food toxicity can also be indirectly picked up by humans. We use huge quantities of insecticides, fungicides, rodenticides and weed killers, which find their way into the tissues of animals, which serve the purpose of our food. We also give hormones and antibiotics and other growth promoting drugs to our livestock which are used as food. We release large quantities of industrial pollutants such as mercury and lead into the waters which are swallowed by the marine animals that land on our dining tables. A few years back, a great alarm was raised when it was found that samples of tuna fish, which are widely consumed, contained mercury levels much higher than those which could be considered completely safe. How the mercury got into the tuna is not quite clear, but it could have come from the industrial wastes dumped into the oceans in large quantities. The residues of DDT are easily traceable in our food crops and animal products. The food and drug laboratories bulletin (June, 1967, New York) stated that each individual in the United States consumes daily 0.08 to 0.12 mg of chlorinated organic pesticide.

By our thoughtlessly widespread use of DDT and other pest killing chemicals, we have created for ourselves a situation which is a potential health hazard for the human population. Sladden *et al.* woefully remarked that "there was no place on the globe so remote from civilization that the creatures living there could escape the tide of DDT and other insecticides which, like a cloud of radioactive dust, now travels through the atmosphere and in the waters of the oceans." Surely there must be some lesson that we must draw from this mode of dangerous living. "Knowledge can teach us to be prudent; but wisdom and experience teach us that in life, whether or not we accept the risk, we can never be absolutely safe. We can only learn, while living dangerously, to behave rationally with as full a knowledge of what we are doing as we can command" (Pyke, 1968).

FOODS AS RELATED TO EATING HABITS

Every nation or community has its own roots in its ancient culture which is responsible for the evolvement of certain food habits, which patronized one kind of food over another. It may be safely assumed that the food habits were formed as a result of local availability, climatic conditions, geographic location and social and political status along with a number of other factors, such as cultural patterns and religious influences. Instances are not rare where nutritious foods have been excluded from the diet in spite of their local availability and foods with inadequate or unsatisfactory nutrition value are elevated socially to the status of super foods. As food habits and food preferences were established, they were passed on to the subsequent generations. Mead rightly described the food habits as "the study of the ways in which individuals or groups of individuals, in response to social and cultural pressures, select, consume, and utilize portions of the available food supply" (Mead, 1945). The key word in the above description is the utilization of the *portion* of the available food supply. This type of food selection has been done by humans all over the world under the direct influence of their society, culture, religion and instincts. Humans differ greatly under the influence of these all-pervasive forces.

Food is not merely a source of satisfying hunger or even providing nourishment for the body. It is a means of discovering one's identity. It represents the individual's culture, religion, social security, prestige and arouses a variety of passions ranging from pleasure, confidence and even violent fanaticism. Foods prepared in a certain manner, dictated by cultural history of the region, have the properties of emotional satisfaction and give the individual a social and cultural dignity. All of us have a certain image of food to which we are linked culturally. The human is not a biochemical engine that will consume anything that will nurture the body in spite of the omnivorous physiology (Lovenberg *et al.*, 1968). Our choices of foods are expressions of ourselves as individuals and as members of a certain cultural group. For example, a man tends to get married to a girl who has a similar cultural background because it tends to preserve his food habits, and the marriage proves harmonious in a number of ways, particularly with respect to the meaning of a particular food and its method of consumption.

When we are concerned with the nutrition and quality of human diet, we are surprised as well as appalled at how some groups of humans adore and eat unsatisfactory foods to the exclusion of those easily available foods which would nourish their bodies better. Basically there are three kinds of diets (animal foods, vegetable foods and mixed foods). The animal sources of foods are habitually eaten by people like hunters and fishermen (Eskimo, Lapp, Samoyed, Fuegian) and pastoral nomads (Khirghiz, Masai, Somali). The plant sources of foods are eaten largely by those overpopulated areas of the globe where animal foods are scarcer (India, Pakistan, Bangla Desh, Burma, China, parts of Southeast Asia and Africa). Mixed diets are eaten by the comparatively well-off countries of Europe, North America, Australia, New Zealand and parts of Asia, South America and Africa (Cuthbertson, 1964).

In this brief discussion we are concerned not so much with the selection of food out of necessity, as determined by availability, but with the selection of certain kinds of foods to the exclusion of others. Numerous instances can be cited where young children suffer from deficiency diseases, not

because of the inadequate means, but because of the tradition-bound, rigidly enforced food habits which fail to support good growth and development during the periods of
their fastest growth. Some of the African tribes (e.g. Akiku-
yus among the Bantus and Kikuyu) live on cereals (maize,
millet, sweet potatoes, plantains) and do not use the game
fish, birds and eggs in spite of their availability. Goats are
used for the purpose of barter as a *currency* rather than a
source of milk or meat (Orr and Gilks, 1931). In Nyasaland,
children are not allowed to eat eggs for fear of bladder disease, and pregnant women are not given eggs for fear of
having bald-headed children. In Ethiopia, a pregnant woman
must not eat roasted meat because it is believed to cause
abortion (Todhunter, 1973).

Cereals are the super foods. Although in most places
in the world, cereals are encouraged and consumed in large
quantities because of the scarcity of animal sources of protein, the fact cannot be ignored that a great degree of unnecessary malnutrition could be avoided only by dispelling
some deep-rooted superstitions and old traditions based on
ignorance and unenlightened nutrition education. A well
known article of high quality food, i.e. milk, is liked in most
areas of the world, but in parts of Thailand it may be rejected
with revulsion as an animal mucous discharge. The Zulus do
not permit milk for the women because of their belief that
their reproductive system somehow hurts the milk-bearing
cattle. (For details the reader is referred to Manocha and Todhunter.) It would require a lot of space to catalogue the human cultural beliefs which prevent the utilization of available nutritious foods around them and compel them to
continue to eat the less nutritious cultural foods.

Hunger, in spite of being the most fundamental driving
force, has not at numerous occasions, prevented the non-utili-
zation of foods by man which are culturally disagreeable.
Think of the Chinese millionaire whose child is dying of beri
beri, or an Indian maharaja whose wife is wearing diamond
necklaces and is suffering from nutritional anemia or maras-

mus, or the rich members of the Masai tribe in Africa who own hundreds of cattle but whose children suffer from severe forms of malnutrition (Hutchinson, 1968). Collis and James rightly put it, "This is a curious reflection on *Homo sapiens*, who in losing the innocence of the animal world seems also to have lost the inherent instinct for correct food."

In the modern food situation, there are two other factors which need to be given some attention. On one side, there is an extra emphasis on animal sources of foods as is done in the technologically advanced countries of the west irrespective of their physiological needs. Not only are seven pounds of grain needed to convert into one pound of meat, but the intake of animal foods beyond a certain level is probably not necessary if the provision of a nutritious well-balanced diet for the promotion of maximum health is the aim. On the other side, there are areas of the world where vegetarianism to the complete exclusion of animal sources of food is practiced, sometimes to the great detriment of the health and welfare of its people, especially the children.

Vegetarianism as a way of religious life has been practiced for thousands of years, especially among some of the Hindu sects, Buddhists, Jains and Zoroastrians. During the recent years, some Catholic orders and Seventh Day Adventists have been practicing it in addition to small groups of individuals and communities all over the world. Most of these vegetarians will include in their diets the milk, in spite of its animal origin, but strongly resist the intake of animal flesh or even eggs. To some, fish is not a meat but to most vegetarians, it is. It is not the intention here to find faults with vegetarianism or excessive nonvegetarianism. The author's intention is only to point out that a variety of vegetables in combination, e.g. a combination of cereals, legumes or oilseeds, fruits, vegetables and nuts can provide all the essential nutrients necessary for good health as well as growth if supplemented with a source of vitamin B_{12}, which must be obtained from a synthetic or animal source (see section on processed foods). A mixed diet consisting of vegetarian sources as well as animal sources is probably the best combination there is to provide an adequately balanced diet.

However, in the present day world, a vast majority of those who are predominantly vegetarians are only cereal eaters, without adequate quantities of other sources of vegetable foods. They are too poor to afford other types of foods and fail to eat a variety essential for good nutrition, if one has to depend on vegetable sources. The richer nations, under the belief that the animal foods are the best foods, are on the other hand continuously increasing their intake of meat and poultry. This is also somewhat wrong from the physiological and practical point of view. Physiologically, people eating large quantities of meat and eggs do not need the high levels of saturated fats and cholesterols accompanying these foods, which manifest themselves in a variety of cardiovascular disorders. When looked at from a practical perspective, it involves the wastage of huge quantities of food grains in order to produce meat. This may be responsible for the apparent food shortages all over the world. It may not be nutritionally irresponsible to try to convince the heavy meat eaters that vegetable foods have their own merits and are not necessarily inferior (Parrett, 1969). At the same time, we must emphasize that animal foods are to some extent essential and desirable, whereas depending upon animal foods for most of the food requirements may not be so. It is quite possible to maintain good health and vigor on a vegetarian diet, but it is not always easy (unless highly educated) to secure the right combination of plant foods to meet the protein needs of desired quality (Todhunter, 1973). Emphasizing too much dependence on either is definitely food faddism. It might not be out of place to present briefly the case of vegetarian food faddists. For example, a physician, Dr. Parrett, believes that the meat diet adds to our body a tremendous amount of waste material which results in poorer health. "As a physician I observed the difference in testing the urine. With a patient on a meat diet I frequently found the total solids double those found in the urine of the patient not eating meat. The solids tend to make a person get tired when doing strenuous exercise. An athlete should increase his endurance by avoiding meat when competing on the field." According to Dr. Parrett, high protein, especially meat protein, adds to the load of kidney wastes, hastens the fatigue point and may well be expected to shorten life, inasmuch as a person dies when any one vital organ is worn out. "Meat is the greatest disease breeder that can be introduced into the human system." As a test for endurance, Dr. Parrett cited a number of athletic competitions in swimming, arm holding, running and other athletic activities. In a deep knee bend test, "the fifteen athletes from Yale dipped up and down from the squatting position more than a thousand times, but could not reach an average of eleven hundred. The rookie vegetarians averaged more than two thousand dips, which was twice as many as the athletes' manager. One man named Wagner made twenty-five hundred dips. He said he could do more but was willing to quit" (*Yale Medical Journal*, 1907).

Dr. Parrett strongly believes that a large number of unnecessary lives are lost to cardiovascular complications resulting from a heavy meat diet. He recommended that if the United States cuts down its high level of meat consumption, it will benefit the people not only in terms of improved health and performance, but it "would cut the sickness rate so substantially that our present doctors and hospital beds might easily meet our needs. The only ones who might suffer would be the morticians, but no one would mind if they had a little more time for vacations."

SOCIO-ECONOMIC AND MARKETING PROBLEMS IN POPULARIZING NEW FOODS

The technologically processed new foods have been formulated, keeping in mind their nutritive value and the role they could play in eliminating the qualitative deficiencies that are obvious in the diets of millions of people all over the world. The family of foods that has received the most attention as fortifiers of cereals are the oilseeds; in a 1971 survey, for instance, 93 percent of the new foods reviewed used an oilseed as a protein base. The oilseeds rightly deserve this honor. They are low in cost, high in nutritive value and are abundantly produced with a lot of potential for improvement. Approximately 110 million tons are harvested annually, mostly in those countries where protein shortage is acute. In 1970, the oilseed production contained about 5 million tons of proteins, which is enough to meet several times over the total protein requirements of the world (Berg, 1973).

At present, most of the oilseeds are used only to extract oil and no significant effort is made to get oil using those modern techniques by which the residue may be fit for human consumption. It is a relatively expensive process over the crude methods used at present, in which case the residue is fit only as animal feed or fertilizer. Ironically, in the protein deficient countries the residue after oil extraction poses a problem of disposal. The residue contains as much as 50 percent protein and can be refined and used as a protein ingredient for human grade foods. Berg explained that this product is extremely attractive economically. "The price of the typical oilseed is 7 cents a pound, of the residue cake 4 cents. From this an oilseed flour can be produced for 12 cents a pound; by comparison, nonfat dry milk costs at least twice as much and other forms of animal protein upward of eight times as much (Berg, 1973).

On paper this is the most ideal situation and given the capital investment to produce on a mass scale these new food products, one could be very optimistic that the nutrition problems of our ever-growing human populations can be satisfactorily solved. In practice this may not be true. First of all, we humans eat food not merely to satisfy our hunger, but our appetite too. Food is a means of satisfying not only our physiological needs, but certain social, psychological and emotional needs as well.

> Food has a profound psychological role to play in society. It is one of the very first means by which we demonstrate our mood and in-

dividuality; thus a baby demands food and then perhaps rejects it; it comes to assert its personality by demanding particular foods and rejecting others. In the same way food asserts itself as an integral part of our culture and many social events in our lives take place around the meal table. More than this, every aspect of our lives is related to it and the intricate network surrounding food is as great whether we live in a sophisticated western society or in a slowly developing poor community (McKenzie, 1969).

We must appreciate that humans don't ingest nutrients, they eat meals which are pleasant looking, palatable and satisfying. Our familiar or traditional foods may be deficient in protein but most of us may not accept eating along with our food as an additive, purified protein which is odorless, tasteless and without any apparent attraction. New foods interfere with our established eating habits. In Germany in 1774, during a grain shortage, people refused to eat potatoes until Frederick the Great ate the potatoes himself in public (Stare and Trulson, 1966). One must not be unwilling to appreciate the nature and extent of social and psychological attributes to food and their impact on the behavior of ordinary individuals (McKenzie, 1969). A United Nations report in 1968 adequately describes the conditions of the success of these new foods.

> The greatest obstacle to the commercial use of new protein foods is not so much in their production in a safe, nutritious palatable and sufficiently inexpensive form, but the requirements for effective marketing and promotion. Excellent products have remained laboratory curiosities because they were not presented to the public in a culturally acceptable manner or were not properly distributed in association with a well-designed educational and promotional campaign.

It has been observed that in the developing countries, school children, even if hungry, refuse to eat nutritionally good foods because of unpopularity or food habits (Ballarin, 1963). All too often the new products have been unpalatable and were formulated based on nutrition and not on their appeal and attractiveness, which often is a major factor in determining the choice of food. It is essential, therefore, that socio-economic and marketing problems likely to be encountered in the process of popularizing new food products be given the same attention, planning or even the investment that are required to overcome the production problems such as suitability of a certain food for human consumption, its nutritive value, local availability of raw material for its production and the capital investment to put the project on its feet.

The key words to the social acceptability of a new food product are education and minimum interference with the established social order. It is only by an all-embracing educational program that one can teach the ignorant masses the nature, source and value of biologically high-quality protein so that they will actively seek, demand and consume the protein-rich foods. School curricula should include a formal education program in nutrition. During this instruction, a firm idea should be developed as to which of all the common foods familiar to the children are the body building foods (rich in protein), energy giving foods (rich in carbohydrates and fats) and protective foods (rich in vitamins and minerals), and that it is essential to eat daily some food of each category in order to insure proper body growth and development.

It may also be important to point out the importance of quality of proteins in terms of their utilization by the body and why the essential amino acids have to be provided in balanced proportions in the foods. This will help to emphasize the importance of technologically processed new foods, which aim to provide all the nutrients in a balanced proportion. In the developing countries, this instruction should also include the methods of nutritionally balancing their traditional diets such as appropriate intake of cereals and legumes and the use of new diets to supplement the traditional ones. Audio-visual aids can also be used to develop a better appreciation of the problems of good nutrition. Studies have shown that children do influence the thinking of their parents and a student could become a nutrition teacher at home. In addition, the education programs must be directed to the adult population as well. This is another form of advertising. It requires a lot of persuasion, canvassing, and coaxing in order to convince people of the desirability of eating the nutritious foods which have been manufactured with the sole purpose of improving the health and welfare of the community. The mass media can play a very important role in this respect. Television is a very effective medium in imparting education by giving visual displays and demonstrations. Unfortunately, this medium has not been widely used where it is needed the most. Efforts should be made to make use of this effective medium of instruction.

However, it must be emphasized that no amount of educational persuasion is going to cut much ice if the marketing and promotion of new food products involves a drastic change in the established eating patterns. The new food products should be designed to supplement existing nutritional intakes, and must never try to replace them. It takes a lot of hard work to get people to change their purchasing and feeding habits. The new food products must fit in as closely as possible with established social customs as well as eating habits (Galliver, 1969). Galliver suggested that for food products to become successful, as a diet or a supplementary food among the masses, a manufacturer should

(1) develop products which are acceptable to the local population and which will fit into their existing or already changing eating habits; (2) ensure raw materials supply; (3) establish sound production methods and quality control; (4) establish a sensible price structure which results in a selling price which the consumer can afford and which offers a fair profit to the producer; and (5) bring the virtues of the product to the attention of the consumer, i.e. promote and advertise.

It is now well recognized that the complementary talents of food technologists, nutritionists and an imaginative food industry are needed to solve the world food problem. In addition, public agencies can help popularize the supplementary foods through an effectively applied nutrition program. Allan emphasized that, in spite of the deeply ingrained food habits in cultures and in families, the new wonder foods must be promoted, after the fashion of commercial products. They must be related to the preferences of taste and preparation of the peoples who need them. They should be made as far as possible from materials locally available and be inexpensive. Their use should be accompanied by programmes of education in nutrition and by national policies integrating nutritional goals with over-all planning embracing many sectors. Greater awareness of the scope and debilitating effects of malnutrition is needed, in both developed and developing lands, in order to generate the necessary support at all levels to meet this world crisis.

It is important, however, to add a word of caution. In our enthusiasm to remove undernutrition and malnutrition or a genuine concern for the unfortunate undernourished masses, we tend to appeal and promote the sales of high protein foods to the members of the low socio-economic groups. This kind of appeal has failed in the past to enthuse the people who need it the most. Here we make a fundamental miscalculation about the image of food. The social prestige carried by a particular food is extremely important for its acceptance. There are numerous examples where the image of a certain food decided its acceptance or rejection. In Britain, a nourishing soup was not accepted until its color was changed from white to brown (Burgess and Dean, 1962).

Nuts may be rich in protein, but if their social image is low they will not be accepted. A new food product, rich in nutrients, may be produced by a subsidy from the government in order to keep its price low, so that people of the lower socio-economic groups may buy it, but it may not be sold because of its poor social image and the belief that this food is meant for the poor people. The same food, if it is accepted by the well-off classes, will be taken by the poorer classes as well. It is unfortunately true that most often the nutritional value is not the major factor determining the individual choices of food. One must understand why some foods of low nutritive value (e.g. soft drinks, white highly milled wheat flour, polished rice, etc.) become popular among the poor classes; it is because they are consumed by the well-off classes. It is precisely due to an unimaginative promotion campaign directed to the poorer classes that some of the wonderful new foods have failed to make a desirable impact on the health and well-being of the undernourished masses. The multipurpose foods in India, Incaparina in South America, Pronutro in South Africa have not proven successes in spite of the blessings and resources of the national governments to their promotion campaigns. In South Africa, the manufacturers of Pronutro directed the product particularly toward the African market, and after satisfactory early selling, sales later declined because the African population believed that a product sold only to them must be inferior to products which were intended for the white population also. It may be very important to give the new food products the image of a valuable food for all the socio-economic classes. If only we succeed half as much as successful commercial operations do, one could be quite optimistic that we are making some satisfactory attempts to solve the world food problem.

This is not to say that we should give up. There are numerous examples which give us an insight into how to promote the new products for large scale use. Pronutro is relatively more successful after the product campaign was revised and directed to the white as well as the African populations. Vitasoy (soy milk) has become commercially quite successful and its promotion directed toward all socio-economic groups. Its packaging is simple, inexpensive, attractive and is distributed through established retail outlets and not through special agencies.

McKenzie outlined the key areas which must be investigated before initiating the sale of a new product:

Area	Type of Information Required
1. Product usage	When is the product likely to be used, and with what foods will it be combined? Will it blend well with these foods?
2. Product competitiveness	With what other foods will the product effectively be competing? Can it successfully demonstrate some acceptable superiority? If the product is a supplement to be added to existing foods during preparation, then can

	methods of justifying this addition be substantiated?[1]
3. Impact on food habits	Does its acceptance require any major or minor modification in eating habits? If so, can these changes in consumer behaviour be successfully achieved?
4. Equipment required	Is any new equipment or cooking procedure necessary? If so, can the housewife be easily persuaded to make this change?
5. Storage	Does the product require any different type of storage arrangements? If so, will these special facilities be available and acceptable?
6. Advertising copy	How can advertising copy be designed to indicate effectively the fulfillment of a need, overcome competitive products, and justify changes in behavior?[2]
7. Name	What from the consumer's viewpoint would be a suitable name for the product?
8. Packaging	What sort of packaging would be most acceptable to the consumer?

[1] The superiority or justification will not be in health or nutritional terms but in terms of appeal based on taste, better fulfillment of psychological needs, etc.

[2] This will imply general knowledge of the consumers' motivations.

The unconventional foods are a great challenge to the food industry, as well as the advertising and communication media. The new foods have to compete with the well established food habits and must be pleasing to the palate, cheaper, and aesthetically more appealing than the already accepted foods. The author has no doubt that the food and advertising industries will rise to the occasion in promoting their acceptance. Regardless of their intrinsic merits, most of the new foods are not likely to be accepted as they are developed or produced. Their production needs, not only a margin of economic profitability, but also a buffer time in which they may be slowly pushed into the market. The pessimism about the prospects of changing the food habits is unwarranted. There is ample evidence that with skill and patience, the acceptance for a new food can be won. It may take weeks, months or maybe a year to do so. Pirie warned that introducing a new food before completing elaborate cooking experiments is to invite its failure. The other way to ensure its failure is by introducing new foods to criminals, orphans or other unfortunates (Pirie, 1968).

There is every reason to believe that as our campaign of persuasion goes on, there will be voluntary changes in food habits for the better. Under certain changed circumstances, individuals or communities change their patterns of food habits and adopt the new foods almost spontaneously. In the beginning stages, the new foods should be encouraged only as small amounts of supplements to the established traditional diets without interfering with the eating patterns. Objections to certain foods may be especially strong regarding foods prepared from materials not considered so far as edible (proteins from microorganisms, protein concentrates from vegetables and fish, unconventional sea foods, etc.). However, much as the people may grumble in the initial stages about using them even as supplements, the steadfast marketing campaign for their promotion will ultimately have a salutary effect and the acceptance of the new foods will be most likely won.

REFERENCES

Allan, D. A.: *UNICEF News*, March, 1972.

Altman, P. L., and Dittmer, D. S. (Eds.) : *Metabolism*. Federation of American Societies for Exptl. Biology, 1968.

Ballarin, O.: *Effects of Processed Foods on the Consumer in Developing Countries*. Presented to World Food Congress, Washington, D.C., June 8, 1963.

Ballester, D., Barja, I., Yanez, E., and Donoso, G.: *Br J Nutr, 22:* 255, 1968.

Bamford, F.: *Poisons, Their Isolation and Identification*. Philadelphia, Blackstan, 1961.

Bender, A. E.: *Food Tech, 1:* 261, 1966.

———, *R Soc Health, 5:* 221, 1969.

Berg, A.: *Population Bulletin, 29:* 1, 1973.

Bhagavan, R. K., Doraiswami, J. R., Subramanian, N., *et al: Am J Clin Nutr, 11:* 127, 1962.

Bigwood, E. J.: *World Health*, April, 1969.

Black, J. N.: *Ann App Biol, 67:* 272, 1971.

Bogorov, V., and Stepanov, V.: *World Health*, April, 1969.

Brown, L. R.: *Population Bulletin, 29:* 2, 1973.

Burger, I. H. and Walters, C. L.: *Proc Nutr Soc, 32:* 1, 1973.

Burgess, A., and Dean, R. F. A.: *Malnutrition and Food Habits.* London, Travistock, 1962.

Calvin, M. E., Knepper, R., and Robertson, W. O.: *N Eng J Med, 270:* 625, 1964.

Carpenter, K. J., and March, B. E.: *Br J Nutr, 15:* 403, 1961.

Center for Disease Control. *Annual Summary on Food Borne Disease Outbreaks,* Atlanta, Georgia, 1970.

Chandrasekhara, M. R., Indira, K., Prasanna, H. A., Ramanathan, G., Jagannath, K. S., Leela, N., Srinivasan, K. S., Vaidehi, M., and Murthy, I. A. S.: *Nutr Rep Int, 6:* 239, 1972.

Chichester, C. O.: In Rechcigl, M. (Ed.) : *World Rev Nutr Dietet,* 1973, vol. 16.

Cloud, W.: *The Sciences, 13:* 8; 6, 1973.

Collis, W. R. P., and Janes, M.: In Scrimshaw, N. S., and Gordon, J. E. (Eds.) : *Malnutrition, Learning and Behavior.* Cambridge, MIT Press, 1968.

Critchfield, R.: *It is a Revolution All Right.* New York, Alicia Patterson Fund, 1971.

Cuthbertson, D. P.: In Beaton, H. H., and McHenry, E. W. (Eds.) : *Nutrition,* New York, Acad Pr, 1964, Vol. 2.

Darby, W. J.: *Nutr Rev, 30:* 27, 1972.

Davidson, S., Passmore, R., and Brock, J. F.: *Human Nutrition and Dietetics.* Baltimore, Williams and Wilkins, 1972.

Dean, R. F. A.: *Sp Rep Series #279.* London, Medical Res Council, 1953.

Doraiswamy, T. R., Singh, N., and Daniel, V. A.: *Br J Nutr, 23,* 1969.

Dovring, F.: *Scientific American, 230:* 2, 1974.

Dreyer, J. J.: *S Afr Med J, 71:* 1304, 1968.

Editorial: *S Afr Med J, 23:* 377, 1968.

Ehrlich, P. R., and Ehrlich, A. H.: *Population, Resources, Environment.* San Francisco, Freeman, 1970.

FAO/WHO Expert Committee on Nutrition: *WHO Tech Rep Ser #97,* Geneva, 1955.

FAO/WHO Expert Committee on Food Additives, 1956.

Filer, H.: *Commodity Year Book.* Commodity Res Bur, Inc, New York, 1972.

Finberg, L., Kiley, J., and Luttrell, C. N.: *JAMA, 184:* 187, 1963.

Food and Agriculture Organization. *The State of Food and Agriculture,* Rome, 1967.

Franke, R. V.: *Natural History,* January, 1974.

Galliver, G. D.: *Proc Nutr Soc, 28:* 97, 1969.

Genigeorgis, C. A., and Reimann, H.: In Rechcigl, M. (Ed.) : *World Rev Nutr Dietet,* 1973, vol. 16.

Gordon, J. E., and Scrimshaw, N. S.: In Bourne, G. H. (Ed.) : *World Rev Nutr Dietet,* 1972, vol. 15.

Gray, W. D.: In Gould, R. F. (Ed.) : *World Protein Resources*. Washington, Am Chem Soc, 1966.

Harris, R. S., and Loesecke, H. Van (Eds.) : *Nutritional Evaluation of Food Processing*. Chichester, Wiley, 1960.

Hein, R. E., and Hutchings, I. J.: *Proc Symp Vitamins and Minerals in Processed Foods*. AMA, Chicago, 1971.

Heller, B. S., Chutkow, M. R., Lushbough, C. H., Siedler, A. J., and Schweigert, B. S.: *J Nutr, 73:* 113, 1961.

Henshall, J. D.: *Proc Nutr Soc, 32:* 17, 1973.

Hollingsworth, D. F., and Martin, P. E.: In Bourne, G. H. (Ed.) : *World Rev Nutr Dietet*, 1972, vol. *15*.

Howe, E. E., Guilfellan, E. W., and Milner, M.: *Am J Clin Nutr, 16:* 321, 1965.

Hutchinson, J.: In McCance, R. A., and Widdowson, E. M. (Eds.) : *Calorie Deficiencies and Protein Deficiencies*. Boston, Little, 1968.

Hutchinson, J. B., Moran, T., and Pace, J.: *Br J Nutr, 13:* 151, 1959.

Jansen, G. R.: *Nutr Rep Int, 7:* 555, 1973.

Jelliffe, D. B.: *Infant Nutrition in the Subtropics and Tropics*. Geneva, WHO, 1968.

Joseph, K., Rao, N., Swaminathan, M., Indiverma, K., and Subramanyan, U.: *Ann Biochem Exp Med, 20:* 243, 1960.

Josephson, D. V.: In Gould, R. F. (Ed.) : *World Protein Resources*. Washington, Am Chem Soc, 1966.

Kuher, M. J.: *Res Commun Chem Pathol Pharmacol, 2:* 95, 1971.

Kwok, R.: *N Engl J Med, 278:* 796, 1968.

Lal, S. B.: *Indian J Med Res, 40:* 471, 1952.

Leela, R., Daniel, V. A., and Rao, S.: *J Nutr Dietet, 2:* 78, 1965.

Liener, I. E.: In Gould, R. F. (Ed.) : *World Protein Resources*. Washington, Am Chem Soc, 1966.

Liener, I. E., and Pallansek, M. J.: *J Biol Chem, 197:* 29, 1952.

Lovern, J. A.: In Gould, R. F. (Ed.) : *World Protein Resources*. Washington, Am Chem Soc, 1966.

Lovern, J. A.: *Proc Nutr Soc, 28:* 17, 1969.

Lovenberg, M. E., Todhunter, E. N., Wilson, E. D., Feeney, N. C., and Savage, J. R.: *Food and Man*. New York, Wiley, 1968.

Manocha, S. L.: *Malnutrition and Retarded Human Development*. Springfield, Thomas, 1972.

Matoth, Y., Elian, E., and Gruenberg, E.: *Am J Clin Nutr, 24:* 226, 1968.

Mayer, J.: *Science, 176:* 237, 1972.

McKenzie, J. C.: *Proc Nutr Soc, 28:* 103, 1969.

Mead, M.: Committee on Food Habits. *Nat Res Council Bull #111,* Washington, 1945.

Meadows, D. H., Meadows, D. L., Randers, J., and Behrens, W. W.: *The Limits to Growth*. New York, Universe Books, 1972.

Mertz, E. T.: *Fed Proc, 25:* 1662, 1966.

Mickelsen, O.: In *Present Knowledge of Nutrition.* New York, Nutrition Foundation, 1967.

Mickelsen, O., and Yang, M. G.: In Wohl, M. G., and Goodhart, R. S. (Eds.): *Modern Nutrition in Health and Disease.* Philadelphia, Lea and Febiger, 1968.

Milner, M.: In Gould, R. F. (Ed.): *World Protein Resources.* Washington, Am Chem Soc, 1966.

Mosher, H. S., Fuhrman, F. A., Buckwald, H. D., and Fischer, H. G.: *Science, 144:* 1100, 1964.

Mustakas, G. C., Albercht, W. J., McGhee, J. E., Black, L. T., Bookwalter, G. N., and Griffin, E. L.: *J Am Oil Chem Soc, 46:* 623, 1967.

Narayana Rao, M. N., and Swaminathan, M.: In Bourne, G. H. (Ed.): *World Rev Nutr Dietet,* 1969, vol. 11.

Narayanaswamy, D., Daniel, V. A., Kurien, S., Swaminathan, M., and Parpia, H. A. B.: *Nutr Rep Int, 7:* 111, 1973.

Nelson, O. E.: *Fed Proc, 25:* 1676, 1966.

Newberne, P. M., Glaser, O., and Friedman, N.: *Nutr Rep Int, 7:* 181, 1973.

Nordfelt, S., Gellerstadt, N., and Falkner, S.: *Acta Pathol Microbiol Scand, 35:* 217, 1954.

Nutrition Reviews, 20: 237, 1962.

Nutrition Reviews, 21: 195, 1963.

Nutrition Reviews, 22: 62, 1964.

Nutrition Reviews, 23: 346, 1965.

Nutrition Reviews, 25: 231, 1967.

Nutrition Reviews, 28: 124, 1970.

Oliviera, J. E. D., and De Souza, N.: *N Arch Latin Am de Nutr, 17:* 197, 1967.

Orr, J. B., and Gilks, J. L.: *Med Res Council Spec Report Ser 155,* 1931.

Paarlberg, D.: In *Food, Nutrition and Health World Rev Nutr Dietet, 16,* 1973.

Parpia, H. A. B.: *Sci J, 4:* 66, 1968.

Parpia, H. A. B., Narayana Rao, M., Rajagopalan, R., and Swaminathan, M.: *J Nutr Dietet, 1:* 114, 1964.

Parpia, H. A. B., and Subramanian, N.: In Gould, R. F. (Ed.): *World Protein Resources.* Washington, Am Chem Soc, 1966.

Parrett, O. S.: *Life and Health,* September, 1969.

Pimentral, D., Hurd, L. E., Bellotti, A. C., Forster, M. J., Oka, I. N., Sholes, O. D., and Whitman, R. J.: *Science, 182:* 443, 1973.

Pirie, N. W.: In *International Symposium on Protein Foods and Concentrates.* Mysore, India, 1968.

Pirie, N. W.: *Proc Nutr Soc, 28:* 17, 1969.

Prasana, H. A., Amla, I., Indira, K., and Narayana Rao, M.: *Am J Clin Nutr, 21:* 1355, 1968.

Pretorius, P. J.: *S Afr Med J, 39:* 495, 1965.

Pyke, M.: *Food and Society.* London, Murray, 1968.

Ramakrishna Rao, M. V.: In *Progress in Meeting Protein Needs of Infants and Preschool Children.* Nat Acad Sci, Publ #843, Washington, D.C., 1961.

Rolls, B. A., and Porter, J. W. G.: *Proc Nutr Soc, 32:* 9, 1973.

Rusoff, L. L.: *J Dairy Sci, 53:* 1296, 1971.

Ryther, J. H.: *Science, 166:* 72, 1969.

Sabry, Z. I.: *Can J Public Health, 59:* 471, 1969.

Sakurai, Y., and Nakano, M.: In *Progress in Meeting Protein Needs of Infants and Preschool Children.* Nat Acad Sci Publ #843, Washington, D.C., 1961.

Sapeika, N.: In *World Rev Nutr Diet,* vol. *16,* 1973.

Sauberlich, H. E., Chang, R. Y., and Salmar, W.: *J Nutr, 51:* 623, 1953.

Scrimshaw, N. S.: *UNICEF News,* March, 1972.

Scrimshaw, N. S., Taylor, C. E., and Gordon, G. E.: *WHO Monograph Ser. #57,* 1968.

Sebrell, W. H.: *U. S. Public Health Rep, 24:* 1175, 1930.

Seu, S. R.: *Modernizing Indian Agriculture,* New Delhi Ministry of Food and Agriculture, 1969, vol. 1.

Shacklady, C. A.: *Proc Nutr Soc, 28:* 17, 1969.

Slade, R. E., Bramscombe, D. J., and McGowen, J. C.: *Chemistry and Industry, 194,* 1945.

Sladden, W. J. Z., Menzie, C. N., and Reishel, W. L.: *Nature, 210:* 670, 1966.

Srinivas, H., Tasker, P. K., Narayana Rao, M., Rajalakshmi, D., Rajagopalan, R., and Swaminathan, M.: *J Nutr Diet, 3:* 126, 1966.

Stapleton, MacDonald, and Lightwood: *Am J Clin Nutr, 5:* 533, 1957.

Stare, F. J., and Trulson, M. F.: *Food and Civilization.* Springfield, Thomas, 1966.

Steinhart, J. S. and Steinhart, C. E.: *Science, 184:* 307, 1974.

Steinkraus, K. H., Van Buren, J. P., and Hand, D. B.: In *Progress in Meeting Protein Needs of Infants and Preschool Children.* Natl Acad Sci Publ #843, Washington, 1961.

Steyn, D. G.: *Pretoria University Publ. #11,* 1960.

Streeter, C. P.: In *India—A Report from the Rockefeller Foundation,* 1969.

Subrahmanyan, V., Sreenivasan, A., Bhatia, D. S., Swaminathan, M., Bairs, G. S., Subramanian, N., Narayana Rao, M., Bhagwan, R. K., and Doraiswamy, T. R.: In *Meeting Protein Needs of Infants and Preschool Children.* Natl Acad Sci Publ #843, Washington, 1961.

Sundaravalli, O. E., and Narayana Rao, M.: *Nutr Diet, 11:* 101, 1969.

Swaminathan, M., Daniel, V. A., and Parpia, H. A. B.: *Ind J Nutr Diet, 9:* 22, 1972.

Symposium on Soybeans: *J Am Oil Chem Society, 51:* pages 1A to 199A, 1974.

Tape, N. W.: Canad Food Industry, 40: 36, 1969.

Tasker, P. K., Joseph, A. A., and Ananthswami, H. N.: Food Science, 2: 173, 1962.

Tasker, P. K., Ananthachar, T. K., Kurup, K. R., Srinivas, H., Narayana Rao, M. Rajagopalan, R., and Swaminathan, N.: J Nutr Diet, 3: 38, 1966.

Tasker, P. K., Srinivas, H., Jay Raj, A. P., Narayana Rao, M., Rajalakshmi, D., Rajagopalan, R., and Swaminathan, M.: J Nutr Diet, 4: 65, 1967.

Todhunter, E. N.: In World Rev Nutr Diet, vol. 16, 1973.

Trustwell, A. S., and Brock, J. F.: S Afr Med J, 33: 98, 1959.

Tudge, C.: New Scientist, March 22, 1973.

UNICEF News, March, 1972.

United Nations: International Action to Avert the Impending Protein Crisis. U.N. Publ. #E68 XIII, 1968a.

United Nations: Report of the Economic and Social Council of the Advisory Committee on the Application of Science and Technology to Development. U.N. Publ. #E68 XIII, 1968b.

Vernon, E.: Bull Min Hlth Lab Serv, 26: 235, 1967.

Wade, N.: Science, 181: 634, 1973.

Waterlow, J. C.: Br J Nutr, 16: 531, 1962.

Wharton, C. L.: Foreign Affairs, 47: 464, 1969.

White, H. S.: Arch Environ Health, 20: 84, 1970.

Wilcke, H. L.: In Gould, R. F. (Ed.): World Protein Resources. Washington, Am Chem Soc, 1966.

Willcox, O. W.: J Agric Food Chem, 7: 813, 1959.

Woodham, A. A.: Proc Nutr Soc, 24: 24, 1965.

Woodham, A. A.: Proc Nutr Soc, 28: 76, 1969a.

Woodham, A. A.: In Bourne, G. H. (Ed.): World Rev Nutr Diet, vol. 10: 44, 1969.

Woodham, A. A.: In Bourne, G. H. (Ed.): World Rev Nutr Diet, vol. 13, 1971.

Woodham, A. A.: Proc Nutr Soc, 32: 23, 1973.

World Health, April, 1969.

Wurster, C. F.: Science, 158: 1474, 1968.

Yale Medical Journal, 13: 205, 1907.

Yudkin, J., and Watson, R. H. J.: Br Med J, ii, 110: 1969.

Zenkevitch, L.: In World Health, p. 31, April, 1969.

Zohary, D., and Hopf, M.: Science, 182: 8887, 1973.

CHAPTER III

FEEDING INFANTS AND

PRESCHOOL CHILDREN

INFANTS—THE NUTRITIONALLY VULNERABLE GROUP

Present Status of Infant Nutrition

THE PRODUCTION OF BABIES and food is very much lopsided on this planet. Whereas the developing countries of the Far East have a population share of 52.9 percent, producing probably two thirds of all the babies born per year, this area produces only 27.8 percent of the total food supplies of the world. This is in sharp contrast to the 28.2 percent population of Europe and North America, which produces 56 percent of the total food supply (FAO, 1963). The birth rates in the developing countries of the Far East are much higher than the developed countries of the West. The possibility of reversing this unpleasant imbalance between population and food supplies is not very promising, at least in the near future.

A vast majority of infants and preschool children in the poor countries of the world is not able to satisfy the requirements for growth and development because of huge populations, unsatisfactory and inadequate food production, and a high incidence of ignorance about nutritional needs and infections of all sorts (Swaminathan, 1968). The per capita income is woefully low, especially among the lower socioeconomic groups, who incidentally, have the largest number of children. Economically, they are so poor that a worker's entire day's wages may not be enough to buy a quart of milk. Socially, they are steeped in ignorance and superstitions and fail to give to their children the locally available protein-rich foods (e.g. legumes) in the belief that it is hard for the infants to digest them. There is a whole constellation of factors that prevents these groups of people from coming out of their hopeless situation. Bennett and Stanfield very aptly explained the whole situation. According to them, the dietary inadequacies among children may be due to:

> small land plot in relation to family food demand, poor occupational status, isolated or neglected adults or children, widows or immigrants, lack of education, poor participation in health education and children's clinics, large family size and poor spacing, bottle feeding syndrome with dilution of milk, poor knowledge of food value and child requirements, poor parental capacity, inadequate frequency of meals, etc., or recurrent infections. The latter are reflected in an unhealthy natural environment, unclean water supply, swamps, etc., traditional attitudes and methods of disposal of excrement, traditional ideas about communicative disease, poverty, immigrants, poor use of health services and immunization, lack of education, etc.

From the above account, a typical pattern of infant nutrition in the economically depressed classes (which comprise about 80 percent of the population) of the developing countries may be summarized as follows: the neonates are born with a low birth weight obviously due to the poor health of the mother, with no improvement in her diet during pregnancy. These infants grow fairly satisfactorily for a period of about six months or less, as long as the mother is able to produce sufficient quantities of milk, after which time their growth pattern deteriorates. In the subsequent period, the quantity of breast milk becomes inadequate and the child is weaned to starchy gruels with no supplements of vitamins or minerals. Lack of adequate nutrition makes these children easy prey to numerous infections, with the result that most of these children are not able to realize their maximum growth potential.

Overcrowding conditions in the developing countries make it difficult to maintain adequate sanitary facilities, and as more individuals live in a small-sized room, the standards of personal hygiene go down and increase the stresses of family life. Such a lack of sanitation encourages the spread of common vectors of disease such as mosquitoes, lice, mites, flies, etc. The children raised in these conditions often become the victims of intestinal and other infections, as well as nutritional deficiencies. DeSilva described that the children of the underprivileged classes in the underdeveloped countries often have potbellies, believed to be due to the preponderance of starches and the low fat content of their diet, resulting in excessive fermentation. Most of the children in these depressed classes are sick. The irony of the situation lies in the fact that neither the children nor their parents realize that they are sick, because they do not know what it is to be well. It is believed that 70 percent of the preschool children in the developing countries of Asia, Africa and Latin America suffer from varying degrees of malnutrition (Manocha, 1972). The dietary deficiencies accompanied by environmental deprivation play a very important role in the development of personality and outlook on life. It is believed that the experiences of the early years lay the foundation for the bodily as well as mental health of the child in his adult life.

The standards of nutrition of the infants and preschool children in the technologically-developed countries are much superior to those of the developing countries described above. There is a well-established industry that produces nutritionally well-balanced baby foods and products for the preschool child. However, in certain sections of these societies, children do not get the nutrition desirable from dietary, biochemical and clinical criteria, in spite of the affluence. The main reasons for these deficiencies are the ignorance of the parents, misuse of the food budget for soft drinks and other beverages, and lack of appreciation of the needs for growth of the children. In numerous instances, physicians and other professional people fail to correct the attitudes of the parents concerned. In those countries where low-cost medical and public health facilities have been extended, especially to the low income groups, the nutritional quality of the children is adequate. For example, a nutritional survey of 1,401 children in socio-economically different strata of Swedish society revealed that fat provided 40 to 42 percent of the calories, protein provided another 13 to 14 percent of the calories, and the remaining were provided by carbohydrates. Boys consumed more food than girls in the same age group, and the energy requirements of rural children were higher compared to urban children (Samuelson, 1971).

Mother's Welfare as Related to Infant Nutrition

One of the main reasons for a very low rate of infant mortality in the technologically developed countries is the standard of infant care. Not only is prenatal care emphasized, but the medical profession carefully prepares the pregnant woman for the responsibilities of infant nutrition after the baby is born. The mother is familiarized with the fundamental principles of nutrition and the common ailments of childhood. There are very few children who do not get the periodic attention of a trained pediatrician. These measures assure the survival of the infant during the initial years of his childhood. Unfortunately, the standards of infant care in the Eastern countries are less than desirable. Most mothers are illiterate and uneducated, and fail to benefit from printed letters in books or magazines. Most of the conceptions are accidental, and prenatal care is of a rudimentary nature. Although the situation has improved to some extent during the last decade, most deliveries take place in homes whose standards of sanitation are terrible. The delivery is assisted by a midwife who, in most cases, is an illiterate, tradition-ridden, superstitious and unclean woman who does not exercise even such principles of cleanliness as washing the hands with soap (Chandrasekhra, 1972).

No wonder the rate of infant mortality in these poor countries is quite high. In a number of cases, the mother, because of her general debility, is unable to survive the trauma of labor and childbirth, leaving the infant in a more vulnerable state for survival because the chances of such an orphaned infant to get sustenance in the absence of mother's breasts is quite remote. Foster motherhood, even when it exists in the family home, can seldom take the place of the *natural* mother, with all her care, attention and instinctive affection. Neonatal deaths in most cases are due to prematurity, congenital debility or congenital malformations as a result of severe and chronic malnutrition of the mother. An infant born to a mother whose diet is extremely poor, and who has no nutritional reserves of her own because of repeated pregnancies and prolonged periods of lactation, has very little chances of survival. Such an infant, who is physiologically in a very poor state, becomes an easy prey to chance accidents or common infections such as measles, whooping cough, diarrhea, bronchitis, pneumonia, influenza, diphtheria, scarlet fever, or gastric, intestinal and respiratory disorders. (The reader is referred to a recent treatise on the subject by Chandrasekhra.) In the technologically advanced countries, the newborns do not go through these traumatic conditions. The nutrition level of a girl is quite adequate so that, during her period of gestation, even if she continues on her regular diet without supplementing it to take care of the extra needs, she would have enough nutritional reserves of her own to bring forth a healthy baby. The obstetrical care is, in general, satisfactory and the child is immunized against most of the infectious diseases during the first year.

High infant death rates in the developing countries lead to a psychology of producing a large number of children to assure some survivors. But higher birth rates also directly lead to higher death rates in the societies where the nutrition level of the mothers and infants is poor. Multiple pregnancies gradually lead to a deterioration of the nutritional state of the mother, especially when she is lactating for most of the period during the two consecutive pregnancies. The latter arrivals (4th or 5th child) have, therefore, much less chances of survival as compared to the earlier ones (1st, 2nd or 3rd child). A statistical survey in the United States between January 1 to March 31, 1950, showed that for a 20 to 24 year old mother, the neonatal mortality rates per thousand are "16.6 for the first child, 18.2 for the second, 22.0 for the third, 24.9 for the fourth, and 35.8 for the fifth child, after which it rises sharply so that the tenth or later children have only half as much a chance of survival as do the second children (*Fetal, Infant and Early Childhood Mortality,* 1952).

As there is a direct relationship between the nutritional status of the mother and the rate of infant mortality, so is the case with the family income and death rate. If the family's income pattern is such that 90 percent of it is spent on food, the nutrition level of its members will be relatively better if the number of children in such a family is small. The death rate among the vulnerable group (infants) will be higher in those families where five children have to be fed on a fixed income, compared to a family that, on the same income, has to feed two children. Based on a study of per capita gross national products of 45 countries, it was estimated "that infant mortality declines sharply from 165 to about 35 as per capita income increases from $75 to $375. The decline in infant mortality is more gradual and smaller from 35 to 22 as per capita income increases from $375 to $775. Thereafter for further increases in income the decline in infant mortality is only nominal (Chandrasekhra, 1972). A similar relationship exists in those poor countries where the per capita income is less than $75.00. Nine-tenths of all infant deaths occur among the poorest 30 percent of families. The poorest live in slum areas where basic amenities of life such as clean drinking water, sanitary facilities, drainage, etc., are the least available. The forceful writing of Lord Boyd Orr makes the relationship between nutrition and infant mortality all the more clear and may be profitably reproduced here.

> It used to be assumed that the poor represented an inferior strain of the population and that the high infantile mortality among the poor was Nature's method of eliminating the unfit. This view, which would absolve us from doing anything to abolish poverty, is not supported by facts. Where the infantile mortality rate is the highest, the survivors are of the poorest physique and vice versa. The factors which make for high infantile mortality seem to be the factors which make for ill-health and poor physique among the survivors. There is no doubt about the importance of heredity but we cannot dogmatize about inherited differences in health and physical fitness between the well-to-do and the poor until the environmental conditions affecting

the health and physique are comparable in both classes. Of these environmental factors, nutrition seems to be of prime importance, because the results of the feeding tests show that when the diet of the children of the poorer classes is improved, making it more like that of the well-to-do, the rate of growth of the children approaches that of children of the well-to-do class, and there is a noteworthy improvement in health and physique.

Nutrition Needs and Scope for Improvement

Infants are at a stage which involves significant changes in body composition day after day, week after week or month after month because of growth. The nutrition requirements of the infants cannot, therefore, be measured by the same yardstick as for adults who have no compulsion of growth. In terms of body weights, the infants need larger quantities of nutrients compared to adults because, in addition to meeting the growth needs, the infants have a higher metabolic rate and a more rapid turnover of nutrients (Holt, 1961; Holt and Synderman, 1968). By a rough estimate, the caloric needs of the infants in terms of body weight are two to three times higher than those of adults. The basal metabolism, as is understood in terms of maintenance under conditions of rest, is very high in the infants and so are the basal heat production and heat losses (Hegsted, 1957). Energy lost in defecation is higher and while crying a baby increases his metabolism by as much as 100 percent. Holt and Synderman calculated that, whereas a placid infant may do very well on 70 calories per kg, a child that cries and is active in kicking and whimpering may need as much as 130 calories per kg body weight. It is important for a proper evaluation of the nutrition requirements of a growing infant, that one must be aware of the growth pattern at different periods of a child's life. For example, a child, on the average, doubles his birth weight during the first five to six months and triples it by the time he is one year old (MacKeith and Wood, 1971; Robinson, 1970). At the same time, he increases in length from about 19 inches to 29 inches (Ebbs, 1966). This momentum of growth is not maintained in the later period, as may be reflected by the calorie requirements per pound of body weight at different ages. Ebbs described that one to six months of age children require 50 calories per pound body weight per day. This need diminishes to 40 calories at eight years and a mere 23 calories at 12 years of age, which would mean that an infant would need more than double calories per pound compared to an adult person (Ebbs, 1966). This makes it all the more important that adequate attention be paid to infant nutrition.

Protein deficiency states among infants and preschool children are widespread in most of the developing regions of the world because of limited supply of proteins as well as calories as related to the population. The main strategy for improvement lies in two areas: 1. discouraging overnutrition in the opulent areas and siphoning part of the animal proteins to the needy regions; and 2. increased production in those areas of the protein rich and protective foods. The children in these areas depend, for their protein supply, mainly on cereals, which are deficient in one or two essential amino acids. Even small supplements of animal proteins to the diets of these children can go a long way in improving the biological quality of available protein. Milk, poultry and fish sources can be developed among the rural communities with relatively small investments (Lovern, 1966, Parpia, 1964), but the greatest scope lies in the production of vegetable sources of protein (Lahery, 1962). The developing countries have a vast potential for producing protein rich legumes and oilseed meals (Swaminathan, 1966; 1968). The other method is to undertake mass scale production of processed infant foods, weaning foods and high protein foods based on judicious blends of oilseed meals (peanuts, soybeans, etc.) and fish flour, and fortified with vitamins and minerals. Trials on feeding these foods to preschool children have been highly successful, and 40 to 50 gm of these special blends used as supplements promote satisfactory growth and can also be used in the treatment of protein malnutrition in the preschool children (Parpia, 1964; Swaminathan, 1966).

Adequate nutrition for a child is essential, but it may be

added that infant feeding does not stop at providing nutrients. The infant requires other essential nutrients which the nutritionists may not care to list but to an infant, they are as important for adequate growth. These are warmth, stimulation, cuddling, and intimate contact with the mother, all of which give him a sense of belonging and influence to a great extent his emotional and social development. Food greatly influences the child's emotional and social development, but his hunger for warmth, stimulation and a sense of belonging is equally strong. Any disturbance can upset him greatly, instilling in him a sense of insecurity, fear and hostility (Odlum, 1948).

NUTRITION OF THE FETUS AND NEWBORN

Nutrition Needs of the Growing Fetus

A pregnant mother goes through a series of metabolic alterations to be able to satisfy the nutritional needs of a growing fetus inside her body. These alterations involve a great deal of stress and strain and raise her own nutritional requirements in a significant manner. Mothers with normal health are able to cope with the demands made by the fetus. The latter is generally regarded as a parasite having priority on the nutrients circulating in the maternal blood stream (Naismith, 1969). In mothers who are not very healthy, as is the case of millions in the poor, developing countries, a physiological adaptation, or adaptive mechanism, becomes operative during the period of pregnancy which facilitates the conservation and maximum utilization of the available nutrients in order to safeguard the developing fetus (Venkatachalan, 1962). This is probably why the chronically undernourished women in the tropical countries are able to produce babies whose birth weights are within the normal range. This is to say that the fetus in such cases acts as a true parasite, being able to grow at the expense of the mother. Similar observations have been made by Naismith in rats. After a careful study, Naismith concluded that the same mechanisms for the protection of the fetus against the adverse effects of poor nutrition operate in man as in the rat (Nai-smith, 1966).

Although the growing fetus has priority over the mother in fulfilling its needs, there is ample evidence to suggest that there is a certain limit beyond which the host-parasite relationship between mother and the fetus fails to operate. If the mother goes through a period of severe and prolonged malnutrition prior to pregnancy or during the pregnancy period, she fails to safeguard a satisfactory growth of the fetus, which may result in premature expulsion of the fetus. In the author's laboratory, squirrel monkeys maintained on 8 percent or less protein in the diet had a significantly high rate of abortion in the latter half of the gestation period (unpublished observations). Several studies from all over the world have pointed to a close relationship between nutritional deprivation of the mother and the incidence of miscarriage, still-births, premature births, or low birth weight (Sharma, 1955; Venkatachalan, 1962). A detailed survey in South India revealed that a large number of women who experienced prolonged episodes of malnutrition before the onset of pregnancy and did not improve their nutrition during the gravid state had an extremely limited ability to nurture a fetus. This was reflected in a high percentage of premature expulsions of the fetus. Even in those who completed their full term, the average birth weight was much less than the World Health Organization's standard of 2,500 grams. Venkatachalan suggested that these small sized, underweight infants, even if they are physiologically and functionally mature and manage to live, probably possess very little nutritional reserves and become potential subjects for the development of nutritional deficiency and its consequences during the early months of life (Venkatachalan, 1962). The reader is also referred to the author's earlier monograph on the subject (Manocha, 1972).

The quantity of blood made available to the fetus determines the rate of growth and finally the birth weight, and when this fact is stretched to different species, the blood supply to the growing fetus determines the differences in rate of growth as well as the birth weight (Table III). In humans, most of the growth takes place after the full establishment of the placenta as a vehicle of transferring blood. Whereas the fetus weighs only thirty grams at the end of three months, it weighs 3,000 grams or more at full term, which indicates the rapid growth in the last six months when adequate nutrition is made available through the umbilical blood vessels. As the gestation period progresses, the nutritional needs of the fetus are progressively increased (Widdowson, 1962; 1969b).

We may discuss briefly how the fetus derives from the mother the various nutrients. Carbohydrates reach the fetus as glucose and the fetus has the ability to synthesize its own glycogen. Glucose crosses the placenta readily by a simple process of diffusion as the fetal blood glucose concentration is about half that of the mother. Not all the glucose is oxidized, and some of it is stored as glycogen in the fetal liver and skeletal muscle (Shelley, 1969). The accumulation of fetal glycogen depends to a great extent on the maternal nutrition and can be lowered by restricting the maternal intake by 20 to 25 percent (Howding and Shelley, 1967).

Nitrogen is provided to the fetus in the form of amino acids, and it is interesting to note that the concentration of free amino acids in the fetal blood is higher than in the maternal blood (Clemetson and Churchman, 1954). Since the

TABLE III

RATE OF GROWTH OF NINE SPECIES BEFORE BIRTH

Species	Length of gestation (days)	Weight at birth (g)	Mean growth rate (g/day)
Mouse	21	2	0.09
Rat	21	5	0.24
Cat	63	100	1.6
Dog	63	200	3.2
Pig	120	1,500	4.2
Man	280	3,500	12.5
Elephant	600	114,000	190
Hippopotamus	240	50,000	210
Blue Whale	330	3,000,000	9,000

From: E. M. Widdowson, *Proc Nutr Soc 28*, 17, 1969.

L-isomer passes through to the fetus more frequently than the D-isomer, it suggests an active transport process.

In the early period of fetal development, the fetus does not lay down any fat stores, except the utilization of essential lipids and phospholipids in the nervous system and cell walls (Wilkinson, 1969). However, as the fetal growth progresses, it is increasingly able to synthesize its own fat from glucose. There is no evidence that fatty acids, except probably linoleic acid, cross the placenta. Hytten and Leitch believe that acetyl coenzyme A, which crosses the placenta, may act as a precursor to synthesize fatty acids and lipids (Hytten and Leitch, 1964). As a final analysis, it seems that, although the fetus has to synthesize its own fat, it accumulates as much as 560 grams of fat by the time of birth. This is next only to water, which in a full term fetus may be as much as 2,400 grams.

Vitamins are made available to the fetus in ample quantities which ensure a satisfactory growth. Vitamin A concentration, as well as carotenoids, is lower in the fetal than in the maternal blood, and large intakes by the mother do not change this ratio (Lewis *et al.*, 1947). Most vitamin B, especially thiamine, folate and B_{12}, reach the fetus quickly through the placenta. Vitamin C is supplied as dehydroascorbic acid as it is better able to cross the placenta as compared to L-ascorbic acid. The mechanism of the transfer of vitamin D is not clear at this time.

Most of the mineral elements are provided to the fetus in generous amounts. Measurements of sodium reveal that 500 to 1,000 times as much sodium reaches the fetus as is required for growth (Cox and Chalmers, 1953). Regarding the calcium and phosphorus requirements, Widdowson calculated that the fetus requires a total of 28 grams of calcium and 16 grams of phosphorus during the last three months of gestation, and this amount reflects as much as 5 percent of the total calcium in the plasma of the mother and 10 percent of the inorganic phosphorus during the last three months of gestation (Widdowson, 1962). Iron, copper and zinc are mainly attached to the specific proteins. Fetal plasma at full term contains nearly three times as much iron as the maternal plasma (Vahlquist, 1941). Whereas the concentration of iron gradually increases throughout the gestation period, the copper concentration falls in the same period. Zinc is higher in concentration in the plasma of babies born prematurely compared to full term babies. However, babies after birth always have a higher zinc concentration than the mother. Zinc, which is attached to the proteins, is transferred to the fetus.

We may mention briefly the process by which the fetus excretes the waste products. The fetus is bathed in amniotic fluid, enclosed in the amniotic membrane. Normally, the fluid has a composition similar to the plasma ultrafiltrate, but as the gestation period comes closer to an end, it becomes dilute, due probably to large volumes of fetal urine added to it (McCance, 1964). The fetal urine is indeed very dilute compared to maternal urine. Whereas the proportion of urea, sodium and chloride is 194:156:154 m-moles/litre in the mother's urine, the fetal urine contains only 17:44:41 m-moles/litre of these elements (McCance, 1953). The human fetus drinks amniotic fluid to as much as one litre per day. As Widdowson explained, "almost the whole of the ingested salts and water must be absorbed by the fetal gut into the circulation. Where and how this takes place in the human fetus is quite unknown, but sodium and water have been shown to be absorbed from the stomach of the rabbit fetus. This is interesting, because the absorption of water and salt is not generally considered an important function of the stomach in adult life (1969b). The fetal intestine is generally filled with sticky material called meconium, which is extruded by the neonate, but occasionally it is also passed out into the amniotic cavity before birth.

Passive immunity is passed on to the young one from the mother, before as well as after birth. The baby is born well-equipped with passive immunity and the concentration of maternal antibodies of the neonate may even exceed that of the mother. After birth, the process of transmission of immunity through maternal milk continues (Brambell, 1967).

It is not easy to say whether or not a fetus could swallow solid objects. Under normal circumstances, it cannot, but the following story published in Time Magazine, June 14, 1968, under the caption of "Unborn Baby Swallows Bullet," would tell otherwise. The incident happened in Brooklyn, New York.

> Mrs. Lucy Ortiz, 20, who was eight months pregnant, was standing at the open window of her apartment at about 1 a.m. on Tuesday morning. An unknown attacker fired a .22 gun at her and the bullet entered the right side of her abdomen. Doctors were unable to find the bullet but when they X-rayed the child, they were astonished to find the bullet lodged in its stomach. They are still trying to decide whether the bullet would work its way out through the child's intestines or whether an operation will be necessary. Police are hunting the attacker. The mother is in fair condition.

Feeding the Newborns

It is evident that, during the last week of gestation and the first week of postnatal life, the human organism passes through a very vulnerable period, and food restriction during that period could have grave consequences in terms of physical and mental development (Davies and Russell, 1968; Dobbing, 1968). This is particularly true of the prematurely born infant who has not yet developed his birth stores and whose maternal supply of nutrients is abruptly cut off. The fetal glycogen reserves indicate that if breast feeding is begun within a few hours after birth, the child may be spared any unnecessary damage.

Some starvation of the neonate is inevitable because some time is bound to be lost from the time of ligation of the umbilical cord and starting to feed. If the period of labor has been quite long, which is sometimes the case, the fetal distress could also prevent the infant from accepting food for some time (Wilkinson, 1969). Most of the time, the neonate is first given a little sugar solution before putting him on milk. In that case, the likelihood of hypoglycemia (abnormally low blood sugar level, which may cause clinically recognizable symptoms such as convulsions, apnoeic attacks, coma, high frequency tremors of limbs, etc.) to develop in a neonate is indeed remote. If some of the symptoms do appear during the forty-eight hours, they may be relieved by intravenous administration of glucose. Cornblath *et al.* calculated that blood glucose levels must be as low or lower than 20 mg/100 ml to produce any hypoglycemic symptoms (Cornblath *et al.,* 1964) .

As a recommendable preventive measure of hypoglycemia, Neligan suggested that a predisposed newborn baby should be given adequate calories in the form of milk and intravenous glucose, if the blood sugar does not rise above 20 mg/100 ml even after four hours of milk intake. Milk may have to be given very early and soon after birth, even if the gastric tube has to be used. Some physicians prefer intravenous feeding compared to gastric tubing. During the brief period of starvation after birth, the neonate mobilizes its own food reserves to meet the growing metabolic needs. After birth, the oxygen consumption is increased because of a much higher rate of activity compared to the fetal existence. Instead of glucose, the fatty acids then play a dominating role in producing cellular energy. The adipose tissue of the neonate not only serves as a source of circulatory free fatty acids, but also to produce heat. It must be emphasized here that, although the amount of free fatty acids as a source of energy may be enough, the fat deposits in the human infant are not sufficient to provide a good thermal insulation (Hull, 1969) . The lowest comfortable temperature for a naked, mature infant is 34° C. Adults at this temperature would feel quite uncomfortable. Below this temperature, the rate of oxygen consumption increases greatly in an effort to produce extra heat to maintain thermal stability. Hull emphasized that infants immediately after birth have lower body temperatures and are liable to catch cold when cold air blows on their wet, exposed skins. It is desirable to keep the baby wrapped in warm clothing, in bed with the mother. This is good for the emotional welfare of the mother as well as the warmth and comfort of the baby (Hull, 1969) .

Breast feeding should be started within a few hours after the birth. The newborn has all the reflexes which help him feed himself during the critical early period of life. First is the rooting reflex, which motivates or causes the child to turn to the breast nipple or any object touching his cheek. The second most important reflex is the deglutition reflex, under the influences of which the posterior two thirds of the tongue, the oropharynx, esophagus, and cardiac sphincter actually help the child swallow the liquid from the breast or bottle. Third there is the extrusion reflex, which helps the child to extrude objects placed on the anterior one third of the tongue. This reflex begins to diminish at about nine weeks, and the child at that time is ready to be fed semisolid foods. (Willis, 1964).

One does not have to go around the supermarkets to look for a nutritious milk formula for the baby that will revitalize the nutritional reserves of the newborn. The first milk from the mother's breasts, called colostrum, is not only nutritious, but is highly concentrated in the vitally-needed vitamins and minerals, besides body-building protein. Although the amount of colostrum available to the baby at each feeding is small, the act of sucking promotes the flow of milk and helps to establish satisfactory lactation. During the first two to three days, the baby loses about half a pound of weight due to partial starvation and loss of water. However, this loss is considered normal because, after the breasts start producing adequate quantities of milk, the body regains weight quickly. Unfortunately in some areas of the world, human superstitions in the form of cultural practices successfully starve and harm a child in its most vulnerable period of growth. Keen described a situation in which a great percentage of Swazi infants die during the first month, due probably to severe forms of malnutrition perpetrated on the child due to a culturally-based superstition that the neonate should not be given breast milk until the umbilical cord drops off (Keen, 1946). This may take as many as five days or more, and during this period the child is given small quantities of soft maize meal. Among the Zulus, the child is deprived of breast milk during the first few days of life under the cultural belief that the colostrum is harmful for the baby (Jali,

1950). In some parts of India, colostrum is considered unclean because of the belief that it has remained in the breasts during the entire period of pregnancy and, therefore, may be harmful to the baby.

Feeding the Prematures or Low Birth Weight Babies

Prematurely born infants have more severe problems of nutrition than full-term babies. It is possible that maternal nutrition before and during pregnancy may be one of the reasons for premature expulsion of the fetus. Other factors that may contribute are type of prenatal care, age and health of the mother, the spacing and complications of pregnancy, and faults of uterine implantation (Ebbs, 1966; FAO, 1957). A neonate born at full term contains 11 to 15 percent lean body mass, 12 to 16 percent subcutaneous fat deposits and adipose tissue, and 73 percent extra- and intracellular water. The percentage of water in a prematurely born infant increases to around 82 percent, which dangerously reduces the proportion of lean mass as well as adipose tissue (Forbes 1962; *Nutrition Reviews,* 1963). A premature infant also has inadequate birth stores of vitamins and minerals; the reflexes that help a full-term baby in feeding itself have not been fully developed; and he cannot suck or swallow normally. By its very word, *premature,* the baby lacks maturity in every way, including the quantum of digestive enzymes which may help him to overcome his deficiencies by making good use of the food offered to him. For details, the reader is referred to some important publications (Cornblath *et al.,* 1964; Crass, 1957; MacKeith and Wood, 1971; Powers, 1948; Richelderfer *et al.,* 1967; Silverman and Sinclair, 1966; Wharton, 1965).

The caloric requirements of the prematures are high, as are their needs of vitamins and minerals. The need for vitamin D and Vitamin E appears to be especially high. It has been suggested that the anemia of prematurity and a syndrome commonly found in prematures consisting of edema, skin changes and platelet count in the blood is due to a deficiency of vitamin E. The newborns weighing under 1,500 grams at birth have almost no fat or glycogen reserves (Widdowson, 1968) and their protein reserves are equally poor. Strictly speaking, there is no expendable protein store in the body of such an infant (Ghadini *et al.,* 1973), and it may be safely said that no patient faces a more critical need for protein than the low birth weight infant in the first weeks of life—anabolic processes must function at maximum rates, enzymes must mature rapidly, while paltry resources are strained to the utmost (Ghadini, 1973). It is probable that the high mortality rate among the premature may be directly related to the problem of nutrition and our ability to cope with it, rather than to any physiological inability. Holt and Synderman believe that it may be that the premature "needs a variety of accessory substances which the mature infant can manage for himself (Holt and Synderman, 1968).

As discussed in a later section, breast feeding is highly desirable and must be encouraged. In the event that a decision has been made by the physician or the mother to bottle feed the baby, it is important to learn in the early neonatal period if the infant is allergic to certain milk. Allergic sensitivity to mother's milk is quite rare, but may appear in certain cases where some forms of protein in the mother's diet may find their way into the milk in an unsplit form and produce certain symptoms of sensitivity in the infant (Holt and Synderman, 1968). It is not rare to find allergic sensitivity to some proteins, such as lactalbumin, in cow's milk (Holt and Synderman, 1968). Holt and Snyderman point out that in rare but dramatic manifestations, a single drop of cow's milk may, within a few minutes, lead to uricarea, asthma, acute gastrointestinal symptoms, and shock in alarming proportions. In these circumstances, the elimination of cow's milk from the diet must be done immediately. Fatalities have also been reported. Goat's milk is often well tolerated by these infants, but at times there is sensitivity to this also, and a milk-free diet must be given. There are substitute soy-base or meat-base formulas which provide adequate nutrients. Such extreme sensitivity is not always permanent.

For a premature or a low birth weight infant, breast milk

may be ideal in terms of its easy digestibility, but a formula containing cow's milk, with higher quantities of calcium and protein, is well tolerated by a premature baby. (Goldman *et al.*, 1962). It may seem that the premature babies could not be able to handle the nitrogen load from the higher protein content of cow's milk, but surprisingly, they seem to be able to do better than the full-term babies in this respect (Gordon *et al.*, 1937).

Feeding the low birth weight infant should be started as early as possible during the first twelve hours after birth, because this will mean increased blood-glucose levels, which will reduce acidosis and ketonia by preventing tissue breakdown. Early feeding will also restore glycogen stores in the liver and chances of hyperbilirubinemia and hypoglycemia are greatly reduced. Babies born to mothers with diabetes are more susceptible and are prone to develop, within the first twelve hours, symptoms of hypoglycemia. This may be prevented by starting oral feeding within a few hours of birth; if there is coexistent respiratory distress, dextrose is given intravenously without delay (MacKeith and Wood, 1971).

Depending on the birth weight and condition of the infant, the doctor will have to decide whether an oral or intravenous method of feeding is more practical. The former may have the problem of regurgitation and inhalation of milk into the lungs. In most hospitals these days, tube feeding is routinely used for prematurely-born infants, in-between giving the bottle a trial (Cornblath *et al.*, 1964). The prematurely-born infant needs more frequent feeding because of his inability to take sufficient quantities at one time.

In the premature infant, the renal excretion and filtration capacity of glomeruli and tubules is also not efficient; edema may be the result of water retention in extracellular confinements. In a full-term infant, solutes as well as water are filtered out, although during extreme conditions such as very hot weather, fever, vomitting, or diarrhea, renal excretion of water may lead to dehydration. It is only after about six weeks that glomeruli and the tubules are able to concentrate urine and conserve water and the infant is successfully able to maintain water balance (Willis, 1964).

DIGESTION AND ABSORPTION OF FOOD
IN EARLY INFANCY

The infant sucks milk from the breasts of the mother or the nipple of a bottle by a sucking process which is, in itself, quite specialized. It involves sealing the lips air-tight and squeezing milk out of the container. The former function is performed by certain eminences (*pars villosa,* or sucking blisters). The milk is squeezed out of the milk cisterns by the infant through an elevation of the dorsum of the tongue, travelling from the front backwards, against the hard palate. The milk then passes through the pharynx to the esophagus, where coordinated peristalsis speeds it on its way to the stomach. The gums then open, the tongue slides forward, its tip often appearing between the gums, and the cisterns refill with milk. The gums then close again and the biting, stripping, and swallowing cycle is repeated (MacKeith and Wood, 1971). The mechanism of sucking milk from the bottle is essentially similar. A cleft lip generally does not facilitate an air-tight mouth so necessary for smooth sucking, and may prevent the baby from sucking sufficiently. The stomach at birth has the capacity to hold only one or two ounces; but it expands quite rapidly as the nutrient requirements of the growing infant increase. By the time most babies leave the hospital to go home, they are taking three to four ounces of milk at a time. However, at this age, the system is somewhat imperfect and the child swallows almost as much air as milk, which needs to be *burped* out after the feeding. The infant from birth to six weeks requires around 3.3 ounces of milk per pound of body weight per day, which is necessitated by the high levels of growth. From seven to eighteen weeks, this milk intake is reduced to 2.5 ounces of milk per pound of body weight per day. This level of milk intake is further decreased to about 2.1 ounces of milk per pound of body weight per day between nineteen and twenty-six weeks (Foman, 1958). The water requirements of the infant are in the vicinity of 2.5 ounces per pound of body weight per day, unless severe conditions such as fever, vomitting or diarrhea increase the need for water.

In the early part of life, only the fluids are allowed to pass through the esophagus, and this is the main reason why milk is the major source of nutrition during the first three months of life. All solid objects are thrown out because of the vomiting reflex. Starting from about three months up to five or six months, the child gradually develops the skill to chew or swallow lumps of food. This is the time when semisolid foods of animal as well as plant origin may be introduced. For example, cookies may be softened with saliva and then swallowed. Saliva by the age of three months increases significantly its starch digesting enzyme, amylase, to the level of being able to contribute significantly to the digestion of starch.

In early infancy the stomach mainly curdles the milk and serves as a regulatory organ for passage to the small intestine, because the whey passes on through the stomach much sooner than the casein part of the curd. The disintegration of the curd does take place to a great extent in the pyloric antrum of the stomach (Platt, 1961). The stomach secretes pepsin which attacks the large protein molecules, and its pH is quite low. Some fats are also split by gastric lipase. It may be safely assumed that up to a period of three months, the stomach does an efficient job of taking care of milk and passing the contents on to the small intestine, where the process of protein and carbohydrate digestion is more active, having mixed with pancreatic and bile fluids in the duodenum. The food in the small intestines is churned and moved forward by the peristaltic movements until, in about three to four hours, most of the stomach is emptied and the residues of food reach the caecum. The villi, or finger-like projections of the small intestine, are the main sites of digestion and absorption, and are equipped with arteries, veins and lymph vessels. The small intestines in the infant secrete amylase and esterokinase, but the pancreatic juice puts small quantities of lipase, a fat-splitting enzyme, and trypsin and chymotrypsin, which split polypeptides into smaller-sized peptides. Amino peptidases further split the peptides into amino acids. Willis explained that "during the first three months, the intestinal fluids contain sufficient proteolytic enzymes for the digestion of 95 percent of human milk protein and similar percentages of protein supplied by processed, soft curd cow's milk. With unprocessed cow's milk, tough curds may form and result in lowered protein absorption." The amino acids are absorbed into the blood vessels through the intestinal villi.

Milk carbohydrates are easily reduced from di- or poly-saccharides to monosaccharides. The disaccharide enzymes (lactase, maltase) split the sugars lactose and galactose to glucose, sucrose to glucose and fructose, and maltose to glucose before they are absorbed at the microvilli level in the small intestines. Amylase is not present in sufficient quantities in the neonatal period, but by nine to twelve weeks, sufficient quantities of amylase are present, which coincides with the period of the child's readiness to take starch-containing semisolid foods.

The fat molecules are emulsified by lipase into mono-glycerides, glycerol and fatty acids. The short-chain fatty acids, e.g. butyric acid, are water-soluble but the long-chain fatty acids are made water-soluble by bile salts. It may be added here that, during the first three months, the quantity of lipase secreted is small, and it is advisable to keep the fat content of the milk as low as possible in formulas. For human milk, sufficient amounts of pancreatic lipase are present to digest 80 percent of the human milk fat at birth, 95 percent at four weeks, and 100 percent by eight weeks (Levin, 1963).

Regarding the sites of absorption of different nutrients, iron and calcium are absorbed in the duodenum. Glucose, some iron, ascorbic acid, folic acid, riboflavin, pyridoxine, some fat and some broken products of protein and lactose are absorbed in the jejunum. The remaining protein, lactose, sucrose, maltose, fats and vitamin B_{12} are absorbed in the ileum. In an infant, it takes about ten minutes for the food to pass through the jejunum and two hours to pass through the ileum (MacKeith and Wood, 1971). As the baby grows, the process of digestion gradually takes on the adult pattern.

The prematurely-born infant experiences a lot of difficulties in ingestion, digestion, and renal excretion compared to a full-term baby. In the former, the ingestive mechanism is underdeveloped and the oropharyngeal muscles as well as the cardiac sphincter are weak, making not only swallowing but also the retention in the stomach more difficult, explaining why premature infants regurgitate more often. The peptic and tryptic capacity of the digestive glands for the gastric and intestinal digestion of protein are indeed very poor (Werner, 1948). The activity of pepsin may be just right at an acidity level created by human milk, which may not be true of cow's milk. The latter raises to some extent the gastric pH and also the proteolytic effectiveness of pepsin (Jean *et al.,* 1958). Renal excretion in the prematurely-born infant is also limited due to the immaturity of the kidneys (Willis, 1964).

The fecal matter of the infants still contains certain nutrients: casein, fatty acids and minerals, in addition to live and dead bacteria. The artificially-fed babies pass stools which may be more foul-smelling compared to breast-fed infants because of the larger quantities of excreted casein and undigested fat. Excessive protein in milk tends to make the stools harder because of casein curds. For proper digestion, it is advisable to give the baby low starch, low fat, and easily curdable protein in the diet.

BREAST FEEDING—ITS IMPORTANCE AND DESIRABILITY

Desirability of Breast Feeding

Breast feeding the newborn is the most ideal and desirable thing to do. This is not to say that artificial feeding is in any way harmful. Everyone knows that bottle-fed babies are healthy and happy children, and there is nothing wrong with raising children on animal milk. It is strongly advisable, however, that the mother should not resort to it on spurious grounds. The decision should be made after a careful evaluation of all factors in the best interest of the baby. Some women make the choice to bottle feed only on the grounds that it will interfere less with their freedom to pursue careers or vocations. The following account is written with the intention of bringing to focus some of the favorable aspects of breast feeding.

Human milk has a composition which enables the infant to derive maximum benefit from its nutrients (Jelliffe and Jelliffe, 1971). It may be said that human milk is most ideal for human children and possesses a certain biochemical composition that is ideal for the growth of the human baby. The enzymes in the digestive system of a human baby are not so effective as to make full use of the higher protein content in cow's milk. The curd made from cow's milk is harder than that made from human milk. The latter is soft and the enzymes of the small intestine break down the protein molecules easily to make amino acids available through the walls of the intestine for body-building purposes. Cow's milk is not that easily processed, and a higher protein content may be of no advantage to the infant. Instances of intolerance to human milk are very rare, and the efficiency with which the infant utilizes protein is much higher than in cow's milk or other humanized formulas (Barnes, 1957). Jelliffe went as far as to say that, try as we may to *humanize* cow's milk, the precise constituents of breast milk cannot be grossly mimicked biochemically (1967). Winnicott believes that breast feeding is one of those natural phenomena that justify themselves, even if they can, where necessary, be bypassed. Davies emphasized that the mineral composition of breast milk is perfectly suited to the newborn kidney and has an important homeostatic effect in the first weeks of life (1965; 1969). In addition, the proportion of proteins, fats and carbohydrates in breast milk are the most appropriate for the needs of the infant (WHO, 1965).

There are certain unique anti-infection properties in human milk that are not found in animal milk (Jelliffe, 1973;

Jelliffe and Jelliffe, 1971). Special mention should also be made of the nutritive value of colostrum, the breast milk secreted during the first few days after the birth of the baby. Not only does it contain higher quantities of protein and fat than milk in the later period, but it is richer in vitamins and minerals as well. Colostrum is alkaline and has a slight laxative effect (Ebbs, 1966). The yellowish-colored colostrum is too good to be wasted either by a deliberate decision to bottle-feed or by keeping the baby on a sugar solution for two to three days until the mother's milk is cleared of colostrum, as is done in some countries in the East. From the nutritional point of view, this practice is harmful, and starves the neonate of his requirements for nutrients, giving him a bad start in life. The intake of colostrum greatly benefits the baby and adds to his birth stores a rich supply of vitamins and minerals.

The ideal method of initiating feeding to the newborn is to give him small quantities of lactose water and to put him to the breast within the first twelve to twenty-four hours. Every effort should be made to ensure that the first breast feeding is a rich and satisfactory experience for the mother and the child. It may be that, because of the inexperience of both partners, the infant gets little or no milk; in any case, the baby should be allowed to try and suck for awhile. Subsequently, the baby may be nursed every four hours around the clock. The baby who is able to suck the quantity of milk which is adequate for his needs is likely to be satisfied, quiet and sleep well, whereas a hungry baby may be restless (*Nutrition Reviews*, 1967).

MacKeith and Wood, while addressing a nursing mother, have given a good account of some of her apprehensions and what to do about them:

Remember that all babies lose weight in the first week of life, and so do not think that because your baby loses weight at first that it means you are not going to have enough milk for him. If he is sleepy in the first few days, it is not necessary to prod or shake him into sucking. Babies often are sleepy for several days, and though they are benefitted by being held close by their mothers, they do not take much milk. This is because milk production only comes on gradually, little being made until the fourth or fifth day. You will probably notice at this time that the breast gets much fuller. Often the start is quite smooth, but sometimes the breasts get over-full and rather tender. If this happens, your doctor or nurse will tell you what to do, and with their advice and help, it will settle down in a few days, and for most mothers, breast-feeding will go on satisfactorily. Most mothers can breast-feed successfully, and by following the advice you get at the prenatal examinations, you will probably be another of the mothers who enjoy breast feeding, and find that it is convenient and gives a good start to the baby.

The supply of milk is generally enough for a neonate in spite of the small quantities of milk produced in the breasts in the first few days. In case you and the doctor think that the baby remains hungry or thirsty because of inadequate lactation, and his weight loss during the first week is unusually large (over 10 percent of the body's birth weight), or if the baby fails to gain about a half an ounce daily in the second week, it may be advisable to give extra water to the baby after or in-between the breast feedings. This water is generally boiled or may be half strength normal saline (one level teaspoon in 500 ml water) or sugar water containing a teaspoonful of sugar in four ounces of water (MacKeith and Wood, 1971).

Breast milk is likely to include certain vestiges of the mother's food, such as alcohol, but most of the drugs eaten by the mother are not excreted in the milk. For example, if the mother is habitually on barbiturates or salicylates, they are unlikely to affect the baby, although excessive alcohol or barbiturates may make the baby sleepy after the feeding. Nicotine derived from smoking may be excreted in the milk, but as some studies indicate, it has no harmful effect on the baby (Perlman *et al.*, 1942). Arsenic finds its way into the milk and may be, to some extent, hazardous to the health of the baby, but it is never given therapeutically these days (Manocha, 1972). Bacteria are generally present in the milk, but unless there is a case of infection of the breast, they are not pathogenic (Illingworth, 1968).

Because of the safety, sterility and cleanliness of breast

milk, breast-fed babies generally experience fewer infections and episodes of illnesses. The incidence of colic, diarrhea and constipation in these babies is considerably less than in babies fed on animal's milk. Colic is particularly common and uncomfortable to the baby (Ebbs, 1966). There are certain factors in breast milk which encourage the growth of *Lactobacillus bifidus,* which in turn causes the bowel contents to be more strongly acid, thereby inhibiting the growth of *E. coli* (MacKeith and Wood, 1971). The stools of the breast-fed baby have also been observed to contain certain hemagglutinating antibodies to *E. coli* (Kenny *et al.,* 1967). Olsen described the stool of a breast-fed infant as being soft, yellowish-green in color, with a low pH (4–6), giving a fermentative odor. The fecal matter of the infant fed on cow's milk in general is firm, yellowish-brown in color, and has a neutral or alkaline pH (6.5–8.7), giving a putrefactive odor (Olsen, 1949). Pathogenic bacteria, which are always putrefactive rather than fermentative, find a more favorable environment for survival in the higher protein, less acid condition present in the intestine of the infant fed on cow's milk (Willis, 1964).

In several countries of Asia, Africa and Latin America, milk is not available in sufficient quantities. In terms of expense, it requires a working man's wages for half a day to buy enough milk to feed a baby, while at the same time, there is no guarantee the milk from the market is sterile, uncontaminated and unadulterated. In these countries, there are generally no refrigeration facilities and no uncontaminated storage places. On the other hand, the mother could provide adequate quantities of milk, if only she is given a little extra good-quality food (Someswara, 1959); then she could provide the most sterile milk in the most convenient containers—the breasts—from which the baby could be fed at any time of day or night with little trouble to the mother (Gopalan and Belavady, 1961). The more times the infant is put to the breast at the onset of the nursing process, the faster and more adequate will be the lactation. In addition, the milk is warmed to temperatures that are ideal and liked by the baby. The only disadvantages of breast feeding are occasional discomfort to the mother because of sore nipples caused by excessive sucking and some restriction in her daily chores due to the fact that she must be available at four to six hour intervals. The former problem can be solved by some care and alternating of the breasts during nursing. As for the latter inconvenience, one or two nursings of artificial milk may be introduced to enable the mother to be away for eight to nine hours, if she is working out of the home. Occasionally, special medication may have to be given to stimulate the production of large quantities of milk. Thorazine may be given three times under the supervision of a physician (Brown, 1973).

Many workers in this field of investigation have listed a number of physiological advantages of breast feeding, which may be usefully mentioned here. It must be emphasized, however, that more work is needed before their validity is fully established.

1) Cow's milk does not contain as much lactose as human milk, and galactose, formed by the hydrolysis of lactose in the intestine, is essential for the synthesis of cerebrosides, which is the main lipid of the myelin of the brain. The human brain myelinates to a great extent only after birth. Lactose also increases the retention of dietary calcium so that the higher lactose content of human milk allows a maximum utilization of the calcium in the milk (Duncan, 1955).

2) Coronary artery lesions observed at autopsies are much fewer in young adults who were breast fed. So is the incidence of dental caries (Davies and Russell, 1968; Osborn, 1968). Even in adolescent life, the beneficial effects of breast feeding seem to persist. A study of the arteries suggests that the arteries of those who were bottle fed were abnormal compared to the arteries of those who were breast fed. Similarly, ulcerative colitis is less common in those adults who were breast fed in infancy (Acheson and Truelove, 1961).

3) Immunoglobins which are passed on to the infant along with breast milk inhibit the growth of harmful bacteria

in the intestine and the body (Kenny *et al.*, 1967), and hence protect the infant from recurring infections.

4) The incidence of sudden unexpected *cot* or *crib* deaths may be lower in breast-fed infants. Protein from cow's milk may be absorbed from the gut during increased permeability in the early period of life, and regurgitation or aspiration of even a very small quantity of milk into the lungs might cause a severe anaphylactic reaction leading to pulmonary edema and death in a sensitized infant. Davies explained that well over a thousand crib deaths in this country every year might not occur if breast feeding were carried out, even if only in the first weeks of life (1969).

5) There are reports in the literature which indicate that the incidence of asthma and eczema are much lower in the breast-fed (Grulee, 1934). Similarly, neonatal tetany occurs only in bottle-fed infants. Widdowson believes that it is due to the high phosphate and unsaturated fat content of cow's milk. Davies reports that fits from hypomagnesemia also occur only in bottle-fed babies (1969), and Strauls and Murphy show that the consumption of human milk should reduce potential radiation exposure (Davies *et al.*, 1965).

In 1934, Grulee studied approximately 20,000 infants and found a greater incidence of morbidity and infection in the bottle-fed as compared to the breast-fed. Similar results were obtained by Robinson in 1951 after a study of 3,266 infants. Whereas this may have been the case in the early fifties, recent studies show that this significant difference in the pattern of incidence of sickness has been greatly reduced due to scientifically-based humanized milk formulas available on the market.

Besides providing the needed nutrients, the emotional and psychological aspects of breast feeding are often overlooked. Breast feeding leads to an intimate physical contact between the mother and the child, and helps to establish a close relationship between them. According to this author, the warmth of two bodies helps the exchange of something that makes breast feeding a rewarding experience for the mother and a source of emotional security and well-being for the infant. Just as close physical contact between adults leads to *love* and emotional attachment for each other, the physical contact between the mother and the child may be the beginning of an emotional security that may ultimately determine the outlook of the growing child towards his fellow beings and to the world. Psychologists emphasize more and more that breast feeding provides certain types of emotional experiences for the mother and child which may prove significant in having a favorable impact on both. Breast feeding may be a very satisfying experience for the mother. Lactation, like coitus, must be physically pleasurable if the race is to continue (Mead and Newton, 1967). The average mother does not deeply analyze her feelings about breast feeding. A few feel intense pleasure comparable to orgasm (Newton); many take satisfaction which may be in having relieved the baby's hunger or having done her duty as a mother, or there may be a deeper satisfaction with a sense of peace and relaxation (MacKeith and Wood, 1971). From the point of view of the mother's health, breast feeding and sucking by the infant help in the healthy regression of the uterus, besides being a rewarding experience.

Some remarks may be made on the breast feeding and the intake of oral contraceptives. As mentioned elsewhere, estrogens do bring about a certain degree of inhibition of lactation. From that viewpoint, it may be advisable to use some other method of contraception during the first six to eight weeks. The estrogens in quantities available in the *pill* do not inhibit established lactation. Suckling on the part of the baby is a more powerful stimulus than the inhibitory action of small amounts of estrogens. If the baby is sucking at the breast regularly, the lactation should be quite successful, but if the mother feels that because of the *pill* her lactation has been adversely affected, she would be wiser to give up the *pill* in favor of some other method of contraception. At this stage of our knowledge, the question is still undecided (MacKeith and Wood, 1971).

Modern Trends

There has been a disturbing trend all over the world away from the practice of breast-feeding in favor of feeding with the bottle. During the last two decades the whole concept of breast feeding seems to have undergone a change in the industrialized countries because of the easy availability of sterile satisfactory substitutes for breast milk. Millions of mothers have resorted to milk formulas made from pasteurized cow's milk and relieved themselves of the routine of breast feeding at regular intervals. Babies fed these formulas show a completely satisfactory pattern of growth and weight gain (Beal, 1969). There are several reasons ascribed to this change. Women are very conscious about maintaining the shape of their breasts because they have become a symbol of sex in the modern world, and many women feel that breast feeding may reduce their attractiveness. The second main reason for this change is the aggressive advertising campaigns of the commercial companies producing milk formulas and baby foods. Day after day they have tried to portray an image of superiority of formulas to breast milk without any counter-suggestion to the mothers on the part of physicians.

To some extent, psychological fears regarding the establishment of successful lactation prevent some mothers from trying to breast-feed their babies. A firm positive approach to breast feeding should be adopted by physicians during the prenatal visits (Applebaum, 1970). The unnecessary fears created by prejudicial attitudes among relatives or friends, including the *old wives tales* should be cleared by the doctor so as to relieve the mother of the fear and anxiety about her own ability to succeed. It has been recorded that, before World War II, 38 percent of the mothers nursed their babies. However, during the war, 90 percent of the mothers breast fed successfully over long periods of time, because artificial formulas were scarce. In most cases, it is evident that insufficient lactation is generally due to the mother's anxiety, so that she switches to the bottle in spite of having initiated breast feeding in the first place. Sixty-eight percent of the new mothers begin breast feeding their babies, but within two months this percentage dwindles to 25 percent or less (Beal, 1969).

Some women make a decision to bottle feed their babies mainly on the grounds of aesthetics. In that case, it may be undesirable to use hormone therapy to inhibit lactation. Vartan, after extensive observation, strongly opposes the idea of giving estrogens for the suppression of lactation. Large doses may inhibit lactation, but could also result in headaches and rebound increase of secretion (MacKeith and Wood, 1971).

Fortunately, in the developing countries, the rate of breast feeding among women has been traditionally quite high. In most Middle Eastern and African countries, breast feeding is encouraged and is continued up to eighteen to twenty-six months. A number of studies in South and Central America reveal that breast feeding is rarely continued for over a year, but in the Far East (India, Pakistan, Burma, Ceylon, Malaysia, Indonesia, the Philippines, Thailand and South Vietnam), a prolonged breast feeding is encouraged, depending, of course, on the ability of the mother to lactate, or its interruption by the next pregnancy. Until a few years ago, breast-feeding in these countries was a cultural must. The ancient Hindu medical text, *Charak Samhita,* has a detailed description of the value of human milk and the practice of breast feeding. Lately, however, there has been a very disturbing trend among the urban women of these countries, which is largely a result of commercial advertising of milk formulas. This has caused a lot of mischief. In the absence of absolutely safe drinking water, refrigeration facilities and sanitary conditions, baby formulas are often the carriers of common infections and, instead of helping infants to maintain their growth tempo, subject them to a variety of infections. A number of reports from the developing countries have brought attention to the increasing prevalence of marasmus in the earlier months of life, which formerly affected only the older children. It is well-known that even the undernourished mothers are able to produce as much as 400 to 600 ml of milk daily for a number of months. In most of the overpopulated developing countries, the general level of sanitation in and outside the home is less than desirable, and a mother who substitutes a bottle for her breasts (unless clinically indicated) is being less than a responsible mother, not acting in the best interests of her baby.

MILK AND MILK SUBSTITUTES FOR FEEDING INFANTS AND PRESCHOOL CHILDREN

Milk for Artificial Feeding

Whereas in the United States, cow's milk is most commonly used, in other countries the milk used to feed infants may have come from buffalo, camel, and even reindeer. Table IV gives the composition of the milk from various animals (see Appendix III). In Europe, North America and other industrialized countries where humanized commercial milk formulas are available, artificial feeding poses no great problem in terms of its composition or sterility. However, in the urban areas of tropical and subtropical countries where artificial feeding is done either as a concern for the shape of the breasts or a simple imitation of Western ways, this may not be the case. In most cases, milk from the market is fed to the infant. In such cases, it is important to understand the value of the fat content of the milk as well as the size of the fat globules, and whether or not they can be properly utilized by the infant. The process of homogenizing milk can be of great value in this regard. In this process, the fat globules are broken into smaller particles which can be easily emulsified in the gastrointestinal tract. Because of this, enzymes acting in the small intestine break up the fat into fatty acids and glycerol with greater ease and are easily absorbed through the intestinal wall.

It is also important to learn the protein content of the milk given to the baby because higher amounts of protein in the milk are of no particular advantage. In India and sev-

TABLE IV

COMPOSITION OF MILK OF VARIOUS ANIMALS (mean values)

Animal	Percentage			
	Water & Ash	Protein	Sugar	Fat
Woman	89	1	6	4
Ass	90	2	6	2
Mare	90	3	5	4
Cow	87	3	5	4
Elephant	68	3	9	20
Buffalo	85	4	4	7
Camel	87	4	6	3
Goat	82	4	5	8
Guinea-pig	86	5	2	7
Pig	85	5	3	7
Sheep	79	7	4	9
Whale	49	8	3	34
Cat	82	9	5	3
Rabbit	71	10	2	17
Reindeer	68	10	2	17
Dog	75	11	3	10
Rat	68	12	3	15
Seal	29	20	1	50
Whale	64	12	2	22

Data from: R. MacKeith, and C. Wood, *Infant Feeding and Feeding Difficulties* (London, J. & A. Churchill, 1971); and P. L. Altman and D. S. Dittmer (eds.) "Metabolism", Federation of American Societies for Experimental Biology, M-1–3, 1968.

eral other countries, infants are given buffalo milk, which is much higher in protein as well as fat content. The human baby does not have the enzymes to take care of the high protein content in the animal milk. In these cases, it is important that the milk be processed before using it for feeding the infant. Boiling the milk or pasteurization and homogenization solves the problem to a great extent. Boiling the milk changes the nature of the proteins in such a manner that softer curd is formed in the infant's stomach which can be easily digested. It causes the lactalbumin to coagulate in fine particles and subsequent coagulation of casein in the infant's stomach results in a curd that is easily digestible (Holt and Synderman, 1968). Homogenization helps to emulsify the fat globules so that they can be more easily converted into fatty acids and glycerol. Processed animal milk is all the more useful for a prematurely-born infant who needs more nitrogen than the full-term baby and can utilize larger quantities of protein (Gordon *et al.*, 1937; Levine and Gordon, 1942). It may be safely said that if the animal milk is properly processed and is uncontaminated by any pathogenic bacteria, the bottle-fed infants grow as well or even better than the breast-fed babies. To ensure optimum growth, an artificially-prepared formula must satisfy the following three requirements:

a. It must meet the nutritional requirements of the infant. The commonly used cow's milk is quite rich in proteins, as well as the needed vitamins and minerals with the exception of vitamins C and D. It will be useful to give the baby citrus juices on a regular basis. The vitamin D requirements can be met by regular exposure to the sun. These days, most of the baby formulas are enriched with vitamins A and D.

b. It must not be contaminated with any pathogenic microorganisms.

c. It must be prepared in such a manner so as to pose no digestive problems due to its curd quality. The last two requirements are always the concern of those who choose bottle feeding in preference to breast milk. A very useful practice is the routine terminal sterilization by bringing the temperature of the milk to the boiling point in the feeding bottle and then allowing it to cool immediately before each feeding. However, this is not as simple as it seems, especially in the poor developing countries where refrigeration facilities are not available to an average income family. The supply of milk is, in general, very low and in the absence of storing facilities, it is extremely difficult to keep it sterile for a regular four to six hours' feeding. The ignorant and uneducated mothers cannot be expected to be as clean and careful as to make sterile milk feeding.

Artificial feeding also has some other problems, which may be trivial but for which a mother's extra care and attention are essential. First is the problem of whether enough milk has been taken by the infant, which requires the mother's knowledge of the caloric requirements of the child, and also her ability to make an intelligent guess as to the amount of milk that should be taken over a twenty-four hour period. The inhaling of air could cause a number of digestive problems including distention of the stomach. Vomitting resulting in the loss of gastric juices is another problem in the artificially-fed babies. It is important for a mother to remember during and after feeding to help the baby *burp* out the swallowed air.

Milk and Milk Substitutes for Preschool Children

There is a general scarcity of milk and dairy products in most of the underdeveloped countries. These are also the countries which need it the most because around four percent of their populations is in the age group of 0 to 14 years, which is an actively growing group and needs high quality animal protein for maintaining a satisfactory pattern of growth. Meat products are all the more scarce. Emphasis should rightly be placed on the judicious use of available milk resources and alternate vegetable sources of producing vegetable milk should be promoted.

Dairy products are available in different forms and each of them has an advantage over the other under certain conditions. Some of these are as follows:

1. Animal milk. This includes milk from cows, buffalos, goats and other domesticated animals. Animal milk should not be given in its raw form to children because it would be harder to digest and could be carrier of pathogenic organisms. The milk may be pasteurized (milk, water and carbohydrates used in desired quantities and boiled), homogenized (fat globules broken into finer particles), skimmed (fat content removed to prevent certain digestive upsets such as diarrhea), or half-skimmed (generally given to obese children who need to be restricted in caloric intake).

2. Evaporated milk. This is made by a method of extracting water by heat and can be reconstituted to whole milk strength by adding water.

3. Dried milk, from which water is spray-dried. In the powdered form, this milk has a long shelf life and can be mixed with water to form whole milk. This is probably the

most ideal form of milk in developing countries where refrigeration facilities are meagre.

4. Condensed milk. This form has a much higher percentage of carbohydrates than protein.

5. Acidified milk, formed by adding lactic, citric, or acetic acid. This form has been occasionally used by doctors to treat cases of diarrhea or indigestion. This form makes a fine curd in the stomach and has an acidic pH and is well-tolerated by debilitated infants.

6. Protein milk, in which the curd has been separated from the whey and dried.

7. Vegetable milks. These specially-prepared milks have a vegetable base such as soybean, peanut, etc. These are milks of the future and may be an answer to feeding children in the densely populated areas of the world where animal reserves of milk and meat are scarce. India is producing a number of varieties of vegetable milks commercially, and experiments in elementary schools have proven their value in promoting growth equal to animal milk. A number of experiments over long-term periods have revealed that babies fed this milk showed absorption and retention of nitrogen as well as growth equivalent to those fed modified cow's milk (Graham *et al.,* 1970). Such encouraging results would usher in a new era of hope for the nutrition of milllions of babies who cannot get animal milk because of its scarcity. These vegetable-based milks also have great potential for those children who are intolerant of milk proteins or lactose.

The provision of biologically high quality proteins to preschool children is very essential to promote satisfactory growth. A vast majority of these children in the developing countries do not get high quality proteins from their regular diet because of their almost total dependence on food grains for sustenance. Their diet leaves them poor in certain essential amino acids, vitamins, as well as iron. The deficiency of the latter is probably the main reason for the high prevalence of anemia in the Eastern countries (Gutelius, 1969). It may be advisable, therefore, to fortify milk and milk products meant for preschool children with iron. Deficiency of iron may be especially pronounced in prematurely-born infants whose needs may be twice as high as in normal infants (*Medical Letter*, 1971). The following is a brief outline of the measures that a typical developing country, e.g. India, may adopt for the benefit of the health and well-being of its vulnerable sections of society:

1. Improved supply of animal milk by implementing modern and improved methods of raising cows and dairying.

2. Milk should be pasteurized and distributed through special centers, which would assure its availability at a reasonable cost so it can reach the poor consumer who needs it the most. In India, the draft report of the Committee on Child Care stressed the need of adopting a policy whereby children under three years of age get their daily needs of milk, even if the government has to resort to rationing the available quantities.

3. Powdered milk is still available on the international market which can be used to supplement the diet of school children by serving it with their lunches.

4. Powdered milk can also be used in small quantities to improve the quality of protein in the vegetable milk mentioned above.

As a result of nutritional research as well as extensive experiments on animals, it has been established that the properly manufactured milk from vegetable sources such as soybeans and ground nuts (peanuts) can be as useful in promoting growth provided their protein quality is improved by the addition of 10 to 20 percent animal milk, usually in the form of powdered milk.

It is strange but true that the confectionary made of milk products is the most popular in Eastern countries. In most instances, the milk is boiled, then split with the help of lemon or citric acid. The casein is used in the preparation of confectionary and the precious whey is thrown away. This is a callous waste of the scarce milk resources of these areas. The author supports the general recommendation of the Indian Committee on Child Care that

in places experiencing milk shortages, the use of whole milk for manufacture of sweets, pastries, ice creams, etc., may be prohibited and use
of whole milk by hotels and restaurants should be rationed and curtailed to bring about a distinct improvement in the supply position of
milk for children (*Draft Report of the Committee on Child Care,*
1961–62b).

SUPPLEMENTARY FOODS FOR INFANTS

The human female can successfully lactate for a number of months, even up to two or three years at a reduced
level of milk production. However, this is the most active
period of baby's growth, and because of ever-increasing
activity and progressively increased expenditures of calories,
the mother's milk may by the fourth or fifth month become
insufficient to satisfy the baby's needs. It seems important
that, starting from this period, some supplementary food
be given to the infant which could provide for his extra
needs (*Nutrition Reviews,* 1967). The extra food must not
only be digestible, but should be given in a form that the
infant can swallow easily. Besides, these foods should supply
extra vitamins A and C, and iron (Jelliffe, 1971); which the
mother's milk may not be able to provide in sufficient quantities. Properly prepared, the average infant can usually di-
gest cereal at $2\frac{1}{2}$ to $3\frac{1}{2}$ months, fruits at three to four months,
vegetables at four to five months, meat at five to six months,
and egg yolk (hard-boiled and grated) at five to six months.
Apart from milk, the addition of meat and egg yolks is the
best method of obtaining good sources of protein (Chandrasekhra, 1972). Table V gives an outline of a suggested
sequence for food additions to the infant's diet.

In Europe and North America, commercially-prepared
strained baby foods (cereals, vegetables, meats, and fruits)
are available in very convenient containers and the baby
can be fed according to his age and needs without difficulty.
In technologically underdeveloped countries of the East,
this convenience is not available to an average mother.
However, with a little incentive and some education as to
the infants' needs, the mother can prepare at home foods
which will be quite suitable for the growing infants (Jelliffe,

TABLE V

SEQUENCE FOR FOOD ADDITIONS TO INFANT'S DIET

Age	Food addition and its nutritive contribution
2–4 weeks	400 I.U. vitamin D from vitamin D milk or from a prescribed supplement.
2–4 weeks	Orange or grapefruit juice of other source of vitamin C; twice as much tomato juice needed; start with 1 teaspoon diluted with boiled water; increase gradually to 3 oz full strength by 3 months.
2–3 months	Cereal for iron, thiamine, calories; mix precooked cereal with formula; given thin consistency at first; increase to 2 to 5 tablespoons by 7 to 8 months.
3–4 months	Mashed ripe banana, applesauce, strained pears, apricots, prunes or peaches; start with 1 teaspoon and increase to 3–4 tablespoons by one year.
3–5 months	Strained asparagus, green beans, carrots, peas, spinach, squash, or tomatoes; start with 1 teaspoon, increasing to 3–4 tablespoons by end of the year.
4–6 months	Egg yolk for iron, vitamin A, thiamine, protein; mash hard-cooked egg with a little formula; use ¼ teaspoon at first.
5–7 months	Strained meats for protein, iron, B complex, sometimes prescribed as early as 6 weeks of age.
5–8 months	Crisp toast, zwieback, arrowroot cookies, teething biscuits.
7–8 months	Baked or mashed potato or enriched pastas for calories and some additional iron and B complex.
9–months	Peeled raw apple.
8–10 months	Chopped vegetables and fruits.
10 months	Whole egg; plain puddings, such as custard, Junket.

From: C. H. Robinson, *Basic Nutrition* and *Diet Therapy* (London, Macmillan, 1970).

1968). A good beginning can be made by boiling rice and making a fine paste of it. Milk can be added to it to make it thinner and this can be fed to the baby. Other cereals and vegetables can be similarly cooked and well-mashed to feed the infant. The poorer communities of the United States may also be in the same predicament for lack of economic power to buy commercially-prepared baby foods.

The nonavailability of supplementary foods in the developing countries is mainly responsible for the high prevalence of kwashiorkor and marasmus among the preschool children. Of these, most infants fail to achieve their genetic growth potential because of lack of food and recurrent infections, which a physiologically weak child cannot fight as well as a healthy one (Orkney, 1966). In numerous instances, the problem is not that of availability of foods, but of ignorance about the child's needs, and of superstition and lack of knowledge about the nutritive value of locally available foods. First, the child is kept too long on breast milk alone, which meets only partially his needs, and then he is abruptly put on adult food, which is harder to digest and is too spicy for the child. There is no provision for the transition period when the child needs extra supplements in the form that is easily digestible and not too spicy, which would irritate his gastrointestinal tract.

It may be useful to give briefly an account of some of the commonly given weaning foods in various countries. In most Middle Eastern countries, legume preparations, which are meant for adults, are given to the infants in a somewhat mashed form. In a large section of African communities, the child is weaned to whole wheat bread, potatoes, or other adult foods, and no eggs, fish or meat are given until the age of two to eight years (Food and Nutrition Board, 1966). In west Africa, the supplementary food is introduced at nine months and upwards, and consists of maize porridge, cooked yams, yam-flour porridge, bread, cooked rice and cassava meal porridge. In central Africa, cassava is the staple food and, as a paste, is given from three months onwards. In east Africa, soft bananas and maize gruels are given at six to seven months of age (Brock, 1952). In south Africa, maize porridge with small amounts of milk is given on weaning (Gillman and Gillman, 1951). In South and Central America, the supplementary infant diet consists of cereal or cereal porridge, cooked cassava or sweet potatoes and small quantities of legumes. Meats and eggs are not given because they are believed to cause digestive disorders (Autret and Behar, 1954; Gomez *et al.*, 1957; Graham, 1966; Waterlow and Vergara, 1956). In the Far East countries, infants are weaned on rice, cereals and wheat preparations with only small amounts of legumes and negligible amounts of milk. In Burma and the Philippines, milk is traditionally disliked.

In Malaya, only the Chinese occasionally give fresh fish and meat, whereas the Malays and Indians give only rice gruels or other cereals. In Indonesia, small amounts of a soy preparation, tempeh, are given, and in South Vietnam, besides rice gruels, small amounts of dried fish, fruits and condiments are also given (Patuardhan, 1964; Someswara *et al.*, 1959; May and Marcho, 1961; Oommen, 1953; Penalta, 1962).

In India, where a large segment of the population is vegetarian, eggs or fish are taboo for the children. Mothers are generally ignorant about the nutritive value of the common foods around them (Chandrasekhra, 1972). Vegetable sources of food, if properly used, can provide all the essential nutrients as effectively as the eggs, meat and other animal sources of food. Since the animal sources are more expensive and produced in smaller quantities, especially in the developing countries, it is a sagacious policy to formulate baby foods on the locally available vegetable sources. Certain quantities of milk in the form of powder can also enhance the nutritive value of these foods (Samsudin and Williams, 1967).

In most places, the cost of the food, whether it is locally available in raw form or is a processed food at the grocer's shelf, determines to a great extent its use by the family as well as the infant. Unfortunately, ready-to-serve processed foods are at present so expensive that a family belonging to a lower socio-economic class cannot afford them, in spite of the fact that it is the children of this class that need such a food the most. The national and local governments need to subsidize or regulate the price of baby foods to ensure that these are consumed by the economically depressed classes. As the process of urbanization increases in the developing countries, the significance of availability of the economically low-cost processed foods is becoming clearer day by day.

More foods must be standardized with respect to their nutrient content so that the consumer is aware of the diluted, over-sweetened, starch-filled processed weaning food that is at present flooding the markets in a number of countries

(Filer, 1971). A government agency must supervise the release of all the baby foods with respect to their nutritional value in view of their consumption by the most vulnerable sections of human society (Hayes *et al.,* 1965).

It is believed that the biggest deficiency in the developing countries is that of calories. The average caloric intake of an actively growing child is woefully low. In formulation of the infant diets, more attention is paid to the provisions of proteins and the caloric needs are often neglected, with the result that some protein is wasted as metabolized energy and an artificially-created protein deficiency appears. Chamberland and Stickney emphasized that, in order to improve children's diets in the developing countries, the processed food must satisfy the protein as well as the caloric needs, even if the whole concept of utilizing vegetable mixtures based on local availability has to be revised. The planner may have to consider the utilization of new products (Chamberland and Stickney, 1973).

The great responsibility that the food industry has towards the health and well-being of children was recently highlighted by Jelliffe (1971) in an article, "Commerciogenic Malnutrition?". While emphasizing the desirability of extending and popularizing the concept of producing in bulk the children's food based on vegetable mixtures, Jelliffe prodded the commercial firms engaged in the business to be responsible for the nutrition of the foods they sell (Berg, 1972). The food industry must realize that it is under the impact of their advertising of baby milk and foods that there is an undesirable decline in the beneficial practice of breast feeding among the lower economic groups of the developing countries (Wong, 1971). Although it is well recognized that the prime concern of the commercial firms is profitability, irresponsiblity towards the welfare of its clients in the name of profit is deeply immoral (Heilbrener, 1972). The trend must be reversed. At present the infant food industry operating in the developing countries is adding more confusion and misery and, as Jelliffe pointed out, the food industry "probably is a deleterious farce in regard to the nutrition of young children in technologically developing countries" (1971).

A word of caution about the salt consumption by infants may be added here. For good reasons, the human breast milk has a very low sodium content. An infant maintained on breast milk gets about 10 m Eq per day, which has proven to be enough for healthy growth (Mayer, 1972). On the contrary, cow's milk has about three times higher sodium content (30 m Eq per litre). A baby kept on cow's milk formula gets a very high level of sodium from the milk. On top of this, baby foods are introduced quite early which further increases the salt intake of the infant. Unfortunately, the housewife as well as the food industry uses the adult standards of food palatability for the infants. There is no indication that, for an infant, a highly salted food is preferable to a bland preparation. On the other hand, there is a lot of evidence that high doses of salts result in a variety of clinical manifestations. The tendency for edema to develop in a prematurely born infant is largely a function of the sodium in the diet (Mayer, 1972). Experimental work on animals shows that high salt intake induces permanent hypertension. Mayer (1969) rightly advised that "a reasonable policy would seem to be to instruct mothers not to add any salt to eggs, cereals or other dishes they prepare for their infants. Pediatricians and their professional societies should try to influence manufacturers of baby foods—who in other respects have tried to conform with sound nutritional concepts—to stop adding so much salt (or for that matter, to stop adding salt) to the foods they prepare. Manufacturers should be invited to participate in educational campaigns directed at the mothers to teach them not to use the same criterion in judging the *salt taste* of food for their infants as for adults" (Mayer, 1969).

DIETARY NEEDS OF INFANTS FOR NORMAL GROWTH

Proteins, Carbohydrates, Fats and Water

Protein is needed to provide for the growth of new tissues and to provide building material for the routine wear and tear. The infant goes through a period of rapid cell growth which characterizes an increased proportion of proteins in the body. The muscle mass is greatly increased and so far the protein requirements of other tissues, resulting in high levels of nitrogen retention. The proportion of body protein is increased from 12 percent in the infant to 18 percent in the adult (Ebbs, 1966). During the same period, the proportion of skeletal muscle increases from approximately 25 percent of body weight in the neonate to about 45 percent in the adult. Infants who do not get adequate quantities of protein suffer a great deal and are not able to realize their optimum growth potential. Breast milk is generally sufficient to provide for all the protein needs of the infant during the first few months.

As the child grows, the requirements of protein per kilogram of body weight surely and slowly decrease even more than the caloric requirements, which in terms of body weight are very high in the young infant as compared to the adult. An FAO study on protein requirements showed that in the older child, the protein needs are not as great as for the infant, whose major function of the body is centered around activity and growth, while maintenance alone does not require additional expenditure of nitrogen (FAO, 1957). The limiting factor in most human diets is not protein, or a particular essential amino acid, but nitrogen (Howe, *et al.,* 1965). Hegsted calculated the protein needs of a growing child as follows:

> The basal metabolism in calories per twenty-four hours multiplied by 12.5 gives the protein requirements for maintenance in milligrams. The gain in weight per day over the same period multiplied by 0.18 gives the protein deposited as tissue. The sum of these values is the amount of absorbed protein needed. An addition of 10 percent is made to account for losses through fecal excretions. The value thus arrived at should represent the need, when the protein eaten has a maximum biologic value of 100 percent. When the biologic value is lower than this, a larger amount would be needed, and the actual requirements would be the estimated maximum × 100 divided by the biologic value.

The infants, particularly, need proteins of high biological

value, i.e. a protein which can replace gram for gram, body losses of protein due to catabolic activity. In other words, the diet should provide the essential amino acids in certain proportions and nonessential amino acids, which may be used directly or to provide nitrogen for synthesizing purposes. Milk and egg proteins from this point of view are close to ideal and are best for promoting satisfactory growth of infants and preschool children (Hegsted, 1957). Chan and Waterlow estimated the protein requirements of infants at about one year's age. They found that, based on nitrogen balance, 100 mg/N/kg/day is the average maintenance requirement. An intake of proteins at the level of 200 mg/ N/kg per day proved sufficient to produce normal growth as well as satisfactory nitrogen retention (Chan and Waterlow 1966).

It may be said that the growth rate of babies goes hand in hand with the protein content in the milk and the total caloric intake, as is evidenced by the growth pattern in different species. In humans the milk contains 1.3 percent protein and it takes a human baby 120 days to double its birth weight. In the case of horses, cows, sheep and dogs, the protein content of the milk is 2.1 percent, 3.5 percent, 5.2 percent and 9.7 percent respectively, and it takes these offspring sixty, forty-seven, fifteen and nine days respectively to double their birth weights (Degwitz, 1969).

In this context, a word of caution about feeding large quantities of protein in the diet may be in order. The above mentioned growth rates are programmed in the species, which cannot be changed by drinking the milk from those animals. If proteins are given in excessive quantities and are utilized for providing energy as well, a number of undesirable effects could be produced, such as slowing growth rate, increase in the level of material requiring detoxification, and excessive calorie expenditure in specific dynamic action of protein metabolism (Willis, 1964). It is imperative that only sufficient calories from proteins be derived in order to promote efficient protein utilization. Excessive protein intake results in high renal solute load, resulting in a reduced margin of expendable water. Human milk to the baby provides approximately 10 percent of the calories from protein, which appears to be sufficient for maintenance of a metabolic equilibrium as well as balanced growth.

Halac's work on rats is interesting in this respect. He fed two groups of rats, beginning from the time of weaning to the period of maximum body growth, with diets containing 27 percent and 64 percent protein. Body analysis of high protein animals revealed higher proportions of nitrogen and lower proportions of fat, showing hypertrophy of the liver and kidney at the same time. The liver in these animals had to deaminate a greater load of amino acids and the kidney had to excrete more urea. Halac, after the experimental period, put both the groups on a protein-free diet and found that both the groups showed a comparable weight loss, but as time passed, the rats on the lower protein diet showed a significantly higher survival rate compared to the group previously fed very high levels of protein (Halac, 1960).

The carbohydrates mainly serve the purpose of providing calories and energy for various activities. Carbohydrates may not be as essential as proteins needed for body-building, or fats as a source of essential fatty acids and carriers of some vitamins, and tests have been conducted keeping infants on carbohydrate-free diets for prolonged periods of time (Chwalibogowski, 1973). Nevertheless, carbohydrates free the proteins for the main task of body-building by providing the energy needed for basal metabolism and physical activity. Also, carbohydrates are a good source of calories, and when a baby is maintained on a carbohydrate-free diet, it is difficult to avoid the development of ketosis. A crying baby needs twice as many calories and energy as compared to a baby that is quiet and resting. Carbohydrates in the form of lactose are found in double the amount in human milk (9.5 percent) as compared to cow's milk (4.9 percent), and are well-utilized by the infant. A baby suffering from infection may be given a sugar solution which, in addition to supplying a ready source of energy, also provides a satisfactory balance in the assimilation of fat and protein (Ebbs, 1966).

As a general rule, carbohydrates should supply at least half the calories needed by the body. Fortunately, starches and cereals which have large amounts of carbohydrates are more easily produced than the foods rich in proteins. In terms of body weight, the energy requirements of infants are much higher than for older children or adults. It has been estimated that about 50 percent of the total caloric intake is spent on basal metabolism, 25 percent on random activity, 12 percent on satisfying the growth requirements, 3 percent for specific dynamic action, and 10 percent is lost in feces and urine or other modes of insensible water loss (Willis, 1964).

Fats are not only a concentrated source of calories, providing nine calories per gram, but are also the source of essential fatty acids (e.g. linoleic or arachidonic acid) so important for a healthy skin (Adam, 1958). A diet deficient in linoleic acid leads to dryness and thickness of skin accompanied by desquamation. Fats are also essential as carriers of fat-soluble vitamins, and it is highly desirable to include certain amounts of fat in the diet of the infant. Vegetable fats such as seed oils, soybeans oil, corn oil, etc., are a good source of linoleic acid and in a more fluid form than animal fats. They may, therefore, be more easily emulsified in the body as compared to animal fats (DeSilva and Baptist, 1964).

Under certain conditions, infants may not be able to tolerate the higher fat content in animal milk; for example, during an episode of infection, particularly if it is accompanied by nausea, vomitting or diarrhea. Even in normal infants, the fats from animal milk are not as efficiently utilized as those from human milk. Kaumer and Weigers estimated that the normal infant utilizes 93 to 97 percent of the fat from human milk compared to 83 to 95 percent from cow's milk. Infants well-fed on breast milk generally show adequate quantities of subcutaneous fat. Some basic principles in feeding infants and children have been summarized by Collipp (1973)

1. The diet should be adequate but not excessive in calories and all essential nutrients
2. The diet and the way it is fed should be conducive to the development of sound eating habits
3. The diet should be readily digestible
4. A reasonable distribution of calories should be derived from protein (7% to 16% calories), fat (35% to 55% of calories), and carbohydrates (35% to 65% of calories).

Water as a principal component of infant food plays an extremely important role in the maintenance of cellular equilibrium; e.g. the electrolytic balance, by maintaining the ionic composition in the intra- and extracellular spaces, in metabolic reactions, especially in maintaining the body heat, and in the regulation of excretion of urea. If the water intake of the infant is smaller than the desired quantity, the body makes every effort to adapt by reducing water losses. A study of water balance in infants reveals that infants can cut down their water losses by as much as 90 percent (Drescher *et al.*, 1962). However, if water deficits persist for a long time, the result may be dangerous, and symptoms of toxicity due to lack of expulsion of metabolic wastes may appear. It is very rare to have a condition in which the infant has been given excessive amounts of water. If such is the case, the result may be edema, hypervolemia, dilution of urine and water intoxication.

The infant is especially susceptible to water loss because of greater water losses through kidney and skin as compared to the adult, and could become dehydrated within a relatively short period of water deficiency. For a healthy infant, seventy-five millilitres per kilogram of body weight may be enough, but it is a good practice to give up to 150 ml/kg body weight in order to provide an adequate margin of safety (Holt and Synderman, 1968). In hot weather, when the loss of water through the skin may be very high, it is desirable to give generous amounts of water.

Vitamins and Minerals

The vitamin needs of infants and preschool children are similar to the adolescents and adults, and a detailed description is given in the next chapter. Table VI also outlines the need for important vitamins at different stages of infant growth. However, some comments about their special needs may be in order. For example, babies are born with very little stores of vitamin K. A complete lack of it can cause hemorrhage. Fortunately, it is customary these days for physicians to give a dose of vitamin K in the first hours of life. Milk contains limited quantities of vitamins C and D. Vitamin C is needed for the formation of connective tissues and some other important functions in the body, whereas vitamin D helps in the utilization of calcium and phosphorus, and is therefore of vital importance.

Orange juice or tomato juice are good sources of vitamin C. Unfortunately, a vast majority of children in the developing countries do not get those foods that are rich in vitamin C. In these countries, children on milk alone do not get enough vitamin D to allow full absorption and utilization of calcium and phosphorus, resulting in skeletal abnormalities, spongy bones, and bad postures. Such children, either through insufficient exposure to sunlight or lack of vitamin D in the diet, are not able to reach their normal height as adults.

In developing countries, where milk is not fortified with vitamin D, it is essential that children be exposed to sunlight or given a spoonful of cod liver oil on alternate days. The importance of sufficient quantities of vitamin B in the diet of children can never be overemphasized. Infants and preschool children are very energetic and expend energy at a much higher rate than adults. They also consume more carbohydrates for getting energy; hence, they need more vitamin B complex because most of these are used for the production of energy; for example, thiamine is used in the

TABLE VI

RECOMMENDED DAILY DIETARY ALLOWANCES OF VARIOUS NUTRIENTS FOR INFANTS AND CHILDREN

	Age[1] (years)	Weight (kg)	Weight (lbs)	Height (cm)	Height (in.)	kcal	Protein (gm)	FAT-SOLUBLE VITAMINS Vitamin A activity (IU)	Vitamin D (IU)	Vitamin E activity (mg)
Infants	0–1/6	4	9	55	22	kg × 120	kg × 2.2[4]	1,500	400	5
	1/6–1/2	7	15	63	25	kg × 110	kg × 2.0[4]	1,500	400	5
	1/2–1	9	20	72	28	kg × 100	kg × 1.8[4]	1,500	400	5
Children	1–2	12	26	81	32	1,100	25	2,000	400	10
	2–3	14	31	91	36	1,250	25	2,000	400	10
	3–4	16	35	100	39	1,400	30	2,500	400	10
	4–6	19	42	110	43	1,600	30	2,500	400	10
	6–8	23	51	121	48	2,000	35	3,300	400	10
	8–10	28	62	131	52	2,200	40	3,300	400	10

	Ascorbic acid (mg)	Folacin[2] (mg)	WATER-SOLUBLE VITAMINS Niacin (mg equiv)[3]	Riboflavin (mg)	Thiamine (mg)	Vitamin B6 (mg)	Vitamin B12 (ug)	Calcium (g)	Phosphorus (g)	MINERALS Iodine (ug)	Iron (mg)	Magnesium (mg)
Infants	35	0.05	5	0.4	0.2	0.3	0.3	0.4	0.2	25	6	40
	35	0.05	7	0.5	0.4	0.3	0.3	0.5	0.4	40	10	60
	35	0.1	8	0.6	0.5	0.4	0.3	0.6	0.5	45	15	70
Children	40	0.1	8	0.6	0.6	0.5	1.0	0.8	0.7	55	15	100
	40	0.2	8	0.7	0.6	0.6	1.5	0.8	0.8	60	15	150
	40	0.2	9	0.8	0.7	0.7	1.5	0.8	0.8	70	10	200
	40	0.2	11	0.9	0.8	0.9	2.0	0.8	0.8	80	10	200
	40	0.2	13	1.1	1.0	1.0	2.0	0.9	0.9	100	10	250
	40	0.3	15	1.2	1.1	1.2	2.0	1.0	1.0	110	10	250

[1] The allowance levels are intended to cover individual variations among most normal persons as they live in the United States under usual environmental stresses. The recommended allowances can be attained with a variety of common foods, providing other nutrients for which human requirements have been less well defined.

[2] The folacin allowances refer to dietary sources as determined by *Lactobacillus casei* assay. Pure forms of folacin may be effective in doses less than 1/4 of the RDA.

[3] Niacin equivalents include dietary sources of the vitamin itself plus 1 mg equivalent for each 60 mg of dietary tryptophan.

[4] Assumes protein equivalent to human milk. For proteins not 100 percent utilized factors should be increased proportionately.

From: Food and Nutrition Board, National Academy of Sciences, National Research Council Pub No. 2216, 1974.

burning of sugar to produce energy. A deficiency of thiamine could produce symptoms like anorexia, wasting, irritability and loss of reflexes (Ebbs, 1966). The deficiency of nicotinic acid may not be manifest as long as the amino acid, tryptophan, is available in the food in sufficient quantities, because the body can synthesize from this source (Holt and Synderman, 1968). Choline is another B vitamin which can be synthesized by the body in the presence of the amino acid, methionine.

Whereas it may be a good practice to give vitamin supplements daily in the form of drops or tablets, it is important to emphasize here that overdoing it may be harmful to the infant. This is especially true of vitamin A and vitamin D. Excessive vitamin A continued over a period of time, has caused cases of mental retardation among children. Hypervitaminosis A leads at first to a severe vomitting condition, but if the dose is continued to the extent of ten times the recommended dosage, it results in tender swellings in large bones, enlarged liver and spleen, kidney involvement, and loss of hair and skin (Ebbs, 1966). Massive doses of vitamin D cause excessive deposition of calcium and phosphorus. Nausea, polyurea and idiopathic hypercalcemia are associated with overdosage of vitamin D. Therefore, it is extremely important to the health of the infant that large doses of these two vitamins not be given in vitamin supplements. The levels of these vitamins that occur in natural foods are not at all toxic.

The mineral needs of infants and preschool children are generally satisfied when given a regular diet containing a generous quantity of milk. These quantities should promote optimum growth, and extra mineral supplements may not be needed. However, some comments may be made about some minerals, the insufficiency of which may have an adverse effect on the health of the infant. For example, babies are born in calcium-poor conditions. For a positive calcium balance, one gram of calcium per day would be needed, and this would require an intake of one quart of milk per day. In most of the developing countries, the average parents cannot afford to give this large a quantity. With a pint of milk, the losses of calcium may exceed intake, thus resulting in growth stunting.

The iodine needs of a growing child are approximately three times those of an adult. Either a few drops of iodine preparation or small quantities of iodized salt may be given, along with the semisolid foods. Iron is another important mineral the intake of which needs to be carefully monitored. In order to maintain hemoglobin levels in normal ranges, it is essential that the growing child be given either iron-supplemented milk or semisolid foods rich in iron. In the young infant fed on breast milk, iron deficiency is a likely possibility. The prematurely-born infant, lacking the normally present birth stores of iron, may be more susceptible to iron deficiency. It is estimated that under one year, the infant requires a daily intake of six milligrams of iron, which increases to seven milligrams between the ages of one and three years, to eight milligrams between the ages of four and six years, and to ten milligrams from the ages of seven to nine years. In the developing countries of the tropical regions, the iron intake is sufficient and may be as much as twenty to thirty milligrams a day, but a major part of this iron is not absorbed by the body because the diet consists of bulky cereals with high contents of phosphates and phytates (De-Silva and Baptist, 1964). Due to warmer weather, the iron losses through perspiration may also be fairly high.

Special mention may be made of the acid-base equilibrium provided by sodium chloride in the mineral requirements of infants. Although no different from adults, infants are more susceptible to the disturbance of this delicate balance because of episodes of vomitting or diarrhea caused by diet or certain other conditions. Losing chloride, such as occurs in vomitting, may result in alkalosis. Too much salt in the food of an infant or in intravenous infusions may exceed renal excretion and result in fever. Sodium and chloride occur chiefly in the extracellular fluids. A salt deficiency, which usually occurs as a result of losses from the gastrointestinal tract, may result in dehydration (Ebbs, 1966).

It is not advisable under normal circumstances to give
mineral supplements, because an adequately-fed infant gets
all the necessary minerals. The pediatrician may do well to
advise the mothers against too much enthusiasm for vitamin-
mineral supplements for the baby. Being available without
prescription at the drugstore, some mothers are likely to over-
load the infant under the belief that extra quantities are always excreted without any ill effects to the baby. Some
mention has already been made regarding the dangers of
giving excessive quantities of vitamins A and D. Excessive
amounts of minerals, either in the diet or taken orally as mineral supplements, could also be detrimental to the health of
the infant because they impose a high renal solute load and
may induce renal hypertrophy. Excessive quantities of minerals can also interfere with cellular osmotic relationships
which will upset the electrolyte balance and obligate large
amounts of water for renal excretion. As renal loss of water
increases, the margin of expendable water is reduced. The
water balance may become critical if there are increased
extra-renal water losses through evaporative cooling, vomitting and/or diarrhea (Willis, 1964).

SOCIO-CULTURAL INFLUENCES AFFECTING INFANT NUTRITION IN DEVELOPING COUNTRIES

Inadequate food supply and rapidly increasing population in the developing countries are mainly responsible for
poor infant feeding, but it cannot be denied that ignorance,
poor environment and traditional cultural beliefs play an
equally important role in perpetuating the misery of a growing child. Poverty is a seriously limiting factor in most of the
developing countries and in large segments of the developed
countries as well. In fact, its impact on the nutrition of infants and preschool children is so obvious that it does not
need any detailed discussion. However, lack of adequate
quantities of the right types of food is not the sole reason for
the prevalent malnutrition. A careful analysis of the food
availability and infant feeding practices would reveal that
much of the misery can be avoided if only the cultural taboos

and superstitions are removed. Among the majority of the rural populations, a scientific knowledge of nutrition and food is conspicuous by its absence. On top of that, poor environmental conditions such as poor sanitation greatly affect the nutritional status of this vulnerable segment of the society. Deodhar explained that the food which may be otherwise adequate, may be rendered ineffective as a result of general or local infections, infective diarrheas, helminthic infestations, etc., by increasing the demand or by reducing the absorption and assimilation of food. In poor environments, infant food may be infected in all possible ways.

Traditional or cultural ideas about food are the main obstacles in any improvement program. Rice in countries of South and Southeast Asia is a superfood. It is considered a symbol of life and is a must for the infants. Other foods are avoided, or at best, given in small quantities. Other protective foods such as eggs are not given because of the cultural belief that they are too *hot* for the children. Fish, a major source of protein, is prohibited to young children in Malaya because it is believed to produce worms. Instead, the toddler is weaned primarily on cereals. In most Eastern countries, where joint family systems prevail and the grandparents live with their children, the grandmother will have absolute authority on how to feed the baby. She takes upon herself this role because she claims to have experience in child-raising, and to all practical purposes, she dictates what the child should be given and what it must not be given. In most instances, this feeding program reflects the cultural influences without any regard for the nutritional needs of the child (Jelliffe, 1966; 1967).

The remarks of Dr. P. C. Sen, as quoted by Jelliffe, describing the Indian situation, may be appropriately reproduced here.

There are elaborate rules prohibiting consumption of various articles of diet on certain days of the lunar month. For example, (i), if patol (*Trichoxanthas dioica*) is eaten on the third day of the moon, the consumer will have the misfortune of increasing the number of his enemies; (ii), radish on the fourth would mean the loss of wealth;

(iii), coconut on the eighth day would make the consumer a dunce; (iv), beans on the eleventh day would lead to sinful acts; (v), gourd and allied vegetables on the thirteenth day might result in the loss of one's son, and so on. The restrictions are minutely recorded in the Hindu calendar and one wonders what could be the reason for such restrictions. They have been designed as an attempt to assure stable conditions of food supply by regulating the distribution of edible fruits and vegetables (Jelliffe, 1971).

It is evident from the above account that an average mother in an underdeveloped country is tradition-bound and culturally biased in raising her child. If she has learned from traditions that potatoes or a starchy pap or rice is the super-food and is good for her baby, she is not likely to listen to any advice that excludes that cultural food to which she is attached. A nutritionist's and his coworkers' duty is to give fundamental education in nutrition to the mother and convince her to use other locally-available foods, along with her cultural super-food, so that the baby can get an easily digestible balanced food. Care should be taken to recommend to her only those foods which she is accustomed to handling in her kitchen for preparing food for her husband and older children, or a food which is cheap, locally available and usable for other members of the family as well. In doing so, the nutrition field worker is not interfering with her cultural background. He may also find her receptive to the occasional use of commercially prepared baby foods (discussed elsewhere) sold in packaged form in the market if she is told that they contain nothing else but the staples that she uses at home, but are prepared in a manner that provides a balanced diet for her baby.

Deodhar believes the growing industrialization in developing countries like India is a contributing factor in poorer nutrition of the children. In rural areas, the farmers who once produced food crops have switched to cash crops because of their demand by the growing industries, and in the process, have deprived the children of the easy supply of nutritious foods close to home. Deodhar described that:

with industrialization, the old and simple production-consumption type of economy is being changed into the more and more complex forms of production-distribution-consumption economy. In this money economy, while the people have lost the traditional adjustments, they have not yet reached the ecological balance in the new setting and have to choose articles of food entirely on the basis of expense and availability. Unfortunately, because of maladjustment the choice has not coincided with the nutritional needs of an infant, resulting in its poor feeding.

In most developing countries, the common infections are rampant due mainly to inadequate food and unsanitary conditions. Most common is the diarrheal disease which is the major cause of depleting the child and precipitating syndromes like kwashiorkor, marasmus, avitaminosis A, measles, whooping cough, tuberculosis and other syndromes which precipitate malnutritional disease. Sanitary surroundings, personal hygiene of those handling the child, especially the mother, feeding the infant from clean utensils and providing uncontaminated water can go a long way in improving the environment of the child. This process of close contact with the disease processes seems to start from the first day of life of the infant. To give only a few examples, in certain areas, cow dung or black clay is applied to the umbilical cord, or it is left unbandaged, which could lead to tetanus or other infections. In other places, sharp bamboo is used to cut the umbilical cord because steel is considered unauspicious, while in still other places, the dried-out cord is used as a charm around the child's neck because of some superstition (Jelliffe, 1968).

The early discomforts or ailments of a child are generally ignored in the belief that they will be corrected by themselves. But when the ailment persists, household remedies are tried without any regard to symptoms or exact nature of the ailment. It is only when high fever persists and the child appears utterly helpless that medical care is sought. By that time, it is generally too late to help the baby. Even without serious illness, the babies are purged regularly with castor oil or other decoctions, with the result that they lose intestinal flora (Burgess and Dean, 1962). The purgative also has an irritating effect on the intestinal wall. In other places, children are branded to cure colics, which could be very painful, even traumatic, for the child. In some communities, a little opium is given to keep the child drowsy, so that the mother will be able to work outdoors (Chandrasekhra, 1972). This is most undesirable.

These are just a few examples of the tradition-ridden ways of infant welfare which, in spite of the best intentions, prove harmful. If the child is uncomfortable, cries and has fever, no household remedies should be tried. Describing the causes of protein malnutrition in South India, Someswara Rao has described that a sick child does not get any better attention. It is also not unusual to find children suffering from various infections—diarrhea, extensive dermatitis or even nutritional edema—being kept at home without proper medical treatment. They are sometimes treated with traditional household medicines or a variety of talismans are tied to them until the disease reaches an advanced state. Except for smallpox vaccination, which is forced on them periodically by the Public Health Department, the children receive no other prophylactic inoculations. This apparent neglect on the part of the parents to pay attention to the personal hygiene or the health needs of the children must be attributed chiefly to their ignorance about the proper methods of care and upbringing, tradition-bound outlooks and superstitions. Poverty and the absence of facilities for medical aid in some villages is also responsible for this state of affairs (Someswara *et al.*, 1959). Jelliffe has rightly remarked that:

> nutrition programmers should be coordinated with other health activities and should use existing health services to the fullest extent possible. They should also be closely tied to national agricultural and economic planning. Nutrition is so intimately related to environmental sanitation and disease control as well as to agricultural production and economic policy that an isolated approach to the nutrition problems of the preschool child is unsound and usually ineffective (1968).

REFERENCES

Acheson, E. D., and Truelove, S. C.: *Br Med J, 2:* 929, 1961.
Adam, S. J. D.: *J Nutr, 66:* 55, 1958.

Applebaum, R. M.: *Pediatr Clin North Am, 17:* 203, 1970.

Autret, M., and Behar, M.: *F.A.O. Nutrition Studies,* Publ. #13, 1954.

Barnes, L. A. *et al.: J Pediatr, 51:* 29, 1957.

Beal, V. A.: *J Am Dietet Assoc, 55:* 31, 1969.

Bennett, F. J., and Stanfield, J. P.: Recent approaches to malnutrition in Uganda. *J Trop Pediatr, 17:* 1, March, 1971.

Berg, A.: *Harvard Bus Rev,* Jan.–Feb., 130, 1972.

Brambell, F. W. R.: *Proc Nutr Soc, 28:* 35, 1967.

Brock, J. F., and Autret, M.: *WHO Monograph,* No. 8, 1952.

Brown, R. E.: *Am J Clin Nutr, 62:* 556, 1973.

Burgess, A., and Dean, R. F.: In *Malnutrition and Food Habits.* London, Travistock, 1962.

Chamberland, J. G., and Stickney, R. E.: *Nutr Rep Int, 7:* 71, 1973.

Chan, H. A., and Waterlow, T. C.: *Br J Nutr, 20:* 775, 1966.

Chandrasekhra, S.: *Infant Mortality, Population Growth and Family Planning in India.* Chapel Hill, U NC Pr, 1972.

Chwalibogowski, L.: *Acta Pediatr, 22:* 110, 1973.

Churchman, J.: *J Obstet Gynecol Br Commonw, 61:* 364, 1954.

Clemetson, C. A. B., and Churchman, J.: *J Obstet Gynecol Br Commonw, 61:* 364, 1954.

Collipp, P. J.: *Am J Dis Child, 126:* 558, 1973.

Cornblath, M., Baens, G. S., and Lundeon, E.; *Am J Dis Child, 102:* 729, 1965.

Cornblath, M., Forbes, M. E., Pildes, R. S., Liebben, G., and Greengard, J.: *Pediatrics, 38:* 547, 1964.

Cox, L. W., and Chalmers, T. A.: *J Obstet Gynecol Br Commonw, 60:* 203, 1953.

Crass, V. M.: *The Premature Baby.* London, J. & A. Churchill, 1957.

Danes, W. L.: *The Chemistry of Milk.* London, Chapman and Hall, 1939; MacKeith and Wood, 1971.

Davies, J. A., Harvey, D. R., and Vu, J. S.: *Arch Dis Child, 40:* 46, 1965.

Davies, P. A.: *Proc Nutr Soc, 28:* 66, 1969.

Davies, P., and Russell, H.: *Dev Med Child Neurol, 10:* 725, 1968.

Degwitz, R.: In Pfaundler, M., and Scholossman, A. (Eds.): *The Diseases of Children.* Philadelphia, Lippincott, Vol. 1, p. 195, 1969.

Deodhar, N. S.: *Indian J Med Sci, 21:* 768, 1967.

DeSilva, C. C., and Baptist, N. G.: *Tropical Nutritional Disorders of Infants and Children.* Springfield, Thomas, 1964.

Dobbing, J.: In Davison, A. N., and Dobbing, J. (Eds.): *Applied Neurochemistry.* Oxford, Blackwell Scientific Publications, 1968.

Draft Report of the Committee on Child Care. New Delhi, Central Social Welfare Board, Ministry of Education, p. 127, 1961–1962.

Drescher, A. N., Barnett, H. L., and Troupkou, V.: *Am J Dis Child, 104:* 366, 1962.

Duncan, D. L.: *Nutr Abstr Rev, 25:* 309, 1955.

Durham, E. C.: *Premature Infants.* Washington, Federal Security Agency, 1948.

Ebbs, J. H.: In Beaton, G. H., and McHenry, E. W. (Eds.) : *Nutrition.* New York, Aladine, 1966, vol. III.

FAO: *Protein Requirements and Nutritional Studies,* No. *16.* Rome, FAO, 1957.

FAO: *Third World Survey.* F.F.H.C. Basic Study, Nov. 11, 1963.

Fetal, Infant and Early Childhood Mortality. New York, United Nations, 1952, vol. 2.

Filer, L. J.: *Nutr Rev, 29:* 55–66, 1971.

Food and Nutrition Board. *Preschool Malnutrition,* Publ. No. 1282. Washington, National Academy of Sciences, 1966.

Foman, S. J., and May, C. D.: *Pediatrics, 22:* 101, 1958.

Forbes, G. B.: *Pediatrics, 29:* 3, 1962.

Gaensbaur, T. J., and Emde, R. N.: *Arch Gen Psychiatry, 28:* 894, 1973.

Ghadini, H., Arulanantham, K., and Rathi, M.: *Am J Clin Nutr, 26:* 473, 1973

Gillman, J., and Gillman, T.: *Perspectives in Human Malnutrition.* New York, Grune and Stratton, 1951.

Gofalam, C.: *J Trop Pediatr, 3:* 3, 1957.

Goldman, H. H., Karelitz, S., Acs, H., and Seifter, E.: *Pediatrics, 30:* 909, 1962.

Gomez, F., Galvan, R. R., and Munoz, J. C.: *Pediatrics, 10:* 513, 1957.

Gopalan, G., and Belavady, B.: *Fed Proc, 20:* 183, 1961.

Gordon, H. H., Levine, S. Z., Wheatly, M. A., and Marples, E.: *Am J Dis Child, 54:* 1030, 1937.

Graham, G. G.: *National Academy of Sciences, Publ. #1282,* Washington, 1966.

Graham, G. G., Placko, R. P., Morales, E., Acenedo, G., and Cordano, A.: *Am J Dis Child, 120:* 419, 1970.

Grulee, C. G.: *JAMA, 103:* 735, 1934.

Grulee, C. G., and Sanford, H. N.: *J Pediatr, 9:* 223, 1936.

Gutelius, M. F.: *Am J Public Health, 59:* 290, 1969.

Halac, E.: *J Fed Proc, 19:* 326, 1960.

Hayes, R. T., Rinna, A., and Soderhjelm, L.: *Acta Pediatr, 54:* 574, 1965.

Hegsted, M. J.: *Am Dietet, 33:* 225, 1957.

Heilbrener, R. L.: *In the Name of Profit: Profiles in Corporate Irresponsibility.* New York, Doubleday, (1972).

Holt, L. E.: In Brock, J. F. (Ed.) : *Recent Advances in Human Nutrition.* Boston, Little, 1961.

Holt, L. E., and Synderman, S. E.: In *Nutrition in Health and Science.* 1968.

Howding, P. G. R., and Shelley, H. J.: In *Intrauterine Dangers to the Fetus.* Amsterdam, Excerpta Medica Foundation, (1967), p. 529.

Howe, E. E., Jensen, G. R., and Gilfillan, E. W.: *Am J Clin Nutr, 16:* 315, 321, 1965.

Hull, D.: *Proc Nutr Soc, 28:* 56, 1969.

Hytten, F. E., and Leitch, I.: *The Physiology of Human Pregnancy.* Oxford, Blackwell, 1964.

Illingworth, R. S.: *The Normal Child.* London, J. & A. Churchill, 1968.

Jali, E. C.: *Leech, 21:* 17, 1950.

Jean, P. C., Wright, F. H., and Blake, F. G.: *Essentials of Pediatrics.* Philadelphia, Lippincott, 1958.

Jelliffe, D. B.: *Courrier, 6:* 191, 1956.

Jelliffe, D. B.: *Pediatrics, 20:* 128, 1957.

Jelliffe, D. B.: *J Trop Pediatr, 13:* 117, 1967.

Jelliffe, D. B.: *Infant Nutrition in the Subtropics and Tropics.* WHO, 1968.

Jelliffe, D. B.: *Food Techn, 25:* 55, 1971.

Jelliffe, D. B.: In Rechciql, M. (Ed.) : *Food, Nutrition and Health. World Rev Nutr Diet,* 1973, vol. 16.

Jelliffe, D. B., and Jelliffe, E. F. P.: *Am J Clin Nutr, 24:* 968–1024, 1971.

Kaumer, Van De, J. H., and Weigers, H. A.: *Fed Proc, 20:* 336, 1961.

Keen, P.: *Leech, 17:* 30, 1946.

Kenny, J. F., Boesman, M. I., and Michaels, R. H.: *Pediatrics, 39:* 202, 1967.

Lahery, N. L.: *Proc Symp Food Need and Resources.* India, National Institute of Sciences, 1962, p. 190.

Levin, S. S.: *A Philosophy of Infant Feeding.* Springfield, Thomas, 1963.

Levine, S. Z., and Gordon, H. H.: *Am J Dis Child, 64:* 297, 1942.

Lewis, J. M., Bodansky, O., Lillienfeld, M. C., and Schneider, H.: *Am J Diseased Child, 73:* 143, 1947.

Lovern, J. A.: In Alschul, A. M. (Ed.) : American Chemical Society, 1966.

Lowenberg, M. E., Todhunter, E. N., Wilson, E. D., Feeney, N. C., and Savage, J. R.: *Food and Man.* New York, Wiley, 1968.

MacKeith, R., and Wood, C.: *Infant Feeding and Feeding Difficulties.* London, J. & A. Churchill, 1971.

Manocha, S. L.: *Malnutrition and Retarded Human Development.* Springfield, Thomas, 1972.

May, J. M., and Marcho, I. S.: *The Ecology of Malnutrition in the Far and Near East.* New York, Hafner, 1961.

Mayer, J.: *Postgrad Med, 45:* 1, 1969.

Mayer, J.: *Human Nutrition.* Springfield, Thomas, 1972.

McCance, R. A., and Widdowson, E. M.: *Proc Roy Soc B, 141:* 488, 1953.

McCance, R. A.: In *The Adaptation of the Newborn Infant to Extra-Uterine Life.* Nutricia Symposium, New York, 1964.

Mead, N., and Newton, M.: In Richardson, A., and Guttamacher, A. F. (Eds.) : *Child Bearing: Its Social and Psychological Aspects.* New York, Williams and Wilkins, 1967.

Medical Letter, 13: 16, August 6, 1971.

Naismith, D. J.: *Metabolism, 15:* 582, 1966.

Naismith, D. J.: *Proc Nutr Soc, 28:* 25, 1969.

Neligan, G. A.: *Proc Nutr Soc, 28:* 49, 1969.

Newton, N.: *Child Family Digest, 1:* 16.

Nutrition Reviews, 21: 113, 1963.

Nutrition Reviews, 25: 225, 1967.

Odlum, S. M.: *Nutr Child Welfare, 3:* 3, 1948.

Olsen, B.: *Studies on Intestinal Flora of Infants.* Copenhagen, Munksgaard, 1949.

Oommen, H. A. P. C.: *Bull WHO, 9:* 371, 1953.

Orkney, J. M.: *Ind Med Gazette, 150:* 81, 1966.

Orr, Lord Boyd: *Nature, 149:* 734, 1939.

Osborn, G. R.: *Colloques int cent Nat Rech Scient, No. 169:* 83, 1968.

Page, E. W., Glendening, M. B., Margolis, A., and Harper, H. A.: *Am J Obstet Gynecol, 73:* 589, 1957.

Patvardhan, V. N.: *Proc 6th Int Conf Nutr,* Edinburgh, Livingstone, 1964.

Parpia, H. A. B., Narayana, Rao M., Rajagopalan, R., and Swaminathan, M.: *J Nutr Diet, 1:* 114, 1964.

Perlman, H. H., Dannenberg, A. M., and Sokoloff, N.: *JAMA, 120:* 103, 1942.

Penalta, F. L.: *J Phillipp Med Ass, 38:* 675, 1962.

Platt, B. S.: *Fed Proc, 20:* Suppl. 7, 188, 1961.

Powers, G. F.: *Pediatrics, 145:* 1948.

Recommended Daily Dietary Allowances of Various Nutrients for Infants and Children. Food and Nutrition Board, National Academy of Sciences, National Research Council, 1968.

Richelderfer, T. E., Levin, S., and McPherson, T. C.: *Am J Dis Child, 114:* 385, 1967.

Robinson, M.: *Lancet, 260:* 788, 1951.

Robinson, C. H.: *Basic Nutrition and Diet Therapy.* London, Macmillan, 1970.

Samsudin, M. D., and Williams, M. L.: *Am J Clin Nutr, 20:* 1308, 1967.

Samuelson, G.: *Acta Pediatrics,* [Suppl] 214, 1971.

Sharma, J.: *Trop Pediatr, 1:* 47, 1955.

Shelley, H. J.: *Proc Nutr Soc, 28:* 42, 1969.

Silverman, W. A., and Sinclair, J. C.: *New Engl J Med, 274:* 448, 1966.

Someswara, Rao K., Swaminathan, M. C., Swarup, S., and Patwardham, V. N.: *Bull WHO, 20:* 603, 1959.

Strauls, C. P., and Murphy, G. K.: *Pediatrics, 36:* 732, 1965.

Swaminathan, J.: *Nutr Dietet, 3:* 138, 1966.

Swaminathan, M., and Parpia, H. A. B.: *World Rev Nutr Dietet, 8:* 1967.

Swaminathan, M.: *World Review Nutr Diet, 9:* 1968.

Time Magazine: Unborn Baby Swallows Bullet, June 14, 1968.

Vahlquist, B. C.: *Acta Paediat Scand,* [Suppl] *28:* 5, 1941.

Venkatachalan, P. S.: *Bull WHO, 26:* 193, 1962.

Vartan, C. K.: *Lancet, 2:* 1022, 1965; *Br Med J, 1:* 50, 1969.

Waterlou, J. C., and Vergara, A.: *FAO Nutritional Studies,* Rome, 1956.

Werner, B.: *Acta Pediatr, 35:* 80, 1948.

Wharton, B. A., and Bower, B. D.: *Lancet, 2:* 969, 1965.

Widdowson, E. M.: *Volding, 23:* 62, 1962.

Widdowson, E. M.: In Asaki, N. S. (Ed.): *Biology of Gestation. The Fetus and Neonate.* New York, Acad Pr, 1968, Vol. II.

Widdowson, E. M.: *Proc Nutr Soc, 28:* 17, 1969.

Widdowson, E. M.: *J R Coll Physicians Lond, 3:* 285, 1969.

Wilkinson, A. W.: *Proc Nutr Soc, 28:* 61, 1969.

Willis, N. H.: *Infant Nutrition.* Philadelphia, Lippincott, 1964.

Winnicott, D. W.: *Maternal and Child Care, 5:* 147, 1968.

WHO: *Nutrition in Pregnancy and Lactation.* Geneva, WHO, 1965, p. 26.

Wong, H. B.: *Breast Feeding in Singapore.* Singapore, University Press, 1971.

CHAPTER IV

FEEDING THE ADOLESCENTS AND ADULTS

CRITERION OF AN ADEQUATE DIET

IT IS A DIFFICULT proposition to establish sound criteria of an adequate diet, keeping in mind the varied eating habits and the varied metabolic needs of the human populations all over the world (Williams *et al.*, 1973). It is neither essential nor desirable to follow a certain pattern of diet for all to insure the adequate intake of all the nutrients. At least fifty different kinds of nutrients are needed which help, not only the maintenance of optimum health, but also promote satisfactory growth among the adolescents in their period of rapid growth. It is indeed fortunate that the essential nutrients are widely dispersed in nature and can be obtained from many combinations of foods with varying ease (Goodhart, 1968). At the same time, it is also an unfortunate truth that a vast majority of the human beings have somehow lost the inherent instinct for selecting foods which would provide them with a balanced diet. There is widespread ignorance, not only about the needs of the body in terms of body building, energy yielding and protective foods, but also about foods that are rich in proteins or calories or vitamins or minerals.

Human beings are the slaves of cultural traditions regarding the choice of foods and most often they vehemently refuse to eat those items which do not agree with their cultural beliefs, in spite of their richness in the desired nutrients. In the same context, nutritionally poor foods become culturally super foods and, as a result, the members of that community suffer from unnecessary malnutrition. It is a strange paradox that all our life, starting from the first breath to the last, we eat food and yet we are so ignorant about our nutrition needs. In most places of the world, the science of nutrition is not a part of elementary or secondary education, which could help to impart a sound knowledge of the body needs and establish good eating habits in the formative years.

Even in highly advanced countries, where the mass media, food industry and school curricula impart very useful knowledge about the needs of our body, insufficient emphasis is laid on developing a satisfactory concept of a balanced diet, or else the appetite killing sweets would not have become as popular as they are.

As adults, we may learn to select foods which satisfy the basic criteria of an adequate diet, but it is the adolescents that pose a dilemma. Young children may be pushed into drinking milk or other useful items of foods, but adolescents generally oppose that kind of pressure. They may tend to eat more carbohydrates to the exclusion of other types of foods. A regular intake of unbalanced diets such as excess carbohydrates in the form of sweets, may lead to anorexia or loss of appetite. The large growth spurt that usually begins sometime between the ages of 11 and 13 years, requires considerable quantities of wholesome foods to meet the nutritional demands of such rapid growth (Thomas and Call, 1973). It is essential that from the early stage in life, the concept of a balanced and adequate diet be developed to promote adequate growth, health and vigor, and prevent obesities, which could lead to a lot of trouble in later life.

NUTRITION NEEDS OF THE ADOLESCENTS AND ADULTS

Calories

During these days we hear so much about obesity, weight reduction and the desirability of controlling the food intake that the word *calorie* has become quite an undesirable word. This is not true in several countries of the world, where a large section of their populations do not get enough calories to satisfy their basic energy needs. Unless the energy needs of our bodies are satisfied, even some of the precious calories from proteins, which may be more usefully employed in body building, may be used up in order to keep the engine functioning. A *calorie* need not be looked down upon. Maybe if we develop a proper understanding of a *calorie* and its sources, it may help us to modify our eating habits and the fears of obesity may leave us for good. To put it in a simple way, one calorie is the amount of heat that may be needed to raise the temperature of 1 gm of water by 1° C. The study of calories is a study of energy metabolism and at no time of life is there a moment when the energy is not being needed and the calories not being utilized.

Basically, calories are needed for two main purposes. One is to maintain the basal metabolic rate or, in a simple language, keep the engine running at an idle speed. In this respect, the human body is no different from an engine which needs fuel to carry on its activities and keep it warm. The other major need for calories is to promote activity and growth. Basal metabolism takes up more than half of the calories and includes functions such as maintenance of body temperature, muscle mass in good tone, and involuntary activities, as breathing, heart beat, blood circulation and metabolic activities of the cells. Wang, *et al.* calculated that basal metabolic needs take up 57 percent of the total calorie intake. If an allowance of 10 percent is made for calories lost in the excretia, only 33 percent of the calories are available for activity, growth and in digestion.

During the early adolescent years (11–14 years of age), boys and girls, in order to maintain satisfactory growth, require 74 percent and 67 percent calories respectively, in addition to those required for maintaining basal metabolism (Maroney and Johnston, 1937). The basal metabolism depends on the body size, muscle mass and skin surface area and, therefore, will require lesser numbers of calories in women as compared to men. Persons with larger muscular development will have a metabolic rate of at least 5 to 6 percent greater than those persons of the same height and weight, but with less muscle mass. An average woman may need 55 cal/hr, or 1,350 calories per day, compared to 70 cal/hr or 1,700 calories per day in men.

However, in children in their growing periods, the basal metabolic rate is much higher. When the growth period stops, the basal metabolic rate also slows down to some extent and, starting from 25 to 26 years through old age, a person will need progressively fewer calories to maintain his basal metabolism. This is the reason why those middle age persons who do not reduce their caloric intake tend to add up weight. During pregnancy, the basal metabolic rate is increased by as much as 20 percent, whereas if a person is starved there is a significant reduction in basal metabolism observed. After a prolonged period of starvation, it may be reduced to as much as 50 percent of the pre-starvation rate (Johnson, 1967). Similarly the process of lactation would increase significantly the demand for extra calories, which may be as much as 1,000 calories per day (Table VIII).

We compared earlier the human body to an engine and the basal metabolism to the rate at which it runs at idle speed. The thyroid gland, through its hormone thyroxine, regulates the rate of this idle speed. When too much thyroxine is produced, the basal metabolic rate is increased and the reverse is true when insufficient amounts are produced. The basal metabolic rate is likely to differ from person to person and no standard formula can be made on the basis of height and weight.

Let us now consider the energy expenditure or caloric needs for our daily activities such as walking, running, doing physical or mental work or other chores which keep us busy. A larger sized person would use up more calories for doing the same act as compared to a lean person. Similar persons with sedentary work habits will consume less calories compared to those who lead active lives.

Hensen estimated that, whereas a one to three year old child may need as many as 100 calories/kg/day, these figures of caloric needs are reduced to 90 calories for ages 4 to 6, to 80 calories for ages 7 to 9, and 70 per day for adolescents 15 years of age or over, which is equivalent to one-half the caloric needs of an infant. On the other hand, the number of calories consumed per day for basal heat metabolism increases from 983 calories for a 4 year old to as much as 1,436 calories for a 12 year old boy (Macy, 1942; Wang *et al.*, 1936) . An FAO study has tried to calculate the caloric requirements of a reference man and a reference woman under certain conditions considered average.

> The reference man is 25 years of age; weighs 65 kg; lives in temperate zone with a mean annual temperature of 10° C; maintains his weight; and has a work program that keeps him active for eight hours each day. About one and one-half hours are spent in recreation or household work, and about one and one-half hours walking. This man is said to require 3,200 calories daily. The reference woman is described in a similar manner, her weight is 55 kg, her age 25 years, and she maintains her home. Her caloric requirement is assumed to be 2,300 calories (1957) .

Based on caloric requirements at 25 years of age, under similar conditions of work, one must reduce his caloric intake by 15 to 20 percent in order to maintain the same weight by 65 years of age. An average 159 lb. man who would need 1880 calories for basal metabolism and a total of 2,800 calories at 25 years, would need 2,600 calories at 45 years and 2,400 calories at 65 years of age. Similarly, a 120 lb. woman who would need 1,500 calories for basal metabolism and a total of 1,950 calories at 25 years, would need, 1,800 calories at 45 years and 1,650 calories at 65 years of age. The problem in the United States is the easy availability of attractively presented diverse foods and the general lowering of activity levels due to automation. A general reduction in energy expenditures is not accompanied by reduction in caloric intake, with the result that today more than 40 million people in this affluent country are classified as obese.

Mention may also be made of the calories that alcohol provides. In the United States, annually 25 billion dollars worth of alcoholic beverages are consumed, which is roughly equivalent to the value of all the food grains produced by

India with a population 2½ times that of the United States. Since alcohol is a source of ready calories, it may be worthwhile to give an idea of the calories consumed by an average social drinker or a heavy drinker. The caloric equivalent of alcohol (ethanol when combusted in a calorimetric bomb) is seven calories per gram. The alcoholic content of beer ranges from 3 to 7 percent. In terms of their caloric content, beer may have about 30 calories per 100 ml, but this may increase to 60 calories per 100 ml in the case of stronger beers, ales or stouts. Wines have somewhat higher alcohol contents, ranging from 8.5 to 10 percent. A 100 ml of wine contains about 75 calories. Some of the American wines contain as much as 90 calories per 100 ml or more, because of the alcohol and sugar which raise the alcoholic content. Whiskey, brandy, and vodka have much higher alcoholic contents (approximately 30 percent), compared to beers or wines, and per 100 ml they contain as much as 225 calories.

If we translate the caloric figures into units in which the alcoholic beverages are consumed, it appears that a 12 oz. can of beer contains 150 calories; a 1.5 oz. drink of rum or whiskey contains 150 and 110 calories respectively; and a 2 oz. drink of manhattan or martini has 160 calories; and a whiskey sour contains 140 calories. The average 4 oz. serving of wine has 160 (dry) to 180 (sweet) calories. It is evident from these figures that a few cans of beer in the evenings, or a couple of drinks, or wine should not be treated lightly as far as their caloric value is concerned. They are mostly empty calories. As Mayer explained, "from a nutritional viewpoint, it is worth remembering that with the exception of small amounts of B vitamins and traces of minerals in wine and beer, alcoholic beverages are the prototype of *empty calories* and are best avoided by those on reducing diets. The idea that calories in alcohol are not fattening has no basis in theory or fact (1970).

Proteins

In addition to covering the basal requirements of catabolism, proteins serve very important functions in anabolic processes as well as meeting the stresses of infections. Proteins are the basic body building blocks. In addition, the regulatory materials of the body including enzymes and hormones, are protein in nature. It is especially important for the growing years of adolescence that generous amounts of proteins be supplied in the diet, failing which they not only fail to realize their full growth potential but their ability to combat infections also decreases (Fisher, 1954; Lynch, 1958). As a rough estimate of the protein needs of growing children, it may be stressed that the skeletal muscle mass of a newborn is about 25 percent of its body weight. By twelve years of age, this percentage is increased to 45 percent (Scammon, 1923), which clearly indicates the need for generous supplies of protein in the diet (Stearns *et al.*, 1958). A detailed study of the protein requirements of adolescents using five different levels of protein intake (10.3, 14.2, 18.2, 22.2, 26.3 percent protein of total calories intake) suggested that the optimum intake of protein for the adolescent should constitute 15 percent of an adequate calorie intake.

There are a few years in the period of adolescence when the adolescents need large quantities of food. One may have to look at the 1955 figures of the FAO more seriously. The FAO study put the protein requirements of infants at 2.25 gm/kg body weight, reducing it to 1.00 to 1.5 gm/kg during the first two years and thereafter gradually decreasing to 0.5 gm/kg for adults (FAO, 1955). The adolescents in general are fairly active, consume a high level of calories, but because of their concomitant growth spurts, it may be desirable to give them generous amounts of protein, more than generally recommended for their age and weight (Stearns *et al.*, 1958). A study reported by Gallagher on 20 boys reveals that the fat among them took 2,600 to 3,500 calories with 130 to 140 gms of protein intake. The thinner ones consumed 33 or 35 w calories and 120 to 190 gms of protein (Gallagher, 1958). A detailed study of Burke and Stuart on the physique, personality and scholarship of children between 5 to 14 years of age revealed

that protein eating habits tend to remain set in childhood, that *85 percent* of the tall children had good to excellent protein intakes, that none eating excellent amounts of protein were fat, and that three quarters of those taking excellent or good amounts of milk (over 24 ounces per day) had on the average 0.40 major respiratory infections per year. Those taking less than this amount of milk suffered from 0.73 such infections per year. These last differences were statistically significant. Also, it was found that 48 percent having good or excellent intakes of protein had above average red blood cell amounts (above 4.6×10^6). Only 11 percent of those with fair intakes had red blood cell counts of this level. These results were found to be statistically significant. This study suggests that protein intake in larger quantities does help in maintaining health and adds protection against infections (Burke and Stuart, 1943).

One must add a word of caution against too much excess intake of protein in the belief that it is good for health. An allowance of 15 percent protein calories in the diet appears generous enough. In general, the protein allowance should be 12 to 14 percent of the total calories. The latter figure of 14 percent has been recommended by the Nutrition Committee of the British Medical Association. At a level of 20 percent or more protein calories, the body may start reacting adversely. Johnston found that when the growing adolescents are fed food with a protein level in excess of 20 percent calories, they may complain of nausea, abdominal discomfort, vomitting and the urine shows excessive amounts of nitrogen (Johnston, 1961). In order to show that we can do with small quantities of protein, the American physiologist, Chittenden, put himself on a diet which contained only 40 gms of protein daily and after a year on this regimen, proclaimed that not only had he maintained his health very well, but often increased his physical and mental vigor. He believed that since extra work is involved in excreting the nitrogen from the unnecessary high levels of protein, it could put extra strain on the kidneys. Over a long period of time, it would cause renal and vascular disease.

It is known that when the diet contains more protein than is needed, nitrogen will be removed from the excess amino acids by the liver, which nitrogen is then excreted out by the kidneys. The remainder of the amino acid molecule is then used as an immediate source of energy or it may be stored in the form of fat. To put it another way, if the diet does not contain sufficient amounts of carbohydrates or fat, the body has no other alternative except to convert the available protein for the purpose of providing energy, rather than for building or replacing tissues. The energy needs of the body always take precedence over the body building needs. So far, there is not much evidence to state clearly that the human kidneys suffer any damage due to high intakes of protein and excretion of N-end products. The Masai warriors take 250 to 300 gms of protein daily in their diets. Eskimos take large quantities of protein in their diets. However, it may be fair to add that, while protein is a scarce commodity, it may be better put to use if its intake is reduced to around 65 gms per day so that the savings can be passed on to those who do not get more than 45 gms. It is evident from a number of studies that human adults can maintain excellent health on approximately 15 percent protein calories in their diets. This does not mean that we have suggested a solution to the problem of human protein requirements. A review by Irvin and Hegsted has quoted 373 papers, only to state the position of some of our contemporary workers in the field.

In terms of quantity, probably most of the human beings all over the world get enough protein in their diet which should be sufficient for health maintenance. But the greatest drawback in the nutrition of about 70 percent of the human population is the quality of available protein which not only affects to some extent the maintenance, but certainly fails to fulfill the needs of growth of the children and adolescents. In most of the developing countries, cereals in the form of rice, wheat, corn or other staples are the main sources of protein. These cereals are deficient in one or more essential amino acids which may be termed as limiting amino acid. For example, tryptophan is the limiting amino acid in corn and lysine is deficient in wheat protein. In such cases, when the available food consists primarily of these cereals, the nitrogen equilibrium cannot be maintained, no matter how complete or excellent the diet may be in other respects. Maximum utilization of proteins can only take place when all the essential amino acids are available simultaneously, in the correct proportions together with adequate quantities of non-essential amino acids or of nonprotein nitrogen. The body must make up this deficiency by the addition of some other food in order to maintain normal nitrogen equilibrium (Davidson, 1972).

The vegetable cereals, although containing quantitatively adequate proteins for human needs, are nevertheless incomplete and unsatisfactory. The processed foods discussed in Chapter II are designed to remove this deficiency of a limiting amino acid. A mixture of cereals and legumes has proven quite satisfactory to improve the quality of a diet based on vegetable sources and these mixtures have proteins of the biological value comparable to good animal proteins. Whereas the cereals contain in terms of energy 7.6 to 13.6 percent protein content, the legumes contain 18.8 percent to 45.2 percent protein (potatoes 7.6%, rice 8%, corn 10.4%, wheat 13.2%, millet 13.6%, peanuts 18.8%, beans and peas 25.6% and soybeans 45.2%) (Brock and Autret, 1952). In large areas of the world, where increases in population have outstripped the available supply of good quality animal protein, the vegetable mixtures based on cereals and legumes are the most useful substitutes. Egg proteins are a standard to compare the biological quality of proteins from other sources. By this statement, it is assumed that the amino acids are supplied in the correct ratio for meeting the needs of the body and no appreciable excess is left over for catabolism. The proteins from vegetable mixtures may not have 100 percent biological value, but they are of sufficient quality to promote satisfactory growth and maintenance.

Proteins in the diet greatly contribute to the muscular ability of a person. Strong muscles are generally associated with high levels of protein in the diet. It is because the muscles are made of protein. When they are generously supplied in the diet, the muscles develop a firm tone and the pull of the strong muscles holds the body erect without conscious effort, but when the diet is deficient the muscles lose the muscle tone and may become soft and flabby. The person gets fatigued even with a small physical effort. When the supply of protein in the diet is inadequate, the gastrointestinal tract also undergoes certain changes which hinder the proper utilization of the available proteins. The walls of the stomach, small and large intestine, are made of circular muscles which cannot maintain their strength and contraction if the diet fails to supply all the essential amino acids. The prolonged intake of unbalanced diets results in the muscles becoming flabby, with the result that the food is not mixed well with the digestive juices and enzymes and remains partly undigested and thrown out with the fecal matter without having been fully utilized. Even the utilization of energy requires to some extent the availability of protein. In a protein deficient person, fewer enzymes are produced which directly affect the physical and physiological processes of the body. Hemoglobin, the iron-containing material in the red blood corpuscles, is largely protein. All the blood vessels and miles and miles of capillaries consist of a protein structure, whose tone greatly depends on the availability of protein in the diet. The amount of blood actually decreases as a result of insufficient protein intake (Fisher, 1954), which could have a disastrous effect on the functioning of the whole body.

Insufficient protein in the body also delays healing of injuries or wounds. Similarly, in the protein deficient persons the surgical incisions are more likely to break open as compared to a person well provided with protein. No wonder protein makes up the largest proportion of the body. A person weighing 65 kg contains 11 kg of protein, which is equivalent to 17.00 percent of the body. This is more than the fat content (13.8%) or carbohydrate content (1.5%) of the body. All this is meant to say that proteins are so essential that life cannot exist without them.

Carbohydrates

Carbohydrates provide the bulk of the food as well as a source of calories. In the absence of appropriate amounts of carbohydrate rich foods, the digestive system will undergo some undesirable changes. Most nutritionists agree that at least 50 percent of the total calories should be derived from carbohydrates. In developing countries of Asia, Africa and Latin America, their proportion in the food is sometimes as high as 80 percent, with approximately 10 percent calories from protein and 10 percent from fat. This is a somewhat unbalanced proportion.

The richest sources of carbohydrates are the vegetable sources of food, as the plants can synthesize carbohydrates from carbon dioxide in the presence of sunlight. Seven eighths of the world population rely mainly on plants as sources of food. The carbohydrate yields 4 calories per gram weight, irrespective of its form or sweetness. Sugars are sweet, whereas starches are not. Fructose is the sweetest, followed by sucrose, glucose, lactose, dextrin and starch. When a banana or some other fruit ripens, starch is changed into glucose. Milk is the only source of dietary lactose. The process of digesting carbohydrates begins in the mouth as the enzyme in the saliva starts acting and exposes the sugar and starches to subsequent action of digestive juices. The prominent ones are amylase, invertase, maltase and lactase. In the lumen of the small intestine nearly all the carbohydrates are broken down and consist of a mixture of sugars such as maltose, isomaltose, lactose and sucrose. Cellulose and other polysaccharides are not easily digested by the enzymes and are passed on to the large intestine, where they form the bulk of the feces (Davidson *et al.*, 1972). Glucose, fructose and galactose are the end products of carbohydrate digestion. These are single sugars and are absorbed by the small intestine. Through the portal circulation, the liver is their destination. Glucose is the form in which carbohydrates are present in the blood. Blood glucose rises after a meal. This stimulates the production of hormone insulin, which helps the tissues to utilize glucose for energy. Insulin also helps the conversion of glucose to glycogen in the liver and also the conversion of glucose into fat. Insulin is a primary regulator of blood sugar.

Carbohydrates are essential not only to provide energy.

A certain amount of carbohydrates in the diet is also essential to maintain physiological equilibrium. During recent years, some physicians seem to disregard the need for carbohydrates in the diet and discourage their intake by those individuals who want to reduce weight. Carbohydrates maintain a certain degree of gastric acidity in the stomach. This is in contrast to proteins (especially those of meat and fish) which have a buffering effect. Decreased proportions of carbohydrates in the diet can lead to relatively low gastric acidity, which is undesirable because certain harmful bacteria may cross the barrier of low gastric pH and reach the intestinal tract. This may be especially true in young children with fever. It may be rather advisable to give high carbohydrate diets to the sick because carbohydrates help to maintain the desired acidity by delaying gastric emptying (Lennard-Jones *et al.,* 1968; Wadsworth, 1968). Total abstinence of carbohydrates from the diet as recommended by Atkins may be extremely undesirable. It has been suggested that carbohydrate deficiency results in losses of water and electrolytes, ketosis and subjective symptoms of fatigue. Carbohydrates perform a very useful function of preventing ketosis, conserving electrolytes, providing ready glucose for the nervous system, and sparing proteins and decreasing the need for high level intake of fat, which may be necessitated to get sufficient amounts of calories. The intake of high levels of fat is implicated in a number of cardiovascular disorders.

Glucose is the main fuel of the nervous system. The nervous system uses a large amount of energy to maintain its mechanism in working order and nearly one fifth of the total basal metabolism takes place in the brain (Davidson *et al.,* 1972). The nervous system does not store energy and constantly depends on the availability of glucose in the blood for continued activity.

The carbohydrates, being the cheapest source of energy, spare the generally scarce proteins from being diverted to maintain the basal metabolism and the activity level. In prolonged fasting or depletion of carbohydrates, the liver utilizes proteins for gluconeogenesis to replenish its stores of glycogen. It is indeed a wasteful use of protein because the conversion of amino acids into glycogen is a process which uses more energy than it liberates; hence, protein energy is utilized less efficiently than the energy derived directly from carbohydrates. It is essential that a diet should contain sufficient amounts of carbohydrates in the diet so that the protein can be utilized for the purpose of body building rather than providing energy for living. Some carbohydrate is also essential for the complete oxidation of fat in the body.

Luckily, carbohydrates are most abundant forms of food and also the cheapest as compared to those rich in proteins or fats. The yield of carbohydrate food per acre is the highest. Most of the carbohydrate foods are highly palatable and are a valuable source of proteins and some fats as well.

The importance of carbohydrates may be emphasized by giving the example of the dependence of the baby on glycogen at the time of birth. Glycogen begins to accumulate early in fetal life and, at the time of birth, most tissues of the body contain high concentrations of carbohydrates, except the brain.

> The heart glycogen is of particular importance because on it depends the ability of the foetus to survive long periods of anoxia during delivery. The glycogen in the liver is also important because it is mobilized to provide the glucose which is essential for the function and survival of the brain. Failure to accumulate glycogen during fetal life may be a cause of perinatal death or brain damage secondary to temporary heart failure or inadequate supplies of glycogen (Wadsworth, 1968).

No specific requirements of carbohydrates have been established. A high intake of carbohydrates, as is done in the poorer countries, may not be essential or desirable but their restriction beyond a certain level may also be highly undesirable. Proteins need to be spared from being utilized as sources of energy. It is believed that "as little as 100 grams per day (400 calories) of carbohydrates can prevent the water and electrolyte loss attendant with protein catabolism, and probably as little as 40 grams per day are necessary to prevent the development of ketosis" (Latham, 1967). Under normal conditions, when there is no compulsion for weight reduction, a balanced diet might contain 70 grams of protein, 80 grams of fat and 500 grams of carbohydrates, which would yield about 3,000 calories, sufficient for a person pursuing an active profession. In terms of percentage, it amounts to 9⅓ percent of calories from protein, 24 percent from fat and 66⅔ percent from carbohydrate (Sinclair, 1964). Of all the people in the world, Eskimos who live mainly on animal food, eat the minimum carbohydrates. A typical Eskimo diet contains 46 percent calories from protein, about the same from fat and about 8 percent from carbohydrates. The Eskimos, however, take enough carbohydrates to prevent the serious complications of ketosis.

Distinction, however, has to be made between starches and refined sugars as sources of carbohydrates. Unfortunately, in the rich countries, the use of refined carbohydrates has greatly increased. The proportion of unrefined complex carbohydrates (starches from cereals or vegetables), which contributes to the intake of many vitamins and minerals, has greatly decreased. The refined sugars are concentrated carbohydrates and are bad for teeth as well as a proper functioning of the digestive system. An association between the intake of refined carbohydrates in the diet and dental caries is well established. It is believed that craving for excessive quantities of refined carbohydrates such as sugar, honey, candies, etc., may be due to a diet unbalanced in other nutrients, especially proteins and fats.

The story of Macy on nutrition and chemical growth in childhood may be related here (1951). In a ten year study she found that, when a ten year old boy was given a basal diet of 1,500 calories, he also ate as much as 750 calories of sugar. When the value of basal diet was increased to 2,250 calories, the boy reduced his sugar intake to 250 calories. When, along with 2,250 calories basal diet, an extra 250 calories were given in the form of milk, the boy cut down his sugar intake to about 100 calories. Macy reported that in her 2,595 days of regular study, the average sugar intake of 29 children was only 10 grams. When we find our children eating large amounts of refined sugars in the form of candies, we must ask ourselves if we are giving them the desired diets. The pattern of food likes and dislikes ultimately transforms itself into food habits which play an important role in the degree of liking for refined sugars throughout life. Lantz and Wood showed after a thorough survey that the *Anglo* children took on an average 49 servings per week of soft drinks, candy bars, candies, cakes, cookies, etc. This is in comparison to 33 such servings by *Spanish-American* children. It is highly desirable that the intake of refined sugars be regulated from childhood.

Fats

Fats are important in the diet and, apart from being concentrated sources of energy (having 9 cals/gm as compared to 4 cals/gm in carbohydrates and proteins) , fats give the general feeling of satisfaction, palatability of food and a sense of well-being. This may be attributed to delayed gastric emptying of fat giving the feeling of satiety for longer hours after a meal. The polyunsaturated fats take longer to digest as compared to the saturated fats. A monounsaturated fatty acid is one in which the molecules are joined by a double band, which means that a hydrogen atom could be added to each carbon chain at the double band. Oleic acid, common in olive oil and peanut oil, is the common fat in this category. A polyunsaturated fatty acid is that in which two or more double bands are present and, hence, can accept more hydrogen atoms. Linoleic acid or arachidonic acids are the common fats in this category. They are also considered as essential fatty acids. The saturated fatty acids are those to which no hydrogen atom can be added. Palmitic and stearic acids are two examples of these fatty acids and are abundant in animal fats. Most of the animal fat contains saturated fatty acids, except for chickens. For example, cow's fat contains 29 percent palmitic and 21 percent stearic acid compared to only 2 percent linoleic acid. The chicken fat contains 25 percent palmitic acid, 4 percent stearic acid and 18 percent polyunsaturated linoleic acid (Sinclair, 1964) . On the other hand, soy bean oil contains 15 percent saturated fatty acids and 60 percent polyunsaturated acids (Reiser, 1973).

The main function of fats, besides providing satiety due to delayed digestion and onset of hunger and providing a pleasant flavor and palatability, is: a) to facilitate the absorption of fat soluble vitamins A, D, E and K; b) to provide a cushion to the vital organs such as kidneys, against injury; and c) to maintain a constant body temperature by providing effective subcutaneous insulation.

It may be appropriate to explain briefly the metabolic process by which fat is digested. The pancreatic and intestinal juices in the upper part of the small intestine contain a set of enzyme lipases, which hydrolyze fat into di- and mono-glycerides and fatty acids. The process of action by the lipases, is greatly facilitated by the bile, which emulsifies the fats. The 12 carbon chain and somewhat longer fatty acids, after they have been emulsified and hydrolyzed, are absorbed into the lymphatic system and transported along with cholesterol, phospholipid and protein. These particles are termed chylomicrons, which are further dissolved by the action of an enzyme lipoprotein, lipase, found in blood and tissue (Latham, 1970). In normal persons fat is absorbed to 95 percent or more, except for fully saturated glycerides, which are poorly absorbed. In its final stages, fat is utilized to: i. produce energy; ii. build body structure as brain and nerve tissue; iii. add temporarily in the liver until used by tissues; and iv. stored as body fat. It is quite normal for the body to deposit certain amounts of fat in the adipose tissue, in order to serve as a continuous supply of energy. It is believed that without any stores of fat in the body, it would be necessary to eat more often in order to provide energy for mechanical work.

The fat intake varies a great deal from person to person and region to region, depending on the food habits and energy needs. In the United States, the average fat intake is around 35 percent or a little above the total calories. This is in contrast to around 10 percent fat calories eaten by millions of people in Africa and Asia. Whereas the fat consumption in the United States may be somewhat high, the fat intake in African and Asian countries is certainly very low and may lead to lethargic activity levels in the absence of any concentrated source of energy. At the same time, low levels of fat manifest themselves in such symptoms as dry skin, red tongue, folliculosis, eczema and skin infections. But unlike the persons eating high fat food, the incidence of atherosclerosis and myocardial infarction is extremely low among people consuming low levels of fat. After detailed studies, Jelliffe recommended that the fat intake for 3 to 6 year olds may be as high as 42 percent because of their very high activity level, but may be slightly reduced (41%) for 7 to 11 year olds and 37 percent for 12 to 15 year olds (boys) (Jelliffe, 1950).

It may be important to comment here on the implications of fat in the disease processes. The most important lipid implicated in several diseases is cholesterol. Although a small amount of it (0.5–1.0 gm) eaten daily is important metabolically (Foman and Bertels, 1960; Mendez *et al.,* 1961), larger quantities of it can be hazardous to health, especially if taken for a prolonged period of time. Cholesterols in small quantities are present in many tissues, especially in the nervous tissue and liver. They serve as a precursor of vitamin D. For example, cholesterol in the skin can be changed into active vitamin D by the ultraviolet light from sunshine. Cholesterol is abundant in animal food such as egg yolk, liver, kidney, brain, animal fat, butter, cream, whole milk, etc. (Table VII). An average American diet provides from 600 to 800 mg daily of exogenous cholesterol (Latham *et al.,* 1970). In excess quantities, cholesterols are especially implicated in the disorders of the blood vessels, in the causation of atheroma and myocardial infarction. Although a number of other factors such as stress, lack of exercise, smoking, genetic background can be listed which also cause these pathological conditions, abundant evidence exists that large amounts of serum cholesterol (of endogenous and exogenous origin) is directly related to these disorders. By reducing the dietary intake of cholesterol it is possible to reduce the incidence of these disorders.

Dietary cholesterols can be reduced by substituting the saturated animal fats with polyunsaturated fatty acids derived from vegetable sources. These sources contain certain essential fatty acids such as arachidonic acid, which lowers the raised cholesterol level until it reduces the complications of vascular disease such as myocardial infarction (Davidson and Passmore, 1966). A New York study showed that when 814 healthy men between the ages of 40 to 49 years were given polyunsaturated fatty acids for seven years, their serum cholesterol levels fell significantly and they had a lower incidence of coronary heart disease compared to 436 men of the same age group who were given no dietary advice (Christakis, 1966). Even persons who suffered from myocardial infarction showed a greatly reduced incidence of recurrence when soybean oil was the main source of fat in the diet (Leren, 1966). The conclusion of the American Heart Association that the reduction of premature coronary heart disease is possible by a systematic restriction of dietary cholesterol intake and substituting, as far as possible, the animal fat with polyunsaturated fatty acids, is based on proven evidence.

The essential fatty acids such as linoleic acid and arachidonic acid, which are abundantly present in vegetable sources of fat, are quite essential for the maintenance of good health, especially a healthy skin. Arachidonic acid, a long chain polyunsaturated fatty acid, is not as abundant as the linoleic acid but the latter can be readily converted into the former. Linoleic acid, therefore, may be considered essential. Absence of these fatty acids in the diet leads to skin disorders and skin lesions in animals as well as human children (MacDonald, 1968). Discussing the wrong pattern of dietary fat, Sinclair described that when there is a tissue preponderance of saturated fatty acids and certain isomers of polyenes over the polyunsaturated fatty acids, the serum cholesterol becomes dangerously high. When the saturated fatty acids predominate over the level of essential fatty acids, the end result will be atherosclerosis and where there is a tissue preponderance of long-chain saturated fatty acids over the

TABLE VII

CHOLESTEROL CONTENT OF SOME FOODS

(mg./100 grams—approximately 3½ ounces)

Egg yolk	1,400
(1 yolk = 240 mg.)	
Butter	300
Lard	110
Cream	140
Beef	100–125
Pork	60–100
Lamb	70
Chicken and Turkey	75
Liver	250–600
Brains	2,000
Cod	50
Halibut	60
Salmon	60
Sardines	70
Lobster	208
Crab	145
Oysters	326
Whole milk (1 cup)	35
Skimmed milk (1 cup)	1
Egg white	0
Vegetable oils	0
Fruits	0
Cereals	0

From: I. MacDonald, *Practitioner*, 201: 292, (1968).

essential fatty acids, the result will be increased thrombosis and/or decreased fibrinolysis which leads to pulmonary embolism and infarction (Reiser, 1973).

Water

For the maintenance of life, water is as important as oxygen. Without water, one cannot survive for more than a few hours. Water is just not lying around in the cavities of the body; it is an integral part of individual cells, tissues, blood and other fluids of the body. Approximately two-thirds of the total body weight consists of water. The lean person contains somewhat more water than the obese one and infants and children have more body water than older persons. About 75 percent of the water in the body is contained in the cells. The remainder is in the form of blood, lymph, and other fluids around the cells and tissues. The importance of water in the body is not well appreciated by a layman and it may, therefore, not be inappropriate to briefly dwell on its function. Most people understand that blood is the flow of life. Without the water in the blood, life will no longer be possible. Water is the solvent for all kinds of materials inside the body. The body fluids contain a precise amount of mineral elements whose concentration is not allowed to be disturbed. The food is digested by enzymes in the digestive juices. It is in solution form that the nutrients are transported across the intestinal walls, across the cell membranes, to the various tissues and organs.

All chemical processes in the body take place in the presence of water. It is in the water soluble form that all waste materials are eliminated from the body. Around a litre or more of water is filtered by the kidneys and excreted out in the form of urine. A considerable amount of water is also excreted through the skin by perspiration and by the lungs as well as with fecal matter. Water is indispensable for the control of body temperature by evaporating the water through the pores of the skin as well as lungs (Latham *et al.,* 1970). As much as 350 ml water is exhaled out through the lungs and perspiration through skin may evaporate double this amount. It is essential, therefore, that adequate amounts of water be given to the body along with the diet because a human being can survive without food but may not be able to survive long without water. Most foods that we eat contain water in varying amounts. Milk contains 88 to 92 percent water, egg 74 percent water, vegetables and fruits contain 75 to 95 percent water, meat contains 50 to 70 percent water and bread contains 30 to 45 percent water. Even the hard nuts contain 5 to 8 percent water. The dietary requirement of water is about 2 to 3 litres. A rough estimate indicates that the body needs approximately 1 ml per calorie of food intake. The infants lose greater amounts of water in proportion to their size and, hence, would need larger intakes as well.

Occasionally the body does not drain out all the water and the tissues retain it, and the condition is referred to as edema. It may occur when the body is unable to excrete sodium in sufficient amounts. This is not unusual in diseases of the heart, when the circulation is impaired, or when the kidneys are unable to excrete wastes normally. Edema also occurs following prolonged protein deficiency because the tissues are not able to maintain a normal water balance. Pregnant women are also known to retain water in their tissues.

Vitamins

Vitamins are chemical compounds of an organic nature which the body requires in small amounts with food and are necessary for life and growth. They facilitate the use of energy nutrients and regulate the building of body structures. The various vitamins needed by the body, as a rule, are not related chemically and differ in their physiological actions. However several of them, e.g. A, D, K, E and B_{12} consist of several closely related compounds with similar physiological properties. In selecting food sources for vitamins, we have to remember that these vitamins are easily available and are directly absorbed by the body. In other words, they are not in bound form from which the body cannot benefit. The foods that contain antivitamins need to be avoided. Several synthetic analogues of vitamins have proven to be highly poisonous because they block the true vitamins at their site of action in enzyme systems (Davidson *et al.*, 1972).

Foods should be eaten in a form that their vitamin content is not lost, e.g. polished rice, which loses its B complex vitamins; wilted vegetables have lost a lot of vitamin A because it is oxidized in the air. Heat destroys vitamin C easily. Riboflavin is sensitive to light. If a food contains a provitamin, it is as good because the body can convert it into the needed form, e.g. carotene is a provitamin of vitamin A. The body also has the ability to synthesize some of the vitamins with the help of bacterial flora of the gut. For example, nicotinic acid, riboflavin, vitamin B_{12} and folic acid can be synthesized as well. The vitamins can be divided into two categories: fat soluble and water soluble. Fat soluble vitamins may fail to be absorbed by the body if the digestion of fat is impaired.

TABLE VIII

RECOMMENDED DAILY DIETARY ALLOWANCES OF VARIOUS NUTRIENTS FOR THE ADULT POPULATION

	Age [2] (years) From Up to	Weight (kg.)	Weight (lbs.)	Height (cm.)	Height (in.)	kcal	Protein (gm.)	FAT SOLUBLE VITAMINS Vitamin A activity (IU)	FAT SOLUBLE VITAMINS Vitamin D (IU)	FAT SOLUBLE VITAMINS Vitamin E activity (IU)
Males	10–12	35	77	140	55	2,500	45	4,500	400	12
	12–14	43	95	151	59	2,700	50	5,000	400	12
	14–18	59	130	170	67	3,000	60	5,000	400	15
	18–22	67	147	175	69	2,800	60	5,000	400	15
	22–35	70	154	175	69	2,800	65	5,000		15
	35–55	70	154	173	68	2,600	65	5,000		15
	55–75+	70	154	171	67	2,400	65	5,000		15
Females	10–12	35	77	142	56	2,250	50	4,000	400	12
	12–14	44	97	154	61	2,300	50	4,000	400	12
	14–16	52	114	157	62	2,400	55	4,000	400	12
	16–18	54	119	160	63	2,300	55	4,000	400	12
	18–22	58	128	163	64	2,000	55	4,000	400	12
	22–35	58	128	163	64	2,000	55	4,000		12
	35–55	58	128	160	63	1,850	55	4,000		12
	55–75+	58	128	157	62	1,700	55	4,000		12
Pregnancy						+200	65	5,000	400	15
Lactation						+1,000	75	6,000	400	15

	WATER-SOLUBLE VITAMINS							MINERALS				
	Ascorbic Acid (mg.)	Folacin [3] (mg.)	Niacin (mg.[4] equiv.)	Riboflavin (mg.)	Thiamin (mg.)	Vitamin B6 (mg.)	Vitamin B12 (ug.)	Calcium (gm.)	Phosphorus (gm.)	Iodine (mg.)	Iron (mg.)	Magnesium (mg.)
Males	40	0.4	17	1.3	1.3	1.4	3	1.2	1.2	125	10	300
	45	0.4	18	1.4	1.4	1.6	3	1.4	1.4	135	18	350
	55	0.4	20	1.5	1.5	1.8	3	1.4	1.4	150	18	400
	60	0.4	18	1.6	1.4	2.0	3	0.8	0.8	140	10	400
	60	0.4	18	1.7	1.4	2.0	3	0.8	0.8	140	10	350
	60	0.4	17	1.7	1.3	2.0	3	0.8	0.8	125	10	350
	60	0.4	14	1.7	1.2	2.0	3	0.8	0.8	110	10	350
Females	40	0.4	15	1.3	1.1	1.4	3	1.2	1.2	110	18	300
	45	0.4	15	1.4	1.2	1.6	3	1.3	1.3	115	18	350
	50	0.4	16	1.4	1.2	1.8	3	1.3	1.3	120	18	350
	50	0.4	15	1.5	1.0	2.0	3	1.3	1.3	115	18	350
	55	0.4	13	1.5	1.0	2.0	3	0.8	0.8	100	18	300
	55	0.4	13	1.5	1.0	2.0	3	0.8	0.8	100	18	300
	55	0.4	13	1.5	1.0	2.0	3	0.8	0.8	80	10	300
Pregnancy	60	0.8	15	1.8	+0.1	2.5	4	+0.4	+0.4	125	18[5]	450
Lactation	80	0.6	18	2.0	+0.5	2.5	4	+0.5	+0.5	150	18	450

[1] The allowance levels are intended to cover individual variations among most normal persons as they live in the United States under usual environmental stresses. The recommended allowances can be attained with a variety of common foods, providing other nutrients for which human requirements have been less well defined.

[2] Entries on lines for age range 22–35 years represent the reference man and woman at age 22. All other entries represent allowances for the midpoint of the specified age group.

[3] The folacin allowances refer to dietary sources as determined by *Lacto-bacillus casei* assay. Pure forms of folacin may be effective in doses less than ¼ of the RDA.

[4] Niacin equivalents include dietary sources of the vitamin itself plus 1 mg. equivalent for each 60 mg. of dietary tryptophan.

[5] This increased requirement cannot be met by ordinary diet, therefore, the use of supplemental iron is recommended.

From: Food and Nutrition Board, National Academy of Sciences, National Research Council Pub No. 2216, 1974.

Fat Soluble Vitamins

Vitamin A is a fat soluble vitamin and has several known functions in the human body. "Vitamin A aldehyde combines with opsin in scoptic vision. The vitamin participates in synthesis of mucopolysaccharides and release of a protease affecting dissolution of the cartilagineous matrix. It also has a role in reproductive processes (Latham *et al.*, 1970). Carotene is a yellow substance and is a precursor of vitamin A. There are several carotenes found in vegetables that act as a precursor and are converted into vitamin A in the walls of the intestine, liver and kidney. Dark green vegetables, cabbage, lettuce, tomatoes, carrots, pumpkin, papaya, etc., are the common vegetables which contain carotene. Vitamin A is measured in International Units. The standard is 0.30 micrograms of vitamin A alcohol, or 0.60 micrograms of beta-carotene as equal to one International Unit of vitamin A (Latham *et al.*, 1970). The recommended daily dose is 5,000 to 10,000 I.U. For a normal adult, 5,000 I.U. are sufficient, whereas during pregnancy and lactation 6,000 to 8,000 I.U. are recommended. Intakes of 1,500 I.U. for infants and 2,000 to 4,500 I.U. for children are recommended.

Good vision greatly depends on adequate supply of vitamin A. The *visual purple* is a substance that is made of protein and vitamin A and a regular supply is essential to enable you to see continuously. Your ability to see in the dark at night, especially, depends on your supply of vitamin A. Driving at night could be hazardous for those who are deficient in vitamin A. The first symptoms of deficiency are sensitiveness to bright light and burning and itching of the eyelids. As a result of prolonged deficiency of vitamin A, symptoms of xerophthalmia (loss of lustre of eyes and extreme dryness of the conjunctiva) could appear. In extreme cases, blindness is the result. Vitamin A deficiency is quite common in the poor developing countries of the world, especially among the children. There is a general scarcity of milk, and breast milk of the weak mothers is very low in its vitamin A content. The administration of liver oils (liver is a storehouse of vitamin A) improves their condition dramatically.

In the developed countries, however, the average diet provides easily the daily requirements of vitamin A, especially when the milk sold in the market is fortified. Under the influence of commercials, some individuals take heavy doses of vitamin A, which must be discouraged because large doses can be quite toxic. The symptoms of excess doses of vitamin A include lethargy, malaise, abdominal pain, headaches, excessive sweating and brittle nails (Latham *et al.*, 1970). Vitamin A, given in doses of 25,000 to 50,000 I.U. daily for several months, has led to loss of appetite, failure to grow, fretfulness, drying and scaling of skin, thinning of hair, swelling and tenderness of long bones and enlargement of liver and spleen. Mickelsen and Yang described the example of a

> 39 year old woman who took large amounts of the vitamin in the hope of improving her vision. For a number of months, this woman had been taking 150,000 I.U. of vitamin A per day. When she began to feel less well, she increased the intake to 325,000 I.U. She sought medical advice when her frontal headaches became acute and she experienced severe pain while walking. The hair on most parts of her body was sparse. There was an itching rash on her arms and legs. A discoloration of her feet and ankles was associated with edema of her feet. Moderate pressure applied to bony prominences elicited signs of severe pain. The concentration of vitamin A in her serum was 874 mg per 100 ml versus 30 to 70 mg in normal individuals. Even after 5 weeks during which no supplemental vitamin A was given, her serum level was 769 mg. At the later date, many of her toxicity symptoms were disappearing.

Vitamin D is also a fat soluble vitamin, which stores itself in the liver in lean times, but if generous quantities are available, it does not store in large quantities. Vitamin D is essential in the absorption of phosphorus and calcium. As calcium is held in the body by being combined with phosphorus, the presence of vitamin D is essential for the maintenance of skeletal structure, especially in the young age for proper growth of bones and teeth as well. Vitamin D also maintains and stimulates the normal capacity of the gastrointestinal tract to absorb calcium and phosphorus by stimulating its reabsorption from the renal tubules. In the intestines, vitamin D or its metabolites influence the gut muco-sal cells directly and brings about the active absorption and transport of calcium (Palmisano, 1973). There is evidence that the metabolites of vitamin D promote the active trans-port of calcium from gut lumen to serum. Ergosterol is a pro-vitamin secreted by the oil glands of the skin which changes into vitamin D after exposure to sunlight, which then is absorbed back into the body.

Exposure of the body to sunlight is highly recommended but after exposure to sun, one must not clean the body with soap and water, because it could wash off all the vitamin D. Vitamin D does not occur in foods. In small quantities it is present in egg yolk, fish liver oils and butter, but never enough to satisfy the body's needs. It is worthwhile to fortify the milk with a synthetic vitamin as is done in most of the developed countries. Loomis discussed the role of skin pigment in the regulation of vitamin D synthesis in man. He suggested that skin color, which is known to be a function of latitude, is an adaptation which provides both for protection against rickets and minimization of excessive vita-min D synthesis in equatorial regions. DeLuca believed that vitamin D is more like a hormone than a vitamin. Vitamin D is indeed a very powerful substance and in large quantities can be quite toxic. The recommended daily dose for normal adults is around 150 to 200 I.U. However, in the growing chil-dren and pregnant women, it may be as high as 300 to 400 I.U. A daily intake of 100 to 400 I.U. will prevent rickets in chil-dren.

In the developing countries, rickets are not very uncom-mon due primarily to a deficiency of vitamin D. It is a strange paradox that something that is freely available (sunlight) is not made use of. The earliest symptoms of vitamin D defi-ciency are irritability, restlessness, sleeplessness and profuse sweating, especially around the head and neck. There is impaired intestinal absorption followed by increased excre-tion of calcium and phosphorus in the urine and feces. As a result of demineralization of bone, osteomalacia occurs in adults and rickets in children. Osteomalacia in women during pregnancy may need special mention because the severe calcium and vitamin D deficiency is reflected in the fetal stores. The condition is seen in a number of developing countries.

Some vitamin enthusiasts, however, take heavy doses of this vitamin in the belief that, if their body does not need it, it will excrete it out. Unfortunately this is not true of this vitamin. Large doses of 20,000 to 100,000 I.U. have severe effects including loss of appetite, vomiting, diarrhea, fatigue, growth failure and drowsiness. The blood calcium level is increased, and calcium salts are deposited in the soft tissues including the blood vessels, heart and kidney tubules. Kidney stones may form. In children an early common symptom of excessive vitamin D is anorexia and vomiting. The child refuses food and is very thirsty. Weight loss and irritability are common and the condition may lead to death (Latham *et al.*, 1970). It is important that this vitamin be investigated more thoroughly (DeLuca, 1971).

Vitamin E consists of a number of physiologically active tocopherols. During the recent years, vitamin E has assumed the position of a wonder drug and food faddists are popularizing it so much that its consumption has increased more than a thousand fold. Some of the claims attributed to vitamin E are, indeed, fantastic with no scientific study having ever proved or disproved them. It is considered a fertility drug.

> It increases sperm count, makes the ovaries feel good, is used to treat symptoms of menopause and can prevent habitual abortion and congenitally deformed babies. It also relieves chronic constipation and certain gastrointestinal disorders—including peptic ulcers. It is valuable in the treatment of leprosy and various skin diseases. It can cure retarded children—even mongoloids and can help cure brain and neurological disorders. It is a good treatment for diabetes, reverses or slows down the aging process, is a protection against cancer and even makes race horses run faster (Trotter, 1972).

These claims are generally based on uncontrolled trials or clinical impressions. If even half of the claims attributed to vitamin E could be true, it would be the biggest breakthrough in the field of nutrition. It is indeed fortunate that excess quantities of this vitamin are excreted out by the body and no toxic effects have been observed after administering daily heavy doses of this vitamin. The normal daily requirements are believed to be between 20 to 30 I.U. per day for adults. The richest sources of vitamin E are vegetable oils, fresh green and other vegetables. Whole grain food products are also good sources. An ordinary diet supplies enough of vitamin E and it is most unlikely that a dietary deficiency of this vitamin ever arises. Only some premature infants may be born with inadequate reserves and may develop anemia. The administration of iron, folic acid and vitamin E helps (Chadd and Fraser, 1970). Dr. Bieri of the National Institutes of Health, says that there is no evidence that anyone needs extra vitamin E. There is no evidence that any deficiency or even a borderline deficiency exists anywhere in the world. The folklore about vitamin E is 90 percent wishful thinking (*Science News*, 1972).

Some people use mineral oil routinely as a laxative. This practice may be to some extent harmful because mineral oil may dissolve vitamin E in the food and deplete the organism.

It may be reasonably concluded that a deficiency state may occur in small premature infants associated with hemolytic anemia. But in normal adults or children, supplements of the vitamin have no established value in preventing or treating any common human disorders (*Medical Letter,* 1971).

Vitamin K is essential for the normal formation of a key substance in blood clotting. It is called prothrombin, and is present in the blood plasma. It is glycoprotein in nature and is synthesized in the liver. Vitamin K in very small amounts is present in all foods but most of its is synthesized by the human bacterial flora in the intestine. Dietary deficiency of vitamin K in adults is extremely rare.

Water Soluble Vitamins

Vitamin C (*ascorbic acid*) is essential for building the

cementing material that holds cells and tissues together. Its intake in sufficient quantities either through dietary sources or by therapeutic administration leads to strong blood vessels, teeth firmly held in their sockets and bones firmly held together. The recommended daily allowance is 55 to 60 mg for adults (*Ascorbic Acid,* 1968), which can be obtained from raw fresh fruits and vegetables. Fruits of the citrus family are especially rich (oranges, grapefruit, tangerines, limes, lemons, etc.). Among vegetables, dark green vegetables are rich, broccoli being one of the richest. Canned and frozen citrus fruits and juices contain as much vitamin C as the fresh ones. Vitamin C is not affected by light, but is destroyed by excessive heat.

The deficiency of vitamin C results in the development of scurvy. The symptoms of scurvy are likely to appear only after the body stores have been completely exhausted, which means a deficiency of vitamin C over a long period of time. A deficiency in mild forms exists widely in poorer countries of the world, whose populations live predominantly on cereals which are very poor in this vitamin. Mild forms of deficiency result in delayed wound healing, probably because of failure of collagen formation in the connective tissues. In a deficiency state, the scars of previous wounds may break down and become open sores again (Davidson *et al.,* 1972).

Vitamin C has a number of extremely vital functions and it is important that care is taken to assure that its intake is sufficient. The very foundation of our bones depends on vitamin C for strength. In a deficiency state, these foundations may break down, causing minerals to be freed. The bones then become spongy and lack the strength of normal bones. Resistance to fracture also depends on the supply of vitamin C. It also aids in the absorption of iron from the intestines. It is needed to convert folacin to folinic acid. It participates actively in the metabolism of certain amino acids. The adrenal cortex of the body contains high concentrations of vitamin C. The adrenal gland needs vitamin C for the synthesis of hormones and the mechanical strength of the blood vessels, particularly the venules, depends on the availability of vitamin C. In the absence of this vitamin, capillary walls lose elasticity and may break down and the blood may be freed into the tissues causing hemorrhage.

Recently exaggerated claims have been made for the efficacy of large doses of vitamin C in the cure of the common cold. For details, the reader is referred to the famous book of Dr. Pauling. There are not many controlled studies conducted in this area. However, it is true that very high doses of this vitamin can be taken without any toxic effects. After saturation is reached, the body merely excretes the vitamin in the urine.

Vitamin B Complex: Vitamin B is a complex of a number of vitamins. The most important vitamins are thiamine, riboflavin, niacin, B_6 and B_{12}, pantothenic acid, pyridoxine, folic acid, biotin, choline and inositol. There is reason to believe that some more members of the vitamin B complex family may not have been isolated yet. The known members of the complex have been synthesized, and can be used up by the body efficiently, but it may not be wise to depend on the multivitamin tablets. Instead, one should rely more on the natural foods.

Thiamine in combination with pyrophosphate, functions in carbohydrate metabolism as a co-enzyme with carboxylase. This enzyme is essential for one of the many steps in the breakdown of glucose for energy. For that reason, thiamine is important in proper functioning of the nerves and a good mental outlook. It is also essential for a normal appetite and good digestion. The rich sources of thiamine are of vegetable as well as animal origin. Pork, liver, eggs, yeast, nuts, legumes, whole cereals and green vegetables are rich. Brewer's yeast and wheat germ are very rich. Ordinarily one should get sufficient quantity even on a poor diet, but among those people who use polished rice as their staple, the deficiency is quite likely, which may lead to the symptoms of beri beri. Mild to moderate degrees of thiamine deficiency manifest themselves in fatigue, irritability, feeling of depression, moodiness, poor appetite, numbness of the muscle and constipation due to poor tone of the gastrointestinal tract.

The requirements of thiamine are proportional to the carbohydrate intake but the recommended daily allowance is 0.4 mg per 1,000 calories. An extra allowance of .02 to 0.4 mg daily during pregnancy and lactation is always advisable. The intake of excessive amounts of the vitamin are known to be nontoxic. The unused part is simply excreted out by the kidneys.

Riboflavin (B$_2$) is a yellow crystalline water soluble substance concerned with tissue oxidation and respiration, playing thus an important role in protein as well as energy metabolism. Like B$_1$, vitamin B$_2$ also aids in the burning of sugar and produces energy. It is an important vitamin and is available in the commonly used foodstuffs of vegetable as well as animal origin. Milk, meat (liver), fish, eggs, yeast, cereals and green vegetables (beets, turnip greens, carrots, broccoli, spinach, mustard, etc.) are good sources. Being soluble in water, it may be lost if cooked vegetables are eaten and the broth or water content discarded. To some extent, it may be lost from the food if it is exposed to the sun too long. For reason of its water solubility, it cannot be stored in the body as well, because then it will be lost in the urine and perspiration. It is important to maintain an adequate supply from food sources. The daily needs are 1.5 to 1.7 mg for adults. Additional allowance of 0.3 to 0.5 mg should be made for pregnant and lactating women.

The deficiency of riboflavin leads to loss of appetite, decrease in energy and loss of weight. The eyes are strained, with redness in the cornea and continuous watering may result in poor vision. The skin problems are more prominent. Pellagra is generally referred to as rough skin accompanied by sore or cracked lips and sore corners of the mouth and eyelids. In the poor developing countries, the deficiency of riboflavin is quite common.

Niacin or Nicotinic Acid or Nicotinamide is another important member of the B complex vitamins. Pellagra or rough skin is the commonest symptom caused by the deficiency of niacin and is a major health problem among the poor sections of the poorer countries who cannot afford to use dairy products, green vegetables and fruits in sufficient quantities. Niacin functions as a component of two important coenzymes in tissue respiration and glycolysis. The human body can convert the amino acid tryptophan into niacin. Approximately 60 mg of dietary tryptophan is equivalent to 1 mg of niacin. In the United States a normal diet contains about 600 mg of tryptophan, but in those countries where people live on cereals as staples, the tryptophan content is as low as 150 mg or even less. Corn protein is poor in tryptophan content and it is believed that some of the niacin in corn is in bound form or may not be available. The daily needs are in the range of 13 to 18 mg, with 5 to 7 mg extra for pregnant and lactating women. The deficiency of niacin is common in the poorer countries. In advanced stages of niacin deficiency, the resulting pellagra may be characterized by diarrhea, dermatitis, skin eruptions, dementia or insanity. The tongue and the whole alimentary tract is sore. Dementia manifests itself in such symptoms as hostility, violence, aggression and depression. Large doses of niacin show dramatic improvement in the condition.

Vitamin B_6 includes three pyridine derivatives which are interconverted metabolically in the human body. B_6 is involved in the amino acid metabolism and is an essential part of glycogen phosphorylase. It helps to break down food to produce energy. Fat elements of the food, particularly, use B_6 to convert into sugar. Whole grain cereals, milk, meat and vegetables are food sources and the daily requirements are approximately 2 mg, with 0.5 mg extra needed for pregnancy and lactation. Pregnant women may develop a deficiency and need B_6 supplementation. Whether or not pregnancy nausea is due to its deficiency is questionable, but the administration of B_6 does help the nausea. As a result of B_6 deficiency, antibody formation is reduced thus exposing the individual to infection. The first signs of B_6 deficiency are bad skin followed by muscular discomfort, weakness and difficulty in walking. There is increasing evidence that B_6 is intimately concerned with the metabolism of the central nervous system. Some of the commercial milk in which the vitamin is destroyed during processing produces convulsion in infants. B_6 responsive anemias have been reported in adults. Progressive deficiency of B_6 leads to anorexia, poor growth, emaciation and death.

Vitamin B_{12} is a vitamin which is available only from animal sources of food. Liver and kidney are rich sources but other meats, muscle and fish as well as milk and egg also contain small quantities. It is generally bound with the protein and is liberated by the digestive enzymes, especially by mucoprotein enzyme generally referred to as intrinsic factor, and is then absorbed. Adults need 5 mg/day, with an additional mg during pregnancy and lactation. B_{12} is one of the most complex of the B vitamins. The trace element, cobalt, is an essential part of its molecule. It is essential for the production of red blood corpuscles in the bone marrow, for the synthesis of protein and for the metabolism of nerve tissue (Darby, 1967).

Because of its presence in animal foods, with very little in the vegetable foods, a deficiency of this vitamin is present among those poor populations who eat strictly vegetable diets over long periods of time. The B_{12} deficiency results in a syndrome of glossitis, anemia, neurologic changes and low serum levels (Darby, 1967).

Folic Acid is essential for the body to produce normal red blood cells, and a deficiency state leads to macrocytic anemia. Dark green vegetables and leaves, kidney and liver are good sources. Ancient Hindu physicians always recommended the use of liver for the treatment of anemia. Of course, they did not know why it was effective. Cooking and storage of food results in loss of the vitamin. Adult requirements are in the order of 0.4 mg, with an additional 0.1 mg for pregnancy and lactation.

Pantothenic Acid is a part of coenzyme A and is involved in the release of energy from carbohydrates, and is very important for proper growth. It is widely distributed in ordinary foods which can easily provide the required 10 mg of pantothenic acid. The deficiency of this vitamin is very uncommon (Latham *et al.*, 1970). The deprivation of this vitamin during pregnancy can be serious. In rats the deficiency results in resorption, abortion and malformation of the fetus.

Biotin is essential for many enzyme systems, but since it is available in many foods and can be synthesized by the intestinal bacteria, a deficiency state is very rare. Experimental deficiency will lead to fatigue, depression, malaise, anorexia, muscle pain, nausea, signs of neuropathy and dermatitis (Latham, *et al.*, 1970). Progressive depletion of biotin leads to failure of growth, loss of weight, emaciation and death.

Inositol also promotes growth and has a healthy effect on the hair and is rich in heart muscle, liver, yeast and oat meal.

Choline is important in transporting fats in the body. Without choline, fat accumulates in the liver. Prolonged deficiency leads to cirrhosis or fatty degeneration of the liver. It is rich in egg yolk and brain.

Paraminobenzoic Acid is known to play an important role in the prevention of gray hair. It is rich in liver and yeast.

It is believed that there may be other members of the B complex, important in human nutrition, which may still be isolated.

Minerals

A chemical analysis of a man weighing 65 kg shows that he contains approximately 4 kg of 15 or more minerals, which account for about 6 percent of his body. Calcium alone accounts for about half of the mineral matter of the body. At least seven of the mineral elements are present and needed in macro amounts. These are calcium, magnesium, potassium, phosphorus, sodium, chlorine, sulphur and iron. The others are found in small quantities and, hence, are labelled as trace elements. The function and necessity of some of them is well understood. These include iodine, fluorine, cobalt, copper, zinc, manganese, selenium and strontium. There are a number of other trace elements such as chromium, molybdenum, tin, nickel, silver, aluminum, etc., which have been analyzed but whose exact function in human nutrition is still not well understood. What is understood, however, is that they are present in extremely small amounts and are probably important in human nutrition (Underwood, 1971). Time has not yet come for human beings to thrive on completely synthetic foods. We must first understand the role of all the trace elements in human nutrition.

In general, the mineral elements function together in building body tissues and in the regulation of body metabolism. The hard tissues such as bones and teeth contain large quantities of calcium, phosphorus and magnesium and small quantities of a number of other minerals. The soft tissues contain a number of minerals such as potassium, phosphorus, sulphur, iron, etc., in their structure. Minerals control and regulate the passage of material in and out of the cell and regulate the transmission of nerve impulses. The acid-base balance, which is quite delicate, is maintained by the mineral content of the body and so is the sodium-potassium balance in the intra- and extracellular fluids. Here we will discuss briefly the needs of a few important mineral elements.

Calcium: The body of an adult contains 1,200 to 1,500 gms of calcium, 99 percent of which is present in the skeleton. Calcium holds the cellular matrix and provides the hard structure of bones and teeth. Most of the mineral part of the skeleton is calcium salt (calcium hydroxyapatite) but there are also present small and variable amounts of magnesium, sodium, carbonate and citrate (Davidson *et al.*, 1972). The amount of calcium in the blood is comparatively extremely small (100 mg/100 ml), half of which is bound to serum albumin and half in ionized solution. The parathyroid hormone governs the correct amount of calcium in the blood. When the blood level of calcium is low, calcium is removed from the bones. When the blood level goes up, calcium is deposited in the bones or is excreted in the urine.

The main source of calcium in the diet is milk, cheese, whole grain cereals, leafy vegetables, legumes and nuts.

Milk (cow's) contains as much as 120 mg/100 ml and is one of the richest sources. The intake of milk should be encouraged for a good supply of calcium. The recommended daily requirements are put at 800 mg/day, however.

The importance of calcium in the diet cannot be overemphasized. Calcium is used by nerves to transport impulses and in a deficient state, the nerves are tense and irritable and the person could be irritated, growling and short tempered. If the level of circulating ionized calcium in the blood serum is lowered much below 9 mg per 100 ml, the motor nerves become oversusceptible to stimuli, producing the clinical picture of tetany—the flaccidity of the muscles sets in. In India, it is a custom to drink warm milk before going to bed at night. It appears logical because that quickens digestion and absorption of calcium which soothes the nerves, and restful sleep follows. In the absence of calcium, the heart muscles cannot relax. Blood coagulation depends greatly on the availability of calcium. The women cannot maintain a prolonged period of lactation while consuming relatively low levels of calcium.

The requirements of calcium vary with age and depend upon the requirements of growth. A low level of calcium intake would depress growth and produce adolescents which are of much shorter heights than would be expected if the calcium intake had been in the normal range (Food and Nutrition Board, 1969). The calcium needs in children of 1 to 9 years of age are around 0.8 gms/day, which is increased to 1.1 gms/day in 9 to 12 year olds. In the adolescent period (12–18 years), the calcium requirements are estimated at 1.3 gms/day for girls and 1.4 gms/day for boys. Johnston suggested that girls should take 1.4 gms calcium and 1,000 to 1,500 I.U. of vitamin D daily for at least one year before the onset of menarche (Johnston, 1947). When the calcium intake falls short of these requirements, the body tries to adjust to this deficit by retaining a high percentage of the total intake. But the normal pattern of growth trajectory is altered by the nonavailability of adequate amounts of calcium and reflects itself in low statures and poor skeletal qualities. In South and Southeast Asia, where the staple food is rice with very little amounts of milk or vegetables, a calcium deficit is always likely. Several experimental studies in developing countries indicate that when milk is provided to preschool children, their growth pattern suddenly improves. Akroyd and Krishnan showed that an addition of one-half gram of calcium lactate in the food greatly improved the height and weight of Indian preschool children. The children of immigrants to the United States from the developing countries suddenly improve their heights due to generous amounts of protein and calcium available in the diets in this country.

It must be added that, under conditions when the dietary calcium intake is low, the body tries to adapt itself to retain a high percentage of the available calcium, but when the available supply is generous, calcium is absorbed with some difficulty. Holmes calculated that when 1 to 10 year old children are fed diets containing 540 to 1,500 mg of calcium per day, the actual body retention (minus losses in feces and urine) is only 18 to 35 percent with an average of about 27 percent. Increasing the intake up to a certain maximum usually results in an increased total retention. It is advisable, therefore, to provide the growing adolescent with generous amounts of calcium and leave sufficient margin for excretion as well as endogenous losses in the gastrointestinal tract. A generous amount of calcium is needed also because there are certain periods in childhood, such as during respiratory infections, colds, etc., when large amounts of calcium are withdrawn from the skeleton or the available calcium is not absorbed, whereas the well fed child maintains a better mineralized skeleton (Stearns, 1950).

Vitamin D has been known to promote the absorption of calcium (see section on vitamin D). Without vitamin D, a large majority of children are unable to absorb sufficient quantities of calcium in spite of its dietary availability.

There is always a period in the life of young adolescents when they start disliking milk, which is the main source of calcium. During this period of rapid growth, this lack of appetite for milk could hurt the growth of the child. An intelligent mother would recognize its need and conceal the milk products in the diet of youngsters by fortifying puddings with dried skim milk, using larger quantities of cheese in different preparations or by offering milk which is tastefully flavored or colored. However, it may be good to add here that chocolate cocoa interferes with the absorption of calcium from the milk. Calcium from plain milk and cheese is more completely absorbed.

Phosphorus: The body of an adult contains 600 to 900 gm of phosphorus, 80 to 85 percent of which is present in the bones in combination with calcium. The remaining phosphorus is chiefly located in the cells. Phosphorus is vital for the proper use of calcium. It gives rigidity to bones and teeth. Phosphate is an important anion in the cells and phosphorus compounds play a central role in the transformation of energy in the body. The quick release of energy in the muscles and nerves is effected by the breaking of high energy phosphate bonds provided by adenosine triphosphate (Davidson *et al.*, 1972). Many of the B group of vitamins are effective only when combined with phosphates in the body. It is only fair to say that probably no other mineral element has more important functions than phosphorus. It helps in building bones and teeth. It is essential for the phospholipids that regulate the absorption and transport of fats, nucleic acids of all cells and the enzymes which are involved in energy metabolism. Phosphorus compounds bring about muscle contraction and buffer salts in the regulation of acid-base balance.

All natural foods are rich in phosphorus and it is present in all living matter, whether it is of plant or animal origin. The deficiency of phosphorus is very unlikely unless and until a person puts himself on refined and processed foods. A good rule of thumb is that if you take care of your calcium intake, phosphorus will be no problem. It must be emphasized that the ability of the body to use phosphorus efficiently depends greatly on the calcium in the diet. Without adequate calcium, large amounts of phosphorus may be excreted out, taking along with them some of the precious calcium in the form of P-Ca salts.

Magnesium: Magnesium is an essential constituent of all soft tissues and an average adult body contains about 25 gms of the metal, which is next only to potassium as the predominant metallic cation of the living cell. The greater part of magnesium is present in the bones in the form of phosphates and bicarbonates. The skeleton seems to provide the body's magnesium stores (Latham *et al.*, 1970). Most of the foods, especially those of vegetable origin (grain, cereals, potatoes, vegetables, fruits) contain useful amounts of magnesium, because it is an essential component of chlorophyll. Magnesium deficiency is not likely under normal conditions unless excessive losses take place due to excessive diarrhea or from an intestinal fistula (Davidson *et al.*, 1972). Magnesium is extremely important for a number of metabolic functions. Cardiac and skeletal muscle tissues depend on a proper balance between calcium and magnesium ions for normal function. Together with other mineral elements, magnesium regulates nervous irritability and muscle contraction. Inside the cells, magnesium is mainly located in the mitochondria and because of that it is an essential part of many enzyme systems responsible for the transfer of energy.

As mentioned above, magnesium deficiency does not occur ordinarily, but if it happens, the typical symptoms may be depression, muscular weakness, vertigo and liability to convulsions.

Sodium, Potassium and Chlorine: Sodium is present in the extracellular fluid and maintains equilibrium between the extra- and intracellular fluid components. Potassium is the main cation of the cells and it is concentrated more in the intracellular fluid than in the extracellular. Sodium and potassium, together with calcium and magnesium, influence the amount of water held in the cells. They aid the cell walls in "choosing" what materials may pass into the cell and what must be kept out. Chlorine helps maintain the amount of water essential to life processes. The acid-base balance of the body is intimately related to sodium chloride metabolism. In diarrhea, without vomiting, the chief electrolytes lost are sodium and bicarbonate. Not much chloride ion is lost. The body fluids tend to be acidic. In severe vomiting, however, the main loss is of the chloride ions and the body fluids tend to be alkaline. In extreme cases, death may occur when chloride decreases too much. In such a case, the administration of common salt can save life.

Sodium chloride usually comes from the salt which is added to the food at the table or in the process of cooking. In animal foods, there is sufficient salt and there is no additional need for it, but in vegetarian diets, the addition of salt is essential. The daily intake of salt is 4 to 6 gms a day. It may be highly undesirable to eat excess salts with the food because of their effects on the cardiovascular function and the evolution of hypertension. It has been suggested that excessive salt intake by infants (along with baby foods) may play a part in the evolution of hypertension in adults (Hilkner *et al.,* 1965). Potassium is present in most commonly eaten foods and its deficiency is not likely to occur under normal circumstances. Cow's milk has three times as much potassium as human milk. Potassium is a part of most vegetables and fruits. The potassium intake in the United States ranges from 0.8 to 1.5 gms per day. However, in cases of severe diarrhea or vomiting, or in association with certain abnormal physiological states (diuretic administration, renal tubular defects, chronic lung diseases with alkalosis, diabetic acidosis and severe protein-calorie malnutrition), potassium deficiency may result in severe complications (Sandstead, 1967). Potassium depletion is the major biochemical change in kwashiokor resulting from protein deficiency. It is believed that an edematous kwashiorkor patient is more depleted of potassium than of protein and it is as essential to introduce potassium in the diet as it is protein. It may be summarized that potassium is the principal mineral element within the cell. It is essential for the synthesis of proteins, for enzyme functions within the cells and for the maintenance of the fluid balance of the body.

Iron: The average iron content of an adult is approximately 4 gms out of which about 2.5 gms are located in the hemoglobin. Some of it is present in myoglobin, whereas the rest is stored in the liver, spleen, bone marrow and muscle in the form of ferritin or hemosiderin. Minute quantities are also present in the respiratory enzymes and in iron binding protein of the plasma. Iron is, therefore, an essential part of the processes involved in the transfer of oxygen at various sites in the body. Deficiency of iron may result in anemia. Under normal conditions, about one gram of iron is stored in the body, chiefly in the liver, spleen and bone marrow in the form of ferritin, which is a complex compound associated with protein. The iron, important as it is, has a great advantage over other minerals. It is not used up or destroyed in a properly functioning body. Only very small amounts are excreted in sweat or urine. The daily loss may be as little as 1 mg of iron. Even the iron which is released by breaking down old erythrocytes is utilized again and again for the manufacture of new red blood cells. The needs of a healthy male and post-menopausal female are therefore quite small.

However, iron needs during pregnancy need a special mention because the needs may not be fulfilled by an otherwise balanced and satisfactory diet. As much as 500 to 600 mg of iron may be lost by the mother to the fetus and placenta and by hemorrhage during the pregnant period. Also total blood volume increases by about 1,500 ml and the amount of hemoglobin in the blood needs to be proportionately increased unless provided by an extra source. The maternal iron reserves may be depleted in the process. The demand for extra iron especially increases in the late pregnancy period and would raise the possibility of clinical anemia. It has been estimated that without adequate iron supplementation, a significant fall in blood hemoglobin concentrates is observed in pregnant women, who are otherwise in perfectly good health. "The fall in hemoglobin concentration is accompanied by a rise in total circulating hemoglobin; the capacity for oxygen transport is therefore increased" (Thomson and Hytten, 1973). However, the indiscriminate increase in iron intake may not be wise because at the present stage of knowledge, we are not certain that excessive or large amounts of iron are entirely harmless physiologically. In the United States, the advertisement industry has oversold the need for iron in women and has given it the status of a tonic. Iron supplementation only in proper amounts is most recommended where general malnutrition exists, the diet is poor in iron content, or clinical anemia is evident. The WHO expert committee on nutrition in pregnancy and lactation concluded that:

> the indiscriminate issue of iron preparations as a routine to all pregnant women in situations where there is no obvious indication for them is to be deplored. It is not merely wasteful; it also impedes research upon the problem and a more rational approach to the prophylaxis and treatment of anaemia.

Iron is present in a variety of foods and an average American diet would contain more than sufficient amounts of iron. The rich sources of iron are meat, egg yolk, beans, peas, green leafy vegetables and whole grain cereals. Milk is not a good source of iron. It is unfortunate that a vast majority of human populations do not get a variety of foods in their diet, and hence, iron deficiency anemia is quite common in the developing countries, especially among the children.

It is not the daily intake but the absorption of iron by the body which is to a great extent more important. There are foods which contain iron in the bound forms and the body is not able to absorb this iron properly. A report suggests that egg yolk, despite its relatively large amount of iron, inhibits the absorption of iron (Symposium, 1968). In general the absorption of iron depends greatly on the physiological needs of the body and is regulated by the state of iron stores in the body and the state of activity of the bone marrow. When the body stores are low and new red cells are being produced, iron absorption is increased (Davidson *et al.,* 1972). It is strange but true that iron is one element that is not as efficiently absorbed by the body from food sources as are the inorganic salts given therapeutically (*Nutrition Reviews,* 1964).

Sulfur: Sulfur is an element present in all protein material. Two amino acids, methionine and cystine, plus some vitamins such as thiamine and biotin, contain sulfur. Additionally, cells containing sulphate ions and free sulphydryl groups are important in some enzyme systems. It is also present in chondroitin sulphate found in cartilage and bone (Latham *et al.,* 1970). The requirement of sulfur or its deficiency has been difficult to assess because of its presence in all the foodstuffs containing proteins. Depending on the biological quality, about 100 gms of mixed protein will supply 0.6 to 1.6 gms of sulfur. The effects of sulfur deficiency may be closely linked with the deficiency of protein.

Trace elements: The minerals needed in small amounts are supplied in adequate quantities in normal diets and the chances of their deficiency to take place are not great and no special dietary precaution is needed. In general, vegetables, especially the green leafy vegetables, whole cereals, meat and seafoods are good sources of most of the trace elements discussed below. The human needs of these trace elements are not known precisely, mainly because the establishment of need depends on the production of a deficiency state and definition of the daily intake which can cure that deficiency. At the present state of our knowledge, those elements that can be considered essential to man are fluorine, vanadium, chromium, manganese, cobalt, nickel, copper, zinc, selenium, molybdenum, tin, iodine, etc. But by no standard can this list be considered complete (Mertz, 1972).

Iodine: The body of an average adult contains 20 to 50 mg of iodine and slightly less than half of this amount is present in the thyroid gland. The iodine is contained in the hormones of the gland and is essential for the formation of thyroxine and triiodothyronine. Thyroxine has a great influence on growth, mental and physical development.

The thyroid gland, which is the main repository of thyroxine, controls the speed of metabolism, heart beat, contraction of the digestive tract and, hence, bowel movements. In a thyroxine deficiency caused by the deficiency of iodine, the physiology is affected significantly. Less sugar is burned to produce energy, hands and feet are cold and bone marrow fails to produce enough corpuscles resulting in fatigue and affected mental agility. A decrease in the circulating iodine-containing thyroid hormones triggers a reaction from the pituitary gland which results in the enlargement of the thyroid. This hypertrophy is merely a mechanism to conserve iodine.

Food and water are good sources of iodine. Seafoods are especially rich. Dairy products, egg and some vegetables may be good sources, too. But the simplest thing to do to prevent goitre resulting from a deficiency of iodine is to iodize the common salt, which everyone takes daily without fail. Iodine is readily absorbed from the intestine. One-third is utilized by the thyroid gland and the remaining salt is excreted in the urine. When iodine is eaten in excess quantities, it may result in showing symptoms of endemic goitre (Suzuki, 1965). It has been suggested that 1 microgram of iodine/kg/day is sufficient in humans suffering no previous deficiency. However, growing children and women during pregnancy and lactation have increased needs (Latham, *et al.*, 1970). In pregnancy, lack of iodine in the mother may fail to supply the fetus. The baby may be more severely affected than the mother. In extreme degrees of deficiency, the growth of the baby may be retarded and mentally dulled. Someone rightly remarked that the intelligence of a person may be judged by the kind of bread he chooses and the kind of salt he buys.

Fluorine: The absolute need for the body physiology is not well established. What has been established is that fluorine ions are helpful in preventing tooth decay. Traces of this mineral are present in bones, teeth, thyroid gland and skin, but there is no evidence to show that it is indispensable. Ingested fluorides are rapidly absorbed and distributed throughout the extracellular fluid in a manner similar to chloride (Davidson, *et al.,* 1972). The main source of fluoride is the drinking water. In some areas of the world, the natural water contains very high levels of fluoride—as much as 10 to 45 parts per million (Latham and Grech, 1967), whereas in others it may be less than 1 PPM. For a satisfactory prevention of tooth decay or dental caries, it is estimated that 1 to 2 mg per day may be quite adequate, which means that if one is drinking water containing 1 PPM fluoride, his fluoride needs for dental care are well taken care of. It has also been suggested that fluoride plays a role in strengthening bone and as a protection against osteoporosis of old age (Bernstein, 1966). This kind of beneficial effect ascribed to fluoride has not been fully investigated and must be considered with reserve. However, in those areas which contain high levels of fluoride in their water supply, fluorosis may result. It manifests itself in the teeth becoming mottled, discolored, weak and brittle. The bones may also be affected, resulting in increases in bone density.

Copper: The total amount of copper in an adult human may vary from 100 to 150 mg. Yet, even in small amounts, copper is considered an essential element in human nutrition. It is required for the formation of hemoglobin as well as the production and survival of erythrocytes. Copper, like iron, has a dual valency, which makes it a valuable catalyst in the oxidation of reduction mechanisms of living cells. Copper is present in every cell in the body, but is mainly accumulated in the liver. The central nervous system is also rich in copper as compared with tissues other than the liver (Gallagher, 1964). Since copper is widely present even in foods that the poorest of humans consume, a deficiency state is only a rarity. Children are born with ample stores which proportionally may exceed the adult body. A normal adult diet can easily provide 2 mg per day, which is sufficient for the body needs of copper. However, excessive amounts of copper may be quite toxic. Wilson's disease, which could lead to portal hypertension and liver failure, may be a result of the absence of a certain liver enzyme without which the extra copper is not excreted out. The details have been described by Walshe.

Cobalt: The need for cobalt in human nutrition appears to be entirely due to its presence in vitamin B_{12} molecules. Its need in the ruminants is well established because of its need to enable the bacteria in their lumen to produce vitamin B_{12}, but its need in human nutrition is not as firmly established because cobalt deficiency has not been observed. If it were essential, as in the ruminants, a deficiency will cause severe anemia, wasting, listlessness and emaciation. Traces of cobalt are present in many foods.

Zinc: That zinc is an essential trace element in human nutrition has been completely established. Zinc is a constituent of a number of metalloenzymes such as carbonic anhydrase, pancreatic carboxypeptidase, alcohol dehydrogenase, alkaline phosphatase, malic, glutamic and lactic dehydrogenase and probably other pyridine nucleotide-dependent metallic dehydrogenases. Deficiency of zinc could be very disastrous, leading to such symptoms as growth retardation and testicular atrophy (Prasad, 1967; Underwood, 1971). Zinc deficiency has been observed to delay normal healing and Hussain found that zinc sulphate in quantities of 220 mg/day given orally accelerates healing of chronic ulcers.

Zinc is present in all living tissues. Most human diets provide at least 10 to 15 mg of this element which is sufficient for body needs. Its utilization appears to be affected by the dietary calcium level. Milk is as good a source of zinc as of calcium.

Chromium: It is believed that trivalent chromium as a trace element is essential for the normal function of carbohydrate metabolism. Chromium is uniformly present in the tissues of infants, the largest concentration being in the skin followed by muscle, blood and fat. The daily requirement of chromium is not well established yet, but normal diets should provide enough quantities. However, in the children suffering from protein-calorie malnutrition, impaired glucose utilization may be due to deficiency of chromium and it may at least be temporarily corrected by its administration.

Strontium: Strontium, like calcium and magnesium, is a divalent metal and its biological behavior is in many ways similar to that of calcium and is present in those foods which are rich in calcium. It is stored in bone in minute quantities. For details, refer to Widdowson *et al.,* and Davidson *et al.*

Manganese: Manganese is present in most of the tissues. Cereals and legumes and seeds are main sources and provide 5 to 10 mg daily, which appears to be sufficient. Manganese is a part of a number of enzyme systems, especially those of oxidative phosphorylation and fatty acid and cholesterol synthesis. For details, refer to Cotzias' review on the need, physiology and biochemistry of manganese. The role of managanese in human nutrition is not well understood but there are experimental indications that the mechanism of manganese and iron absorption are similar.

Selenium: Selenium appears to be essential as a trace element in the nutrition of ruminants, but its role in human nutrition is not well understood. It is believed that selenium prevents the effects of vitamin E deficiency. Levander described it as an unusual mineral in that natural foods can contain either so much of the element that a toxic effect may be produced or so little that a deficiency occurs. It is believed that selenium deficiency might be a complicating factor in certain types of kwashiorkor. Two Jamaican children suffering from protein malnutrition, who did not gain weight after overcoming the initial acute phase, responded immediately after receiving a daily supplement of 25 mg selenium (Schwartz, 1961).

Molybdenum, tin, nickel, silver, aluminum, silicon, arsenic, bromine, vanadium and zirconium are other trace elements which are considered somewhat essential in human nutrition. Man's requirement for molybdenum is inferred by the presence of this cation in xanthine oxidase and flavorproteins. A deficiency in humans has never been demonstrated. Tin is found in human tissues, especially in the liver, brain and thyroid. Small quantities of tin do not seem to have a bad effect on the health, although its requirement in human health is not well established. Nickel has been shown to be present in human liver and pancreas. Its function is not yet well understood. Silver occurs in blood, liver, sex glands, heart, spleen, kidney, thyroids and tonsils. Its function is not known, although physicians in Indian medicine prescribe it in minute quantities as a cure for anemia and general debility. Aluminum and silicon are too insoluble to be absorbed by the body. Even large amounts of aluminum injected into veins have caused no damage. As yet, they have no known nutritional significance. Arsenic in its natural state is nontoxic, and is rapidly excreted by the kidneys, but the industrially produced trivalent form is toxic if allowed to accumulate in the tissues. Bromine is present in the human blood. The section of the pituitary gland which affects growth contains 10 times more bromine than any other part of the body. Vanadium seems to influence the lipid metabolism and is a constant component of human serum, whereas zirconium is present in brain tissues. Their exact nutritional significance is not yet well understood.

NUTRITION NEEDS OF ATHLETES AND DURING EXERCISE

Nutrition and Physical Performance

Physical activity has been categorized as: i. very light work such as desk work in an office, which may consume as few as 2.5 calories per minute; ii. light work, which involves some movements of the body and limbs but does not require exertion (leisurely walking, painting, etc.) and may consume 2.5 to 4.9 calories per minute; iii. moderate work, which requires some exertion and effort such as cycling at slow pace, brisk walking, going up and down stairs at a fast pace and may consume 5.0 to 7.4 calories per minute; iv. heavy work such as skating, high speed bicycling, running, etc., which may consume 7.5 to 9.9 calories per minute; and v. very heavy work such as high speed running, swimming, sharp climbing, which may consume 10 calories or more per minute (Mayer, 1972). The level of nutrition in terms of energy intake must be established from the type of physical work involved rather than weight on a person or his age.

It has been argued, however, that the larger sized persons spend more energy in performing a particular activity compared to smaller sized persons (Malhotra *et al.*, 1962). The growing children need calories for meeting the growth requirements as well as activity and, since younger persons happen to be more active, their total intake may be as much as 50 percent more than the average adult. Similar allowance can be made for pregnancy and lactation. Over a nine month period a pregnant woman needs approximately 80,000 extra calories but in terms of physical performance for normal adults, the nutrition intake should be strictly in accordance with the physical performance. The individual needs to learn to adjust his appetite so that at his regular level of physical performance, he neither burns away reserves nor has to accumulate the excess in the form of fat. It is well established that among the obese, the level of physical activity and exercise is significantly below the average. Mayer described that only 18 percent obese boys and 22 percent obese girls showed a level of physical activity in the normal range. Whether it is the cause or the effect of it, it is clear that physical performance among the overweight persons is not in proportion to their food intake and, as they keep on accumulating excess weight, the desire for exercise and athletic activities decreases.

> I am convinced that inactivity is the most important factor explaining the frequency of *creeping* overweight in modern western societies. Natural selection, operating for hundreds of thousands of years, made men physically active and resourceful, well prepared to become hunters, fisherman or agriculturists. The regulation of food intake was not designed to adapt to the highly mechanized sedentary conditions of modern life, just as animals were not created to be caged (Mayer, 1972).

It must be emphasized, therefore, that our bodies are built and well prepared for hard physical work. A sedentary inactive life could easily start a degenerative process. A sedentary existence could lead to obesity, which would further promote the beginning of diabetes, heart disease, osteoporosis, and a number of clinical complications. It is imperative that, irrespective of the luxuries that modern scientific age has put at the command of man, he must exercise or indulge in vigorous physical activity in order to remain healthy.

It is not very difficult to imagine what will happen if one continues to lead a sedentary life. Volunteers who submitted to complete bed rest for several weeks showed skeletal decalcification, reduced blood volume, reduced muscular mass and impaired ability to take up and transport oxygen due to reduced stroke volume and cardiac output (Astrand, 1972). In these individuals, not only is the heart rate very high at rest but the heart rate goes very high with only a minor physical activity. The strength of the heart muscle is greatly reduced due to less efficient regulation of blood circulation. Such a person may not have the capacity to climb the stairs in a two story building. The human body is truly a working machine. It needs a lot of nutritive care. It dislikes emotional and psychological stress, but it flourishes on a moderate but regular exercise. Our organs and systems are designed to function better and better if their muscles are kept in good tone. This is especially true of the heart muscle. With physical training larger amounts of blood can be pumped through the heart with lesser strokes. When the body is at rest and no work is being performed, the heart pumps about 5 liters of blood every minute, while at the same time 5 to 8 liters of air are being inhaled by the lungs. However, the heart's construction permits it to pump 15 to 20 liters or more of blood per minute and pulmonary ventilation may exceed 100 liters per minute. The nervous system can also be said to be dominated by the body's demand for motion (Astrand, 1972). Regular exercise is like lubrication in good car care.

The likelihood of an active person surviving the first heart attack is immensely more as compared to a person who has a sedentary mode of living. Investigations on animals and observations on men have revealed that physical training or a vigorous life style can open up more blood vessels in the arterial tree in the heart muscle, that is collaterals may develop in the coronary arteries. Similarly collaterals may develop in peripheral arteries. A narrowing or occlusion of a vessel due to arteriosclerosis in such an individual will not mean the same catastrophe if there are other vessels than can take over the transport of blood with its oxygen and nutrients to the tissue peripheral to the damaged vessel (Astrand, 1972).

To the adult persons who are not interested in modern athletics or who do not want to spend money on special exercising equipment, Mayer strongly advised running as an exercise.

> Running is cheap and requires no partner or special equipment. Early in the morning, before breakfast, is a good time of day for running, particularly in suburban neighborhoods; however, it may be more convenient to do it at the end of the day, and this is not harmful. In fact, at this time muscles will be somewhat *warmed up* by the normal activities of the day. Exercise before supper, particularly if vigorous, will usually decrease rather than increase appetite. There are also psychologic advantages of a *break* at the end of the day (Mayer, 1966).

Exercise is an ideal method for maintaining weight. In the early twenties, when the process of growth has been completed, most men do not tend to recognize that they no longer need extra food to satisfy the requirements of growth. The rate of basal metabolic rate also has reached its plateau and is going to taper off from age 25 onwards, which means the only way to continue to eat on the old pattern or to maintain the old food habits, is to consume the extra calories by vigorous physical activity. The preferred thing to do will be to reduce somewhat your food intake and exercise regularly at the same time so that the weight at the age of 25 could be maintained over the middle age years and onwards. Eating is one of the great pleasures of human existence.

Besides the desirability to exercise or perform vigorous

physical activity for the sake of maintaining weight, one has to be aware of the creeping disease process. For example, there is a direct relationship between exercise and blood cholesterol levels. Physical activity on a regular basis reduces the serum cholesterol levels. Several studies have shown that persons who take on high fat regimens but maintain a high level of physical activity have serum cholesterols lower than those who eat an average fat diet but lead a sedentary life. It is well known that individuals with a higher concentration of cholesterols and triglycerides in the blood or a combination of these, run a higher risk of death from cardiovascular diseases than those active persons who have a low cholesterol level. A direct relationship is, therefore, observed in the exercise and the incidence of coronary disease.

In investigating a relationship between the level of physical activity necessitated by occupations and the incidence of coronary heart disease, Morris and his coworkers found among the London bus operators, the incidence is much greater among the sitting drivers than the bus conductors, who in the two-level buses do a great deal of stair climbing during their working hours. A similar relationship was observed among the mail men. Mortality from the coronary diseases was significantly higher among the sitting mail men as compared to the walking mail men who delivered the mail from home to home. Active physical performance is not only essential for the young and middle age persons. The older persons can greatly benefit from a physical training program. The detailed studies of DeVries on the physiological effects of an exercise training regimen upon ages 52 to 88 showed that the trainability of the older persons is greater than what had been suspected so far and does not depend upon having trained vigorously in youth. It is believed that the improvement in muscular function among the old is more due to the improvement of central nervous system activities than muscular hypertrophy.

Influence of Diet on Muscular Work

The human is, strictly speaking, a biochemical engine

which utilizes energy at a rate at which it has to do mechanical work, except for the constant amount of energy which is needed to maintain the idling speed. It is quite expensive in terms of energy to maintain the idling speed or the basal metabolic rate. A 24 hour bed rest costs as much energy as would be needed in walking 20 miles at a speed of 3 mph (Astrand, 1973). For athletic performance or vigorous physical activity, the muscles have to work overtime. It is important, therefore, that we have some understanding of the physiology of the muscular work. Briefly, adenosine triphosphate (ATP) is the carrier of chemical energy and is responsible for its transformation into mechanical energy. The ATP is broken down into a diphosphate compound (ADP) during the process. For a continuous maintenance of muscular activity as would be required in running or swimming, the ATP must be rapidly restored from ADP and the high energy creatine phosphate. Under normal circumstances only a small amount of ATP and creatine phosphate is stored in the muscles, but the latter store a large quantity of energy supply in the form of glycogen and fat. It is estimated that a 75 kg healthy person with 20 kg of muscles can store 1.5 k cals of ATP, 3.5 k cals of creatine phosphate and 1,200 k cals of glycogen. The same person could deposit the equivalent to as much as 50,000 k cals of fat. If oxygen supply is available, the glycogen can be broken down to supply a large source of available energy, as only a fraction of glycogen can be utilized anaerobically, i.e. without oxygen. The key to the great energy stores in the body is oxygen and the aerobic phosphorylation by mitochondria (Astrand, 1973).

Why some individuals can perform heavy muscular work for long durations and others cannot is not a simple question to answer. Astrand is a well known authority in this area. He believes that "It is still an open question as to what extent one can, by training, increase the stores of ATP and creatine phosphate and improve the ability to utilize these stores. The so-called white muscle cells are specialized on anaerobic work and the red muscle cells are more aerobic in their metabolism. These muscles are innervated by different types of motoneurones and have also different mechanical properties (Granit, 1970; Guth, 1968). In man, the number of muscle fibers in a muscle group is probably finally established after the embryo has reached the age of 4 to 5 months. It appears that the proportion between white and red muscle fibers is most likely established by the genetic code, which may mean that one can only, to a limited extent, modify the inborn quality and the quantity of the muscle mass. It is probably why some individuals are by endowment sprinters, and others are long distance runners doomed to perform poorly in a 100 m dash.

A prolonged sustained muscular work or athletic work requires glycogen stores and oxygen to utilize them although the recent work of Brodan, *et al.* (1973) indicates the role of an aerobic metabolism during exhausting exercise. The oxygen uptake of the individual is directly proportionate to his ability for energy utilization which, in turn, reflects, the individuals's ability to do heavy prolonged work. Different diets provide different amounts of stores of glycogen in the muscle and hence influence mechanical performance. The larger the quantity of glycogen available, the heavier and more prolonged muscular effort the individual can make. For athletes, therefore, the amount of stored glycogen in their muscle at the time of their athletic performance is of paramount importance. The intake of protein as well as carbohydrates and fats is as much essential for an athlete as for an individual engaged in other types of work. However, it is important to point out that the protein needs of athletes are no different than those of other persons not engaged in heavy work. A standard 1 gm/kg protein daily is sufficient for persons of all professions. Extra amounts of protein intake may be desirable in those persons who are either growing or building muscle mass by training.

It will be interesting to compare the effect of carbohydrates and fats as sources of energy in the process of supporting heavy athletic work. Christensen and Hansen did classical experiments in 1939 which still have not been repudiated. They found that when a person is engaged in a type of exercise requiring aerobic metabolic processes, 50 to 60 percent of the energy was supplied by fat. When a person is engaged in heavy work which requires the participation of anaerobic metabolic processes, the carbohydrates play a major role in providing the energy. A prolonged type of work can be sustained more readily from the energy from carbohydrates in the form of glycogen. Lewis and Gutin stressed that the availability of carbohydrates could become a limiting factor in prolonged endurance work. In designing diets and training regimens for endurance sports, the means by which the stores of this fuel may be built up should be given careful consideration (Lewis and Gutin, 1973). In this respect the investigations of Bergstrom *et al.* (1967) on the synthesis of muscle glycogen and the relationship between diet muscle glycogen and physical performance are of great importance. They found that when an individual is given a normal mixed diet, before the performance, the muscle glycogen content is 1.75 gm per 100 gm wet muscle. Such a person could perform at maximum work load up to 115 minutes. If a person is kept for three days on a high fat-protein diet, the muscle glycogen content is reduced to 0.63 gm per 100 gm wet muscle, with the result that the individual cannot sustain a work load for more than 57 minutes.

On the other hand, after a three day rich carbohydrate diet, the glycogen content of the wet muscle is increased to 3.51 gm per 100 gm wet muscle and the person could increase his performance level to 167 minutes, which further proves the importance of muscle glycogen in sustaining heavy work for prolonged periods of time. Astrand suggested a method of increasing the glycogen content of the muscles still further. If the glycogen depots are emptied first by heavy prolonged exercise and then are maintained at a low level with a low carbohydrate diet, then a few days before a performance a rich carbohydrate diet could supply the glycogen at a high level of more than 4 gm/100 gm wet muscle and the maximum work time can be increased to as much as 4 hours or more.

While we are discussing the importance of glycogen for sustaining prolonged heavy work, we must add a few sentences about the blood glucose. With a normal level of 1 gm/litre glucose in the blood, the total amount of blood sugar is around 5 to 6 gms. If this source of energy were available for heavy exercise, it could be depleted in a very short time. For example, 3 gm of carbohydrates are utilized every minute of heavy exercise. Since the central nervous system solely depends on glucose for its supply of energy, nature has very wisely kept the blood glucose off-limits for utilization in maintaining heavy work. The exact mechanism of this phenomenon is not clear. In explaining the phenomenon, Astrand believed that to prevent a marked decrease in the blood glucose concentration, some sort of a barrier must exist to prevent the glucose from entering the muscle cells and being used up in their metabolism (Astrand, 1973). The permeability of the cell membrane for glucose depends on the plasma insulin concentration which falls during heavy exercise (Hunter and Sukker, 1968; Pruett, 1970). Secondly, phosphorylating enzymes are necessary for the uptake of glucose across the membrane. One such enzyme, hexokinase, is inhibited by products from the breakdown of glycogen (Hultman, 1967). Therefore, glycogen is a more readily available substrate for energy production in the working muscle cell than the exogenous glucose. This fact is an advantage for the central nervous system which might otherwise suffer from lack of glucose.

One may conclude that carbohydrate is a better fuel for sustained energy than fat or protein (Lewis and Gutin, 1973). In order to get the maximum out of one's endurance ability it is advised that exercise should be tapered off at least 48 hours before the athletic performance and that the athlete will do well to take a 24 hour rest before the event. The last meal before the performance should be one rich in carbohydrates. There is some misunderstanding with respect to the need for protein. It must be emphasized that the optional diet for an athlete is no different from that of any other person engaged in other activities. Extra protein is needed for growing and for increasing muscle mass, but for maintenance the protein needs of an athlete are not elevated in any way.

As a matter of fact, the protein intake should be reduced to a minimum as the athletic event approaches, since proteins are a source of fixed acids, which can be eliminated only by urinary excretion. The problem of the need for urinary excretion during an athletic event could be quite serious (Karlsson *et al.*, 1971).

Diet of the Athlete

The caloric consumption of the athletes is at a much higher level than that of those who lead a sedentary or even an active life. Whereas the latter may consume around 3,000 calories, an athlete may use up to 4,000 or 5,000 calories a day. There have been recent reports in the literature that vegetarians have greater endurance as compared to non-vegetarians. Most of the apes (chimpanzee, gorilla, orangutan) are traditionally vegetarians and yet, pound per pound of muscle mass, the apes are four to five times stronger than humans. With these reports in mind, a few athletes tend to be vegetarians except for the taking of milk (lacto vegetarians). Whereas it may be true that vegetarians could be as athletic or muscularly strong as nonvegetarians, the former may have to eat large bulks of vegetable foods in order to provide the desired quantity of protein as well as calories. Also, there are few vegetables which are good sources of vitamin B_{12}.

While studying the meal habits and their effects on performance, Hutchinson showed that frequent meals improve the overall performance of the athlete, as more frequent breaks in a routine increase efficiency. Similarly, skipping a meal such as omitting breakfast, decreases the maximal work output and increases the reaction of tissue and muscle tremor. Otherwise there is no special requirement for an athlete's diet. Essentially the athlete eats the same thing as anybody else, but with greater caloric intake. An Olympic athlete takes as much as 4,500 calories a day (Jokl, 1964). For the purpose of increasing calories, carbohydrates prove to be a better fuel than fat. It may be advisable to provide a diet which contains protein, fat and carbohydrate in the ration of 1:1:4 (Williams, 1969).

It appears that there is no particular need for extra fat in an athlete's diet. In a normal diet some amount of unsaturated fatty acids are essential, as they are carriers of fat soluble vitamins, but for an athlete who needs heavier doses of calories there is no reason why fat content of the diet should be increased. For example, 4 ounces of sucrose are absorbed from the gut in a 2-hour period, whereas a pint of raw milk with more than 10 percent fat content will take as much as 6 hours to be absorbed (Bourne, 1968). Regarding the desirability of extra vitamins for the athletes, there is no clear-cut answer. As a matter of fact, there is a lot of confusion in the literature on this score as has been reviewed by Bourne. A number of studies have indicated the desirability of substantially increasing the intake of vitamin B_1 by the athletes. This could be because vitamin B_1 aids in carbohydrate metabolism and mediates the decarboxylation of pyruvic acid. Bicknell and Prescott stated that the needs for vitamin B_1 may be increased to as much as 15 times in severe exercise. This appears to be a very exaggerated figure or else most athletes would be deficient in this vitamin. Similar claims about enhanced requirements of vitamin C have also been made because vitamin C is concerned with the elimination of lactic acid after exercise. Numerous studies have shown that larger quantities of vitamin C allow greater physical endurance for longer periods of time (Van Huss, 1966). More recently, extra quantities of nicotinamide and vitamin E have been added to the list as beneficial to prolonged physical performance. It is probable that nicotinamide helps by being related to its pharmacodynamic effect in causing capillary dilation, but vitamin E is quite controversial. Some believe that in addition to vitamin E there is some factor in wheat germ oil, which improves physical performance, as wheat germ oil has been found to be more effective in improving physical performance than corn oil or cottonseed oil with synthetic vitamin E. The reader is referred to an excellent review by Bourne, who summarized the nutrition needs of athletes in a very beautiful manner:

It seems that the best diet for an athlete is one based on fresh fruit and fruit juices, vegetables, milk, first class protein (such as that found in meat, fish, cheese and eggs), and whole wheat bread, in other words, the type of diet that is recommended for good health for the rest of the population. An athlete who bases his diet on such a nutritional basis will probably find that extra vitamins will have no effect on his performance or his recovery from it; and it seems likely that only in those athletes whose diet is already defective is a special vitamin supplement likely to be beneficial.

NUTRITION NEEDS DURING PREGNANCY AND LACTATION

Preparation for Pregnancy

The level of nutrition during pregnancy is of great importance in order to nurture a healthy baby. But feeding the mother during pregnancy is only a part of the story. Numerous studies have given conclusive evidence that the ability of a woman to nurture a healthy fetus (physically, physiologically and mentally) depends to a great extent on her own nutritional state, not only during pregnancy but during her whole preconceptional life. Extensive study in South America also revealed that the nutritional status of the mother before pregnancy is as important in determining the birth weight of the infant and the outcome of pregnancy as is the maternal nutrition during pregnancy (Habicht *et al.*, 1973; Stott, 1973). Good nutrition results from lifelong habits of good diet. Consider for a moment, the nutritional status of the families of the economically depressed classes. A female child born in that family is growing up in poverty with marginal nutrition because the family does not have the resources to adequately nourish the infant. In these circumstances, she is unable to struggle herself out of these poor situations, grows poorly and produces children who are equally handicapped. A condition of poverty is perpetuated from generation to generation and if the female descendant of such a family is to conceive, she is least equipped nutritionally to go through the stress of pregnancy. Being poorly developed with little or no nutritional reserves she may have a hard time in meeting the demands of the growing fetus. It has been rightly remarked that "by the time a woman is pregnant, it is too late to improve her nutrition; perhaps supplements should be given before pregnancy or in childhood" (Rosa and Turshen, 1970).

On the other hand, a woman who had adequate and well-balanced food before her pregnancy, may have an inadequate diet during her gravid state and still may be able to nurture a healthy baby because of the nutritional reserves in her tissues. Thomson has done extensive work in this area. He feels that the females who are nutritionally deprived during their own growth period fail to achieve their genetically determined height and therefore remain short statured through their life (Thomson, 1959). If the dietary deficiency because of poor socio-economic conditions continues into the succeeding generation, the off-springs are also not likely to achieve their full growth potential in terms of tallness. Taking only tallness as a criterion, assuming that short women have not been adequately nourished, Thomson and his group found that the tall women produce healthier, heavier and taller and more active babies as compared to the short ones. They studied more than 26,000 births and concluded: "it is evident that whatever the nature of the delivery, the fetus of the short woman has less vitality and is less likely to be well grown and to survive than that of a tall woman" (Thomson and Hytten, 1973). A significant percentage of small statured women, whose growth has been stunted because of their undernutrition in early life, show abnormal pelvic shapes conducive to disordered pregnancy and delivery.

Baird noted during a study of 13,000 deliveries that fetal mortality rates were more than twice as high in women five feet one inch tall or less as compared to those five feet four inches tall or more. The shortness, whether it is induced by genetic stunting or inadequate nutrition during the periods of growth, seems to have a similar effect on the child-bearing ability (Thomson and Hytten, 1966). Thomson and Hytten aptly remarked that "the gradient of perinatal mortality with stature seemed to be just as steep in the well-to-do as in the poorer social classes. This was unexpected, since it seems reasonable to suppose that shortness in well-to-do women is more likely to be genetic than due to stunting, whereas the opposite may be true among the poor" (1973). On the grounds that short women always seem to be at a disadvantage compared with tall women, from the point of reproductive efficiency, Thomson speculated that the genes which determine the efficiency of growth might somehow be concerned with physiological functioning as a whole. This hypothesis is difficult to support or refute and carries with it the uncomfortable implication that short women are innately inferior from the point of view of physiological functioning, so that the *defect* could only be eliminated by selective breeding.

That the preconceptional nutrition of the mother is relatively important in terms of reproductive efficiency has been shown by another study conducted in England. The Indian and Pakistani immigrants (pregnant women) took full advantage of the maternal and child welfare facilities available in that country along with their local British counterparts. The Asian women were well-fed during their entire gestation period. The postnatal infant death rates between 1 and 11 months were similar in the two groups under study (the immigrant women and the local British sample). However, the study revealed that the neonatal death rate among the immigrant group was 2.4 times greater than the British group. The investigators concluded that the preconceptional nutritional health status of the immigrant mothers was poorer as compared to that of the British girls. The former went through greater stress of pregnancy, encountered more clinical problems, and the birth weight was generally lower. After the babies survived their neonatal period, both groups took equally good care of them (Akyroyd and Hussain, 1967).

A well grown woman is most likely to have tissue reserves which can be diverted to meet the nutritional needs of the fetus, even if the mother's own dietary intake is less than desirable. However, when a poorly nourished adolescent conceives, she becomes a reproductive risk. Her pregnancy is more frequently disturbed and her child more often of low birth weight. Such a child is at increased risk of neurointegrative abnormality and of deficient I.Q. and school achievement (Birch, 1972). When this child, if female, grows through adolescence and becomes a mother in her own time, the reproductive risk is not only greatly increased but the chances of the child being intellectually retarded are greatly enhanced.

A large percentage of adolescent girls in the overcrowded developing countries enter the state of pregnancy without any nutritional preparation for it. These girls in most instances did not get enough nutrition to satisfy the requirements of their own physical growth while they entered the nutritionally hazardous path of pregnancy. Such as unusual nutritional strain not only hinders her own growth, but seems to age her prematurely. As most clinicians would testify, these undernourished adolescent mothers undergo a great amount of physiological adaptation and successfully produce, without nutritional supplementation, live, healthy and adequately grown babies whose birth weight is in the normal acceptable range. In this process, the pregnant mothers make lots of compromises on their own health. It is well known that a healthy pregnant woman has to produce, in about nine months, 5 or 6 kg of complex new tissue, while at the same time prepare herself physiologically for lactation in the postpartum period, capable of supporting equally rapid growth for several months more. Consequently, nutritional requirements must be raised long before the episode of pregnancy. From such a point of view, a woman before pregnancy should form a nutritionally vulnerable group of great importance.

Nutrition During Pregnancy

Nutritional needs during pregnancy are by no means a settled subject. There are many gaps in our knowledge, which only intensive research and an open mind to analyze the evidence can solve. Many of us are so completely wedded to established classical concepts that sometimes it is hard to analyze and interpret the evidence objectively and in a straight-forward manner. It is, however, heartening to note that maternal concerns, prenatal care, the pre-pregnant weight as well as weight gain during pregnancy—all exert strong influences on the outcome of pregnancy (Habicht *et al.,* 1973; Jacobson, 1973; Martin, 1973; Light and Fenster, 1974).

Only to give a brief preview of the nutrition needs during pregnancy, it may be safely assumed that in the early stages of pregnancy the nutrition needs of the fetus are small and can be met from the maternal stores, but as the fetus grows not only is extra food needed to supply the baby, but the *maternal stores* also have to be taken care of. Together, the nutritional needs of the pregnant woman greatly increase, especially during the mid-pregnancy. For a better understanding of the nutritional needs of the pregnant mothers, we may analyze how the total weight gain during pregnancy is distributed between the fetus and the mother. Under normal circumstances, a woman who is healthy in the pre-pregnancy period, if allowed to eat according to her appetite, will add approximately 12.5 kg.

These days, an average weight gain of 24 lbs is considered desirable. The fetus (baby) plus the placenta and amniotic fluid (the fluid in which the fetus is bathed) weigh on the average 4,850 gms. What happens to the rest of the gain in baby weight? This is where *maternal stores* come into the picture. The maternal stores are not meant for the mother and are not intended to make the mother *fat,* as erroneously thought, but are a source of nutritional protection for a few months after the baby is born. After all, the mother's responsibility of feeding the infant does not finish at giving birth to it. Nature does not recognize the availability of pasteurized milk formulae at the supermarkets. Instead, the mother is nutritionally prepared, starting from mid-pregnancy onwards, to store nutrients for the care of the baby after birth. We must also recognize that the nutritional needs of the baby after birth are a lot more than when it was inside, cramped in a small space. The infant outside the mother's body cries, kicks, and uses extra energy not used by him in his *in utero* existence.

For the first few months, the baby has to depend on the

mother for its nutritional needs. It is then, that the mother's stores are useful. In addition to the 4,850 gms taken up by the fetus, placenta and fluid, approximately 1,500 gms are utilized in increasing size of the mother's uterus and the breasts. The blood volume of the mother also increases by at least 1,500 ml during pregnancy. The body also stores a large quantity of protein in the maternal tissues as some nitrogen balance studies show (Hytten and Leitch, 1971; Macy and Hunsicker, 1934), as well as fat. Hytten and Leitch estimated that a woman during her pregnancy stores approximately 3.5 kg fat or a reserve of approximately 30,000 k cals. This fat is deposited merely as a ready source of energy for use in the postpartum period under the influence of progresterone and usually disappears within a few months after the delivery of the baby. This energy deposit is extremely important from the point of view of protecting the baby, especially during late pregnancy and early postpartum period.

To summarize, the weight gain during pregnancy may be divided as follows: the weight of the fetus, seven lbs. or more being desirable; 2 lb. uterus; 2½ lbs. placenta and membrane; 2 lbs. breast tissue; 5 to 7 lbs. fluids; and increases in blood volume by about 15 percent, especially in the latter part of pregnancy. In addition, much nitrogen, calcium and phosphorus are stored in preparation for delivery and lactation (Robinson, 1970).

It is evident, therefore, that during pregnancy not only the quantity, but the quality of food intake is important. In addition to the calories, the mother needs a larger quantity of better quality protein to facilitate or ensure adequate fetal growth and maintenance (Munro, 1974). It is estimated that an average pregnancy needs 900 to 950 gm of protein in addition to the amount normally needed by the woman before she becomes pregnant (Chandrasekhra, 1972). The state of pregnancy leads not only to enhanced need of body building proteins, but also extra calories, calcium, iron, vitamin A, vitamin D, thiamine, riboflavin, niacin, folate, vitamin B_{12} and ascorbic acid. In addition, during the entire period of pregnancy, appreciable quantities of amino acids, vitamin C, folate, etc., are excreted out. The exact reason for this wastage at a time when they could be most usefully utilized is not known. In terms of extra calories, it has been estimated that an average woman weighting 55 kg needs 40,000 calories over the nine months period (FAO, 1957; FAO-WHO, 1970). (Table IX).

TABLE IX

DAILY RECOMMENDED ALLOWANCES FOR NON-PREGNANT AND PREGNANT WOMEN DOING LIGHT WORK

	United Nations		U. S. A.		United Kingdom	
	Non-Pregnant	Pregnant	Non-Pregnant	Pregnant	Non-Pregnant	Pregnant
Weight, kg	55	....	58	....	55	....
Weight gain, kg	....	10 ± 2	....	11	....	12.5
Energy, kcal	2,300	40,000 per pregnancy	2,000	2,200	2,200	2,400
Protein, g	56	65	55	65	55	60
Calcium, g	0.4–0.5	1.0–1.2	0.8	1.2	0.5	1.2
Iron, mg	14–28	14–28	18	18	12	15
Vitamin A, IU	2,500	2,500	5,000	6,000	2,500	2,500
Vitamin D, IU	100	400	none	400	100	400
Thiamine, mg	0.9	1.0	1.0	1.1	0.9	1.0
Riboflavin, mg	1.3	1.4	1.5	1.8	1.3	1.6
Nicotinic acid, mgEq	15.2	16.5	13	15	15	18
Vitamin B_6, mg	–	–	2.0	2.5	–	–
Folate, μg	200	400	400	800	–	–
Vitamin B_{12}, μg	2.0	3.0	5.0	8.0	–	–
Ascorbic acid, mg	30	50	55	60	30	60

From: A. M. Thomson and F. E. Hytten, *World Review of Nutrition And Dietetics*, Vol. 16 (1973).

No wonder that most women react to pregnancy by an increased appetite, with a small percentage either not increasing the appetite or decreasing it in their early part of the pregnancy. What is generally not understood is the significant increase in appetite in the early stages of pregnancy when the energy requirements of the fetus are very small and the maternal basal metabolism has not significantly increased. Cuthbertson explained that it may be a process of internal storage in preparation for the anticipated heavy demands of the fetus as its growth progresses (Cuthbertson, 1971).

The calorie needs are especially increased during the last

trimester. The precise amount may depend on the living pattern of the pregnant woman, but unnecessary restriction of the food intake as has been practiced in numerous cases in the United States and elsewhere is not looked upon favorably any more. The revised edition of the recommended daily allowances suggests strongly that pregnant women can benefit from an additional 10 grams over the recommended 65 grams of protein as well as larger amounts of calories (Committee on Maternal Nutrition, 1971 & 1973). It is now believed that an allowance of 65 grams of proteins during pregnancy is not adequate to permit maximum protein storage during the third trimester in young women (King *et al.,* 1971). If the caloric content of the diet is low, some of the needed protein may be utilized for providing energy (Kaminetsky, 1973). The situation can be corrected by increasing calories if protein intake is sufficient. When both calories and proteins are in short supply, it may result in a serious reduction in body proteins—muscles, cells, serum, enzymes and hormones (Hunscher and Tompkins, 1970). If the protein deficiency is severe, the nutritional rehabilitation may necessitate the intake of as much as 120 grams of protein per day along with appropriate increases in calories. In addition, daily supplementation with 30 to 60 mg of iron and with 200 to 400 mg of folic acid seems warranted for most pregnant women. Needs for other vitamins and minerals are also increased and those needs ideally are met through diet (Jacobson, 1973). The abnormalities in metabolism and functional capabilities caused by undernutrition during the critical period of pregnancy can persist long after an adequate supply of nutrients has become available (Roeder and Chow, 1972).

It appears that nutrition standards during pregnancy have been set to a great extent arbitrarily and the actual requirements still need to be worked out in detail. This is all the more true of the adolescent or teenage girl who gets pregnant while still needing extra nutrition to complete her own growth processes (Jones *et al.,* 1973; Working Group, 1971). Hillman and Hall have summarized some of the obvious difficulties in assessing precisely the optimum nutritional needs of gravid state and may be usefully reproduced here.

(1) The ethical, moral and legal limitations of investigating the human subject are compounded by the need to consider the interests of the child (and of the father) as well as of the mother.

(2) Animal studies, characterized by species and strain differences, cannot readily be extrapolated to human experience.

(3) Intra- as well as inter-individual variations preclude simple and valid conclusions from limited observations. Since not only the mother, but also the fetus and the placenta must be regarded as distinct biologic entities, the number of nutritional combinations appears infinite.

(4) The metabolic interdependence and interaction of at least half a hundred essential nutrients precludes simple identification of the precise role of each of these dietary components.

(5) Factors such as parental age, birth rank, and birth interval, influence the outcome of pregnancy, albeit not always as independent variables.

(6) The mother's pre-conception diet (and possibly that of *her* mother) is important. The adult woman is the outcome of growth, enhanced, warped, dwarfed and mutilated by the adventures of life.

(7) The ability of the human organism—and almost certainly of others—to adapt to suboptimal intakes (sometimes with subsequent impaired ability to utilize desirable increments) of dietary essentials complicates the problem of establishing optimum quantities and proportions of these substances. Metabolic mechanisms peculiar to pregnancy also seem to sustain successful reproduction in the presence of nutritional adversity. Together with superimposed, special demands, conception appears to generate equally special resources for meeting them.

(8) Nutritional deprivation typically is most severe where a wide range of non-nutritional adversities concurrently dispose to maternal and fetal complications. Clinical and epidemiologic studies have been comparatively unsuccessful in dissociating nutritional factors from other elements of the socioeconomic environment with which variations in perinatal experience are also closely identified. Psychologic factors, in particular, are being implicated in the causation of untoward effects.

(9) Assessment of the outcome of pregnancy obviously is a function of the criteria adopted. A wide range of indices—maternal and fetal, early developing and late appearing—represent not only a convenient battery of parameters for evaluating reproductive experience, but, unfortunately, also an equal number of opportunities for incon-

sistent and even incompatible interpretation. Nutrition considered optimum in respect to one aspect of reproduction is not necessarily optimum in respect to every other, and, moreover, is not necessarily optimum in respect to nonreproductive aspects of individual health and survival.

While we still have to answer some very important questions about the nutrition needs of pregnancy, the Nutrition Action Group in San Francisco, headed by Dr. Tom Brewer, has been very active in propagating their views of the nutritional implications of the gravid state. They have been advocating a generous amount of balanced diet, rich in protein as well as calories, throughout pregnancy. This group has strongly criticized the reducing diets on which a number of physicians put their patients throughout their prenatal period, for which there is no justification. Lowe, Higgins and Brewer have urged in the strongest terms that there is no justification of restriction of weight gain during pregnancy through low caloric regimen, restricted salt intake or by the use of diuretics (Brewer, 1973; Higgins, 1972; Lowe, 1972). Brewer has termed such a restriction in food intake as "Thalidomide II" because such a regimen could lead to the mental retardation of the child born to a mother whose diet in the last trimester is seriously reduced under the orders of her physician.

Vedra strongly criticized the practice of prescribing diuretics for the pregnant woman showing signs of preeclampsia. He emphasized the potential danger of these drugs and suggested complete bed rest for a woman whose blood pressure reaches 140/90 and shows signs of proteinuria. She should at the same time be given a wholesome diet. Insufficiency of calories and proteins when her metabolic demands are fairly high can lead to a state of semi-starvation which could be a direct cause of large volumes of fluid retention. This may be erroneously interpreted as a gain in fat and the patient may be advised to reduce further the caloric intake, resulting in disastrous consequences (Jones *et al.*, 1973).

Several studies have shown that improved nutrition of the mother during pregnancy has a profound effect on the infant's birth weight, its chances of survival as well as learning abilities (Manocha, 1972). This is in spite of the fact that the metabolism of the mother during gestation becomes more economical. From catabolic it becomes anabolic (Giroud, 1973). During early pregnancy, often before the woman is even aware that she is pregnant, critical development of the fetus takes place. A woman poorly nourished prior to pregnancy is much more subject to complications of pregnancy such as toxemia, hypertension, anemia and premature birth as also shown in animal studies on monkeys (Roberts *et al.*, 1974). It can be safely said that the orderly sequence of fetal development and growth, the mechanism for nourishment of the fetus, the storage of nutrients in anticipation of labor and delivery, and the development of mammary glands represent a level of anabolism unequalled in any other time of life (Robinson, 1970) Birth weight of the infant may not be a conclusive index of the physical and mental health of the baby, but does provide a reliable parameter for assessing the physiological make-up of the baby in terms of survival and functioning abilities. WHO figures show that of

every 1,000 infants born live and weighing 1,000 grams or less, 912 will die shortly after birth. Of the 1,000 babies between 1,000 gm and 1,500 gm, 512 will quickly die, while in the group between 1,500 and 2,000 gm, 180 will not survive. And, of 1,000 weighing between 2,000 gm and 2,500 gm, 41 will die soon after birth. In the group between 2,500 to 3,000 gm, only nine of 1,000 will soon succumb. The best chances for life are found in the group over 3,000 gm, where just four of every 1,000 will die (Symposium, Nutritional and Fetal Development, 1972).

In the poorer sections of the developing countries where women subsist on meager nutrition (as low as 1,400 cals and 30–40 gms of protein), they show a high percentage of premature termination of pregnancy. In a survey carried out in India, the poorer women gained around 6 kg during pregnancy, starting with an initial weight of 42 kg. This is extremely low in terms of desirable weight gain, which is 25 percent of the initial pregravid weight (Venkatachalam, 1962). The low birth weight of the babies is mainly due to the poor nutrition of the pregravid and gravid mothers (Rajalakshmi, 1971). Similar reports from many parts of the world have illustrated a general association between low birth weights, high fetal and infant mortality rates and diets of poor nutritive value of the gravid mothers. It seems reasonable to conclude that undernutrition and malnutrition among mothers, especially in the developing countries, contribute towards impaired maternal, fetal and infant health and vitality (*Nutrition in Pregnancy and Lactation,* 1965). The learning potential of the child is most likely determined by the brain composition at birth and during the first few months of life, when the child depends on the mother for growth, development and cellular differentiation. Pregnancy, therefore, is no time for watching weight or watching the proportion of a female figure. The mother needs adequate food to nourish a rapidly growing baby inside her. Butler, in a recent symposium, gave an excellent description of an ideal mother in these words.

> If I were a baby and were given the chance to choose my mother, I would certainly look for a tall girl in her early twenties, from a well educated family with adequate level of good nutrition, who would neither smoke tobacco or marijuana nor drink alcohol or use drugs. I wouldn't mind if she were a little plump, provided she had normal blood pressure.

Certainly, time has come to recommend in the most unequivocal terms that a good diet be given to the pregnant and lactating mothers. Chow emphasized that within a limited food supply situation, the woman during her period of gestation and lactation may be given a priority status.

In most developed countries, the caloric intake of the pregnant woman ranges from 2,400 to 2,700, which is an increase of at least 300 to 400 k cal over the normal nonpregnant state. Unfortunately, this is not the case in most developing countries, especially among the lower socio-economic group. While a majority of the population in these countries belongs to this group, the figures could have a very undesirable effect. In India a study of the low income pregnant women showed an intake of 1,390, 1,520 and 1,650 k cals during the first, second and third trimester of pregnancy respectively (Shankar, 1962). This is way low from the recommended level of 2,300 k cals. Another study of a similar socio-economic group revealed that the average daily intake of the pregnant woman was a total of 1,408 k cals with 38 gm protein (animal protein 6 gm), 315 mg calcium and 18 mg iron (Venkatachalam, 1962). In India a caloric intake by pregnant women of 1,400 to 1,500 cals and 40 gms of protein results in nearly 20 percent of pregnancies terminating in abortions, miscarriages and stillbirths. This figure may well be an underestimate and may not include abortions in the early stages of pregnancy (Gopalan, 1962). That the nutrition needs of the pregnant mothers are always satisfied in the developed countries is as untrue as the statement that all women in developing countries subsist on 1,500 calories per day during pregnancy. Calorie or protein intakes of women of low to moderate incomes in Tennessee were found to be as low or lower than averages reported for poor women in Mexico City and Chile (Thomson, 1959; Thomson and Hytten, 1973).

Improving the nutrition of the mothers directly improves the birth weight of the baby. Iyenger reported a significant increase in birth weight among babies born to poor Indian women who, during their third trimester, were given a qualitatively and quantitatively superior diet (Iyenger, 1968). A somewhat similar finding has also been reported by Venkatachalam. It has been estimated that for every 10,000 extra calories given to the mother, the fetus adds 50 gms of its weight (Habicht *et al.*, 1973). A random sample of women belonging to low socio-economic groups in India was admitted to the nutrition ward of a hospital during the last four weeks of gestation due to malnutritional states. During their stay in the hospital, they were given an adequately balanced diet, containing nearly 85 grams of protein and over 2,500 calories per day. In addition, they were able to enjoy complete physical rest. The mean birth weight of the babies born to these women was 2,986 ± 86 grams. This is in contrast to the expected birth weight of around 2,000 grams from women of that particular socio-economic group. This greatly highlights the need for improved nutrition during pregnancy.

One might make a brief mention of the varied drugs that are ingested by pregnant women, especially in the developed countries. Over the last two decades, tablets have become a part of the regular food of a large segment of the population. Women carry at least 2 to 3 different varieties of tablets in their purses in anticipation of their need. They are generally aspirin, multivitamin tablets or iron tablets or antihistamines. The drug ingestion syndrome does not disappear with pregnancy. What effect this drug eating behavior has on the growing fetus inside their bodies is not completely known and needs a comprehensive study. A detailed study of Dr. Forfar on 911 pregnant women and by Dr. Hill on 156 pregnant women belonging to middle to high socio-economic groups is quite revealing. These investigators found that on the average, a pregnant woman in the United States consumes 10 different kinds of drugs. The analgesics (pain killing medicines) are the most frequently used, followed by antihistamines, diuretics, antacids, sedatives and iron tablets (Hill, 1973).

TABLE X

DRUG INGESTION BY GRAVID WOMEN

Drug	Forfar: 911 patients (%)	Hill: 156 patients (%)
Analgesic	63	64
Antihistamine	7	52
Diuretic	18	57
Antibiotic	16	41
Antacid	34	35
Sedative	28	24
Antiemetic	16	36
Iron	82	41
Vitamin supplement		25
Hormone	4	20
Appetite suppressant	1.2	10
Hypnotic	1.4	9
GU antibiotic		6
Narcotic		5

From: R. M. Hill, *Clin Pharm Therapeut 14*, 654, 1973.

Some of these drugs are quite potent in their effect on the physiology of the mother and may affect the growing baby inside the mother adversely (Desmond *et al.*, 1972; Loughnan *et al.*, 1973; Mirkin, 1973) .

Nutrition Needs of Lactation

It is not generally appreciated that the demands made by lactation on the mother are greater than during pregnancy. During pregnancy, the mother has to supply the needs of a growing fetus of 2 to 3 kg weight. The movements of the fetus are almost insignificant and calorie consumption is of a low order. A lactating mother, on the other hand, provides food for a vigorously active, crying, kicking baby with a higher consumption of calories and at the same time, the baby is growing at a rapid rate. This is a strain of a considerable magnitude on the nutrient supply of the mother. If the pregravidic health of the mother is good and she has been getting adequate diets during pregnancy, she will have accumulated a store of nutrients in readiness for satisfactory lactation. If she continues to get a diet richer than her own body needs, she can maintain a satisfactory lactation for a fairly long period of time. Unfortunately, this is not true of most women in the developing countries where the necessity to maintain adequate lactation is all the more important in the absence of well-prepared, easily digestible baby foods. Unfortunately, these are the girls who themselves have sustained underfeeding while in their childhood, which may have impaired the development of adequate mammary tissue (Gunther, 1968). These girls fail to lactate as well as a girl who was adequately nourished in her childhood.

The situation can be compounded if the mother is in her adolescent years. In that case, the stress of pregnancy and lactation has been superimposed over her own period of maximum growth and development. In most of the developing countries, a pregnant woman does not consume more than 1,500 k cals compared to a desired 2,300 k cals. If such a woman continues to live on 1,500 k cals in the postpartum period, it only means that while she has freely drawn upon her own tissues to provide for the growing fetus inside her body, she will continue to do so to feed her infant outside her body. In India a diet survey of lactating mothers revealed that only a small percentage of them were using milk in their diets. In some cases, the problem of providing a good quality diet to the lactating mother is that of ignorance, but in most cases it is the poverty that stands in the way of obtaining reasonably good nutrition.

Also, while there is some appreciation throughout the world that a pregnant mother needs to eat more because of the prevalent belief that she has to eat for two (herself and the baby inside her), there is unfortunately little appreciation of the rather considerably increased needs of a lactating mother. According to one estimate, 1,000 food calories are needed to produce 600 calories of breast milk (WHO, 1965). The energy in milk should ideally be derived from the diet, but in its absence it is subsidized by catabolizing maternal tissues because the quality of a milk, whether it is produced by a well nourished woman or a poorly nourished one, has to be maintained. If the latter is substantially under-nourished, her milk may show some deficiencies of vitamins and minerals, but not a whole lot. Little or no information exists on how women in developing countries (who often have to undertake hard physical work while lactating) meet the energy costs of lactation (WHO Chronicle, 1965). The fortunate thing is that a lactating mother is a very efficient milk producing machine. It is assumed that the energy supplied in the diet may be used for milk production with an efficiency of at least 80 percent (*Nutrition in Pregnancy and Lactation,* 1965). If the lactating mother is given extra quantities of food, she produces larger amounts of breast milk.

To summarize, it is desirable for a lactating woman to have an additional 10 gms protein daily over the quantity recommended for her during her gestation period (20 gms more than the adult allowance). A lactating mother should have no less than 75 grams protein per day. A woman weighing 128 lbs may need as much as 98 gms of protein daily

(McWilliam, 1967). The same is true of caloric intake. Eight hundred calories more than the prenatal diet is needed for lactation. It may sound high, but a lactating mother will do well on an intake of about 3,000 calories which will help her to produce 850 ml or 30 ounces of milk. Human milk contains 20 calories per ounce. Approximately 600 calories are needed for supplying the baby's needs in milk and about 400 calories are needed by the mother for milk production, which puts the additional needs of lactation at 1,000 calories per day (Williams, 1969). A woman in the developing country taking a total of 1,400 to 1,500 calories per day cannot be expected to lactate successfully.

It has been reported that drinking water in amounts beyond the natural inclination of thirst impairs lactation, which may be due to an inhibitory effect on posterior pituitary secretion because of water logging (Illingworth and Kilpatrick, 1953).

There is another aspect of lactation that may be fascinating. In a number of Eastern countries there is a prevalent belief that, while a mother is lactating, she is unlikely to become pregnant. For curious reasons, they look to lactation as a contraceptive. It could also be that they believe nature could not superimpose another pregnancy while she is lactating and feeding one infant. So, a prolonged period of lactation and breast feeding is greatly encouraged. The result may be quite harmful to the mother from a nutrition standpoint, because most often she does become pregnant again. As Chandrasekhra put the Indian situation, the mother continues to nurse the first baby until the new one arrives and occasionally even after the birth of the new baby. "The Indian woman is thus in an almost continuous state of lactation—however meagre—throughout the childbearing period of her life." For such a woman, it is the nonpregnant and nonlactating state from 15 to 40 years of age that is exceptional. The nutritional burden of pregnancy and lactation on these females is so heavy that it results in a process of rapid aging. A thirty-five year old woman after 6 to 8 deliveries on diets of marginal nutritive value appears to be in her early or late fifties.

Picas and Aversions to Food

One must mention certain abnormal eating behaviors of certain adults, which may not be rationalized in any way. This is especially true of the pregnant and lactating women. Picas refers to eating clay, plaster, ashes, charcoal, etc., and they have been observed throughout the world (Cuthbertson, 1964). There is every possibility that certain nutritional deficiencies induce certain individuals to eat these articles. Eating earth and clay by children in India is fairly common, especially those who show intestinal parasites. Pregnant women, especially in their early period of gestation, also eat clay in India. In Nyasaland, pregnant women eat clay and rubble in the belief that their unborn children will be helped by this practice.

A closer examination reveals that most of these women who impulsively eat earthy substances and clay, generally get a diet which is insufficient in calcium. It is probable that the inclination to eat clay is under a physiological demand for calcium, especially in the case of pregnant women. The clay may provide significant amounts of iron and calcium. Among the rural women of southern United States, it is not uncommon to find persons ingesting clay and maize starch. Sometimes the clay may be baked before eating, whereas the maize starch is generally eaten uncooked. Cuthbertson explained that maize starch

> may serve as a substrate for enhanced microbial activity and vitamin biosynthesis in the cecum and colon, and thus lead to increased absorption, particularly of B vitamins. In South America, especially in Mexico, maize is cooked in lime water and eaten. This may be a strange way of cooking maize, but it certainly would provide calcium to the body in the absence of adequate consumption of milk and dairy products (1964).

The pregnant women all over the world have been known for this kind of abnormal eating and craving for unconventional objects. Not only clay, but objects like coal, soap, toothpaste, plastics, chalk, etc., may be liked and eaten as well. No satisfactory biochemical and physiological explanations are available at this time. A number of hypotheses varying from deficiency of calcium, iron or other nutrients to hormonal changes in the body due to pregnancy are put forward. The pregnant women, especially in their early stages, undergo a profound change in their sense of taste and smell. Certain favorite foods suddenly become unattractive and tasteless and certain pleasant objects start giving a foul smell. These aversions and cravings are generally corrected by themselves as the course of pregnancy progresses into the 2nd or 3rd trimester and a normal or even increased appetite for common foods returns.

SPECIAL CONSIDERATIONS

The nutrition needs under special circumstances such as environmental stress, injury, surgery, convalescence or obesity greatly vary from those of the normal individuals who lead at least moderately active lives. The nutrition needs in the course of obesity resulting either from physical inactivity or any metabolic disorder have been discussed at length in Chapter VI. The effect of cold environment on the nutrition needs of an adult is somewhat controversial. Nevertheless, there is agreement on changed needs in the person living in arctic and tropic climates. There is a belief that the energy expenditure for a given task is greater in the cold than in the warm climates because of the need for more heat and to maintain thermal equilibrium (Johnson and Karle, 1947). The reader is referred to a detailed review by Shils, who concluded that working in the cold climate results in increased need for calories. Sufficient clothing is needed to maintain the body temperature, but more frequent meals containing larger than normal amounts of fat would also help. There appears to be no significant increase in the need for vitamins in the cold climates beyond that associated with increased caloric expenditure (Shils, 1968).

In the hot climates, the nutritional needs are altered to some extent but mainly those associated with the dissipation of heat. The need for sodium chloride and water are enhanced. In an attempt to maintain normal temperature,

the body secretes sweat, the evaporation of which removes
heat. No ill effects on the health are probable if water and
salt are periodically replaced. In its absence, though, undesirable effects ranging from decreased physical and mental activity to death could take place. Many observations
have confirmed that the physical status and performance of
persons doing hard work in hot climates deteriorates within
a few hours if water is withheld. When the heat load is high
and continued, thirst may fail to insure an adequate intake
of water. It is recommended that men working in the heat
replace the water lost in sweat by hour to hour intake of
water in quantities sufficient to keep thirst quenched at all
times.

In physical injury or a major surgical operation, there is a
significant loss of tissue, which is accompanied by increased
urinary excretion of nitrogen as a result of breakdown of proteins. A negative nitrogen balance in the order of 12 to 15
gm/day may result because of a loss of 350 to 450 gms of
muscle and other lean tissues (Cuthbertson, 1971). Potassium
is also lost from the cells and may, in a severe injury, be higher
than the corresponding nitrogen losses (Davidson *et al.*, 1972).
If the progress in convalescence is satisfactory, the body does
not suffer any real physiological damage. Davidson *et al.* explained that

> the tissue breakdown in response to injury or surgery is almost cer-
> tainly due to an increased secretion of cortical hormones by the adrenal
> glands. This is part of the normal physiological response to stress and
> is mediated through the pituitary gland and increased secretion of
> ACTH. It is not possible to prevent this loss of tissue by dietary
> measures and, insofar as it seems to be a physiological response, there
> is little justification for attempting to do so. However, the loss must
> be made good when convalescence is established.

In chronic illnesses, especially those associated with
sepsis, the problem of adequate nutrition is likely to be compounded. First, the fever (a natural response of the body to
infection) may raise the metabolic rate as well as the energy
needs so that larger quantities of essential food elements
may be needed. But the associated toxemia may result in an

impairment of the appetite so that not enough food may be eaten in spite of the awareness for its need, resulting in a drastic reduction of weight and a general state of undernutrition and malnutrition. It has been estimated that when a big area of the skin is destroyed by a septic burn, the direct loss of protein from the burned surface may be as much as 50 gm/day (Davidson *et al.*, 1972).

The operative procedure has a direct as well as indirect effect on the nutrition of the individual. Indirectly, the anxiety of the procedure may depress the appetite and reduce the desirable food intake. As a direct influence, the operation is a nutritional stress resulting in loss of tissue and it is most advisable that a patient should be well nourished before undergoing an operation. A diet rich in protein, energy as well as protective foods (vitamins and minerals) is essential. Special requirements of vitamin K may be indicated because of its association with bleeding. An operative procedure is also known to increase the utilization of vitamin C due probably to the increased activity of the adrenal cortex. Surgery on an obese person involves bigger risks of nutritional imbalances than surgery on an average, healthy one. The chances of diabetes in an obese person are much more than the chances in a leaner one. The nutrition aspect during convalescence is probably the most important one and must be paid adequate attention. The body's losses of protein reserves can be made good only by a generous supply of biologically high quality proteins in the diet. A thin and lean patient may be better off when put on a high calorie diet. "The patient's appetite may be fickle and the inclination to eat reduced. Every art of the dietician may be needed too tempt his jaded appetite" (Davidson *et al.*, 1972).

REFERENCES

Akyroyd, W. R., and Hussain, M. A.: *Br Med J, 1*: 42, 1967.
Akroyd, N. R., and Krishnan, B. G.: *Indian J Med Res, 27*: 409, 1939.
Atkins, R. C.: *Dr. Atkins' Diet Revolution.* New York, McKay, 1972.
Ascorbic Acid, Recommended Daily Allowances. NAS-NRC Publication #1694, Washington, 1968.

Astrand, P.: *Health and Fitness.* Stockholm, Skandia Insurance Co., Ltd., 1972.

Astrand, P. O.: In Rechcigl, M. (Ed.) : *World Rev Nutr Dietet* Vol. 16, 1973.

Baird, D. J.: *Pediatrics, 65:* 909, 1964.

Bergstrom, J., Hermansen, L., Hultman, E., and Saltin, B.: *Acta Physiol Scand, 71:* 140, 1967.

Bernstein, D. S.: *JAMA, 198:* 499, 1966.

Berstrom, J., and Hultman, E.: *Nature (Lond), 210:* 309, 1966.

Bicknell, F., and Prescott, F.: *The Vitamins in Medicine.* London, Heineman, 1945.

Birch, H. G.: *Am J Public Health, 62:* 773, 1972.

Brewer, T.: *Medical Tribune,* October 24, 1973.

Brock, J. F., and Autret, M.: *WHO Monograph Series #8.* Geneva, WHO, 1952.

Brodan, V., Kuhn, E., Pechar, J., and Honzak, R.: *Nat Rep Int, 1:* 611, 1973.

Bourne, G. H.: In *Exercise Physiology.* New York, Acad Pr, 1968.

Burke, B. S., and Stuart, H. C.: Physique, personality and scholarship. *Society for Research in Child Development, Monograph #34.* Washington, NRC, 1943.

Butler, N.: In *Symposium on Nutrition and Fetal Development.* New York, November 13, 1972.

Chadd, M. A., and Fraser, A. J.: *Int Z Vitamin Forsch, 40:* 604, 1970.

Chandrasekhra, S.: *Infant Mortality, Population Growth and Family Planning in India.* Chapel Hill, U NC Pr, 1972.

Chittenden, R. H.: *The Nutrition of Man.* London, Heinemann, 1909.

Chow, D. F.: *Nutr Rep Int, 7:* 247, 1973.

Christakis, G., et al.: *Am J Public Health, 56:* 299, 1966.

Christensen, E. H., and Hansen, O.: *Skand Arch Physiol, 81:* 160, 1939.

Committee on Maternal Nutrition of the Food and Nutrition Board. Washington, Natl. Academy of Science, 1971 and 1973.

Cotzias, G. C.: In Comar and Bronner (Eds.) : *Mineral Metabolism,* Vol. 2. New York, Acad Pr, 1962.

Cuthbertson, D. P.: In Beaton, H. H., and McHenry, E. W. (Eds.) : *Nutrition.* New York, Acad Pr, 1964, Vol. 2.

Cuthbertson, D. P.: *Proc Nutr Soc, 30:* 150, 1971.

Darby, W. J.: In *Present Knowledge of Nutrition.* New York, Nutrition Foundation, 1967.

Davidson, S. A., and Passmore, R.: *Human Nutrition and Diabetes.* Edinburgh, Livingstone, 1966.

Davidson, S., Passmore, R., and Brock, J. F.: *Human Nutrition and Dietetics.* Baltimore, Williams and Wilkins, 1972.

DeLuca, H. F.: *Nutr Rev, 29:* 179, 1971.

Desmond, M. M., Schwanecke, R. P., Wilson, G. E., Yasunega, S., and Burgdorff, J.: *J Pediatr, 80:* 190, 1972.

DeVries, H. A.: *J Gerontol, 25:* 325, 1970.

FAO: *U.N. Transactions.* Rome, Italy, 1955.

FAO: *Nutritional Studies, #15,* 1957.

FAO-WHO: *FAO Nutr Meetings Report,* Series #230, 1962; #301, 1965; #362, 1967; and #452, 1970.

Fisher, R. B.: *Protein Metabolism.* London, Mathues, 1954.

Foman, S. J., and Bertels, D. J.: *AMA J Dis Child, 99:* 27, 1960.

Food and Nutrition Board: *Recommended Daily Allowances.* Natl Academy of Science, NRC Publ. #1146, 1969.

Gallagher, G. H.: *Nutritional Factors and Enzymological Disturbances in Animals.* Crosby, Lockwood & Son, 1964.

Gallagher, J. R.: *Ann NY Acad Sci, 69:* 900, 1958.

Giroud, A.: In Bourne, G. H. (Ed.) : *World Rev Nutr Dietet,* Vol. *18,* 1973.

Goodhart, R. S.: In Wohl and Goodhart (Eds.) : *Modern Nutrition in Health and Disease.* Philadelphia, Lea and Febiger, 1968.

Gopalan, C.: *Bull WHO, 26:* 203, 1962.

Granit, R.: *The Basis of Motor Control.* London, Acad Pr, 1970, p. 346.

Gunther, M.: *Proc Nutr Soc, 27:* 77, 1968.

Guth, L.: *Physiol Rev, 48:* 645, 1968.

Habicht, J., Yarbrough, C., Lechtig, A., and Klein, R. E.: *Nutr Rep Int, 7:* 533, 1973.

Hensen, A. E.: In Nelson, W. T. (Ed.) : *Textbook of Pediatrics.* Philadelphia, Saunders, 1959.

Higgins, A. C.: Address 4th Int. Congress Endocrinology Symposium, June 23, 1972.

Hilkner, D. M., Wenkam, N. S., and Lichton, L. J.: *J Nutr, 87:* 371, 1965.

Hill, R. M.: *Clin Pharm Therapeut, 14:* 654, 1973.

Hillman, R. W., and Hall, J. E.: In Wohl, M. G., and Goodhart, R. S. (Eds.) : *Modern Nutrition in Health and Disease.* Philadelphia, Lea and Febiger, 1968.

Holmes, J. O.: *Nutr Abstr Rev, 14:* 597, 1945.

Hultman, E.: *Scand J Clin Lab Invest,* [Suppl] *19:* 94, 1967.

Hunscher, A. A., and Tompkins, W. T.: *Clin Obstet Gynecol, 13:* 130, 1970.

Hunter, W. M., and Sukker, M. Y.: *J Physiol (Lond), 196:* 110, 1968.

Hussain, S. L.: *Lancet, 1:* 1069, 1969.

Hutchinson, R. C.: *Nutr Abstr Rev, 22:* 283, 1952.

Hytten, F. E., and Leitch, I.: *The Physiology of Human Pregnancy.* Oxford, Blackwell, 1971.

Illingworth, R. S., and Kilpatrick, B.: *Lancet, 265:* 1175, 1953.

Irvin, M. S., and Hegsted, D. M.: *J Nutr, 101:* 1, 1971.

Iyenger, L.: *Am J Obstet Gynecol, 102:* 834, 1968.

Jacobson, H. N.: *JAMA, 225:* 634, 1973.

Johnson, O. C.: *Nutr Rev, 25:* 257, 1967.

Johnson and Karle: *Science, 106:* 378, 1947.

Johnston, J. A.: *AMA J Dis Child, 14:* 489, 1947.

Johnston, J. A.: *Nat Acad Sci, R.R.C. Publ. #843:* 319, 1961.

Jokl, E.: *Nutrition, Exercise and Body Composition.* Springfield, Thomas, 1964.

Jolliffe, N.: In N. Jolliffe, F. F. Tisdall and P. R. Cannon (Eds.): *Clinical Nutrition.* New York, Hoeber, 1950.

Jones, P. H., Tillack, W. S., Melton, R. J., and Smith, J.: *Health Serv Rep, 88:* 187, 1973.

Kaminetsky, H. A., Langer, A., Baker, H., Frank, O., Thomson, A. D., Munves, E. D., Opper, A., Behrle, F. C., and Glista, B.: *Am J Obstet Gynecol, 115:* 639, 1973.

Karlsson, J., Diamant, B., and Saltin, B.: *Scand J Clin Lab Invest, 26:* 385, 1971.

King, J. M., Galloway, D. H., and Morgan, S. In *Proc West Hemis Nutr Cong III.* Mt. Kisco, Futura, 1971.

Lantz, E. M., and Wood, P.: *J Am Diet Assoc, 36:* 138, 1958.

Latham, M. C., and Grech, P.: *Am J Public Health, 57:* 651, 1967.

Latham, M. C., McGandy, R. P., McCann, M. D., and Stare, F. J.: *Nutrition Scope Manual.* Kalamazoo, Upjohn, 1970.

Lennard-Jones, J. E., Fletcher, J., and Shaw, D. G.: *Gut, 9:* 177, 1968.

Leren, P.: *Aetna Med Scand,* [Suppl] 466, 1966.

Levander, D. A.: In *Present Knowledge of Nutrition.* New York, Nutrition Foundation, 1967.

Lewis, S., and Gutin, B.: *Am J Clin Nutr, 26:* 1011, 1973.

Light, H. K. and Fenster, C.: *Am J Obstet Gynecol, 118:* 46, 1974.

Loomis, W. F.: *Science, 157:* 501, 1967.

Loughnan, P. M., Gold, J., and Vance, J. C.: *Lancet, 1:* 10, 1973.

Lowe, C. V.: *Am J Clin Nutr, 25:* 245, 1972.

Lynch, H. D.: *Ann NY Acad Sci, 69:* 895, 1958.

MacDonald, I.: *Practitioner, 201:* 292, 1968.

Macy, I. G.: *Nutrition and Chemical Growth in Childhood.* Springfield, Thomas, 1942.

Macy, I. G.: *Nutrition and Chemical Growth in Childhood.* Springfield, Thomas, 1951.

Macy, I. G., and Hunsicker, H. A.: *Am J Obstet Gynecol, 27:* 878, 1934.

Manocha, S. L.: *Malnutrition and Retarded Human Development.* Springfield, Thomas, 1972.

Malhotra, M. S., Ramaswamy, S. S., and Ray, S. N.: *J Appl Physiol, 17:* 488, 1962.

Maroney, J. W., and Johnston, J. A.: *AMA J Dis Child, 54:* 29, 1937.

Martin, H. P.: *Am J Clin Nutr, 26:* 766, 1973.

Mayer, J.: *Postgrad Med, 40:* 6, 1966.

Mayer, J.: *Postgrad Med, 47:* 5, 1970.

Mayer, J.: *Human Nutrition.* Springfield, Thomas, 1972.

McWilliam, M.: *Nutrition for the Growing Years.* New York, Wiley, 1967.

Medical Letter, 13: 97, 1971.

Mendez, J., Scrimshaw, N. S., Ascoli, W., and Guzman, M. A.: *Am J Clin Nutr, 9:* 143, 1961.

Mertz, W.: *Ann NY Acad Sci, 199:* 191, 1972.

Mickelsen and Yang: In Wohl and Goodhart (Eds.) : *Modern Nutrition in Health and Disease.* Philadelphia, Lea and Febiger, 1968.

Mirkin, B. L.: *Clin Pharm Therapeut, 14:* 643, 1973.

Munro, H. N.: *Am J Clin Nutr, 27:* 55, 1974.

Nutrition Committee Br Med Assoc: *Br Med J, 1:* 542, 1950.

Nutrition in Pregnancy and Lactation: WHO Tech Rep Series *302,* 1965.

Nutrition Reviews, 22: 306, 1964.

Nutrition Reviews, 25: 100, 1967.

Palmisano, P. A.: *JAMA, 224:* 1526, 1973.

Pauling, L.: *Vitamin C and Common Cold.* San Francisco, Freeman, 1970.

Prasad, A. S.: *Am J Clin Nutr, 20:* 648, 1967.

Pruett, E. D. R.: *J Appl Physiol, 28:* 199, 1970.

Rajalakshmi, R.: *Trop Geogr Med, 23:* 117, 1971.

Reiser, R.: *Am J Clin Nutr, 26:* 524, 1973.

Roberts, J. A., Hill, C. W., and Riopelle, A. J.: *Am J Obstet Gynecol, 118:* 14, 1974.

Robinson, C. H.: *Basic Nutrition and Diet Therapy.* London, Macmillan, 1970.

Roeder, L. M., and Chow, B. F.: *Am J Clin Nutr, 25:* 812, 1972.

Rosa, F. W., and Turshen, M.: *Bull WHO, 43:* 785, 1970.

Sandstead, H. H.: In *Present Knowledge of Nutrition.* New York, Nutrition Foundation, 1967.

Scammon, R. E.: In Abt, I. A. (Ed.) : *Pediatrics.* Philadelphia, Saunders, 1923.

Schwartz: *Fed Proc, 20:* 666, 1961.

Science News, 101: 44, 1972.

Shankar, K.: *Ind J Med Res, 50:* 113, 1962.

Shils, M. E.: In Wohl and Goodhart (Eds.) : *Modern Nutrition in Health and Disease.* Philadelphia, Lea and Febiger, 1968.

Sinclair, H. M.: In Beaton, G. H., and McHenry, E. W. (Eds.) : *Nutrition.* New York, Acad Pr, 1964.

Stearns, G.: *JAMA, 142:* 478, 1950.

Stearns, G., Newman, K. J., McKinley, J. B., and Jeans, P. C.: *Ann NY Acad Sci, 69:* 857, 1958.

Stott, D. H.: *Dev Med Child Neur, 15:* 770, 1973.

Suzuki, H.: *Acta Endocrinol, 50:* 161, 1965.

Symposium, Iron Deficiency and Absorption. *Am J Clin Nutr, 21:* 1138, 1968.

Symposium, Nutrition and Fetal Development. New York, November 13, 1972.

Thomas, J. A. and Call, D. L.: *Nutr Rev, 31:* 137, 1973.

Thomson, A. M.: *Brit J Nutr, 13:* 509, 1959.

Thomson, A. M., and Hytten, F. E.: In Beaton, G. H., and McHenry, E. W. (Eds.) : *Nutrition.* New York, Acad Pr, 1966.

Thomson, A. M., and Hytten, F. E.: *World Rev Nutr Diet,* 1973, Vol. 16.

Trotter, R. T.: *Science News, 101:* 44, 1972.

Underwood, E. J.: *Trace Elements in Human and Animal Nutrition.* New York, Acad Pr, 1971.

Van Huss, W. D.: *Nutrition Today,* March, 1966, p. 22.

Vedra, B.: *Med World News,* November, 1973.

Venkatachalam, P. S.: *Bull WHO, 26:* 193, 1962.

Wadsworth, G. R.: *Practitioner, 201:* 297, 1968.

Walshe, J. M.: *Proc Nutr Soc, 27:* 107, 1968.

Wang, C. C., Kancher, M., and Wing, M.: *AMA J Dis Child, 51:* 801, 1936.

WHO Chronicle, 19: 326, 1965.

WHO, Expert Committee on Nutrition in Pregnancy and Lactation. *WHO Tech Rep* Series 302, 1965.

Widdowson, E. M., McCance, R. A., Harrison, G. E., and Sutton, A.: *Lancet, 2:* 1250, 1963.

Williams, R. J., Heffley, J. D., Yew, M. L., and Bode, C. W.: *Persp Biol Med, 17:* 1, 1973.

Williams, S. R.: *Nutrition and Diet Therapy.* St. Louis, Mosby, 1969.

Working Group on Nutrition and Pregnancy in Adolescence. *Clin Obstet Gynecol, 14:* 367, 1971.

CHAPTER V

NUTRITION NEEDS OF OLD AGE

A N ELABORATE STUDY into the nutrition requirements of old age is most desirable because in our modern society, the age composition of its members has changed considerably during the last few decades (Hayflick, 1973). The number of old people in our society has progressively increased due to a worldwide control of communicable diseases. Whereas some infants still die in their infancy, more and more people are living into old age. At present, at least 10 percent of the world population can be classified as aged and retired (Riley and Foner, 1968), and every year their population is growing in most countries of the world because of improved living standards and medical care in middle age. During the years 1940 to 1960, the U.S. population of persons 65 years old and over increased 84 percent; from 9 to 17 million persons. At the same time, the number of people 75 years old and over increased 115 percent; from 2.6 to 5.6 million (Theur, 1971), and the numbers have grown significantly since then.

DEFINITION AND PROBLEMS OF OLD AGE

The onset of old age, although arbitrarily put at 65 years of age, varies so much from person to person that it is hard to define an aged person. Judging from external manifestations of age on the face and body, and certain degenerative symptoms, one person at 45 years of age may be old enough to the extent that another person may be at the age of 60 or more. While discussing the nutrition requirements of the old, one may be well advised not to take into account the chronological years, but rather certain degenerative characteristics.

In that context, we may usefully think of three kinds of aging: physical aging, social aging and psychological aging. Different people may experience these at different periods within their life and these aspects should have a direct bearing on the nutrition needs of the individual. It is indeed possible to be physically aged in the forties, while at the same time socially middle-aged and psychologically young. A college professor who is keen of mind, at the height of social involvement, but with little physical activity, may fit this category. It is equally possible to be physically middle-aged in the seventies, socially young and psychologically old. A vigorous golfer with many friends and few social responsibilities, whose thinking has become rigid and slow, would fit this combination. At another extreme, it is possible to be physically alive but socially and psychologically dead. This is true of old and not-so-old patients in mental hospitals and nursing homes. This is also the case in many older people living in their children's homes and having no social role or function there (Tuttle *et al.,* 1957).

The nutrition needs of these different categories of old people will be greatly varied. The purpose of a nutrition program for the aged must, therefore, keep in mind the physical and social, as well as psychological needs. It has to be something more than meal-planning based on nutritional requirements. It must be prescribed in relation to social involvement which facilitates choice of foods based on the individual's tastes as well as social background and psychological needs.

The sudden mandatory retirement of individuals at the age of 65 (in some societies, the retirement age is 60 or less) from their professions suddenly imposes a socio-economic and psychological strain which greatly influences the whole outlook of the individual on life as well as nutritional care of his body. Unless an individual is highly qualified in some special way, the person over 65 years of age has extreme difficulty in relocation (Fishbein, 1973). The elderly are thus left with no other choices except to live on their past savings, social security or the benevolence of their relatives. It is often not easy to live on one's achievements or past savings. Not all elderly persons think of the past as a period of achievement and draw satisfaction out of it. Many of them have had a long life of psychological and economic struggles which, on retirement into old age, are not any solace but rather a burden which they carry along into old age with shrunken income, shrunken social involvement and shrunken body. Economic insecurity, especially, creates pressures, although psychological handicaps such as a decreasing sense of acceptance and accomplishment could be as harmful.

Good nutrition in old age cannot add years to life but may be able to add some life into years, making other social and psychological adjustments somewhat less difficult. It is in this light that we must study the nutrition needs of old people and strive to give them comfort after they have contributed many long years to the service of their community. Williams gave an excellent description of old age:

> Depending on one's resources at this point, there is either a predominant sense of wholeness and completeness or a sense of distaste, of bitterness, of revulsion and of wondering what life was all about. If the outcome of life's basic experiences and problems has been positive, the individual arrives at old age a rich person—rich in wisdom of the years. Building on each previous level, his psychological growth has reached its positive human resolution.

Some people have come to believe that most of the old people live in institutions and that they prefer to live there. The management of institutions take it upon themselves to provide balanced nutrition to these people. The actual fact is that 96 percent of all the old people live in the community in which they have lived in the past (Fishbein, 1973). They face all the uncertainties that accompany an unproductive life, an unsatisfactory level of fixed income and continuous increase in the cost of living. At least 15 percent of the old people cannot keep a house (Fishbein, 1973). Subsistence on a marginally adequate income and nutrition for long periods of time could be an invitation to malnutrition and frank pathological processes. Social security payments are not adequate enough to afford a decent standard of living, with the result that most of the old (except those who have income from their properties or investments) are poor and do not have money to provide adequately for their diets and physical comforts. They are compelled by the limited resources to cut down on the foods they have been eating for a lifetime, and not every time is such a cut sagacious and based on optimum nutrition (Evans and Stock, 1971).

Their lack of initiative, physical energy and ignorance also leads to tremendous wastage of food. The amount of food entering their kitchens does not give a true representation of the food that is actually available to the cells in their bodies. When the aged are involved in preparation of food, it suffers considerable and valuable losses of nutrients, particularly vitamins. Losses in storage and washing out of water soluble components in the kitchen and during cooking are also colossal (Marks, 1969).

In any program of improving the nutrition standards of the old, adequate attention must be paid to correcting their social and psychological sources of trouble, such as social isolation, desertion by dear and near relatives, and getting over financial or other worries. In most cases, after these problems are taken care of, the elderly will feel a desire to eat well. However, if appetite needs to be improved, it may be worthwhile to give the elderly person several small meals a day so that the food is better utilized and absorbed.

BODY CHANGES IN OLD AGE

The onset of old age from the vigorous middle age is a slow process of physiological changes which make the body sensitive and somewhat less tolerant to environmental stress. The process of aging, like the wear and tear of a man-made machine with time, can lead to so much exposure to disease, stress and infections that at a ripe age it may produce a picture of a human being which is quite complex and confusing.

This picture varies from person to person depending on the degree or severity of the above-mentioned exposures.

It is difficult to minimize the misfortune of such exposures to environmental stress, but it may be added that the quality of nutrition can either accelerate the process or slow it down. One person, having taken good nutritional care of himself, may be young at the age of 70, whereas the others, having gone through similar environmental stresses, ignored nutrition at the same time and could be aged and senile by age 50. Watkin stressed that, practiced with care, sensible nutrition from age 40 onward will go far in ensuring a vigorous and long life by deferring the development of disease processes (Watkin, 1966).

Old age leads to a general slowing down of metabolic processes and a concomitant modification of eating habits is desirable (Williams, 1969). The food habits acquired during the life of vigorous activity cannot continue into old age without discomfort and ill effects. The athletic ability, especially the speed of doing things, decreases significantly in old age. The other physiological processes that may show signs of loss are the vision, sexual powers, general vigor and probably intelligence. The last one is quite controversial. Numerous studies indicate that with advancing age, intelligence decreases proportionately (Birren, 1959), but a longitudinal study of Eisdorfer reveals that there is no significant drop in intelligence level before the age of seventy.

The composition of the blood in old persons with respect to acidity, volume, osmotic pressure, glucose, hemoglobin and protein content is maintained within normal limits as compared to middle aged persons (Solomon and Shock, 1969). This is not the case with different organs of the body; their performance deteriorates to a certain extent depending on the functional demands (Shock *et al.*, 1963). Solomon and Shock described such changes taking a standard of a 30 year old person and giving him a performance score of 100 percent. By these measurements, the rate of conduction of impulses in the ulnar nerve diminishes by 15 percent between the age of 30 and 90 years (Solomon and Shock, 1969), whereas renal blood flow is reduced by 50 percent, resting cardiac output by 30 percent (Branfonbrener, 1955) and maximum breathing capacity by 40 percent (Shock, 1962). Although the rate of degradation of thyroxine is significantly reduced in old men, (Gregarman, *et al.*, 1962), their thyroid glands are quite capable of responding to exogenously administered TSH (Baker *et al.*, 1950). Muscle strength decreases with age so that a 90 year old is about equivalent to a 15 year old (Fisher and Birren, 1947). Loss of muscle strength is attributed to the loss of muscle fibers. The other change with advancing age is a decrease of intracellular water. In a glucose tolerance test it takes much longer for an aged person to return the blood sugar level to normal compared to a young person and so is the case with respiration rate after a mild, moderate and hard exercise.

The loss in the number of functional cells is particularly evident in the tissues, which do not have the ability to regenerate, e.g. the nervous system, skeletal muscle, cartilage, heart, kidneys, etc. The kidneys invariably show a loss of renal functions which is a direct reflection of the loss of its functional units (Shock, 1961). This leads to a reduced or inefficient performance of these organs as the aging process continues. A few comments may be made on performance of the nervous system in the advanced years of life. There are more and more indications that, whereas improper nutrition may affect the different organs of the body adversely, the nervous system remains essentially unchanged and a person at 70 years of age may be as intelligent, alert and capable of additional learning as a middle aged person.

However, there are certain aspects of nervous function that do deteriorate (Rudd, 1973). Most prominent among these impaired functions are decrement of reaction time, visual acuity, organization, rate of conduction of impulses in motor nerve fibers, slower alpha rhythms in electroencephalograms, etc. (Birren, 1959; Fridenwald, 1952; Norris *et al.*, 1953). Some of the anatomic changes include loss of neurones in the cortex, together with changes in the Nissl substance of remaining cells, pale staining nuclei, and irregular cell outlines (Rothschild, 1947). Other changes include hypertrophy among astrocytes, the formation of argentophile placques, and an increase in intracellular lipid-containing pigment (O'Leary, 1952). It is not clear how much functional impairment the above mentioned changes bring about in the nervous system. It is probable that some of the changes connected with aging affect the speed of performance. Otherwise the older persons are mentally quite alert. Certain behavioral changes may be attributed to decrement in sensory process (Weiss, 1959).

MEAL PLANNING FOR THE AGED

Meal planning for the aged is no different from a similar program for the middle aged adults. Old age is necessarily a continuation of the past life, along with likes and dislikes about certain foods. It may be advisable to encourage an old person to continue to eat his favorite foods if they have been modified to some extent, keeping in view the changed physiology, changed activity level and changed social interrelationships. While we talk of certain modifications in food intake, we have to think about the established food habits through long periods of time. The old people are known to be most rigid in their food habits as compared to any other age group. For example, if men and women are used to consuming large quantities of fried foods, rich desserts, highly seasoned foods and strongly flavored vegetables in their middle age, it is difficult to dissuade them in their ripe age to restrict their use. They may prefer to omit proteins, vitamin, or mineral rich foods in order to continue to eat their favorite carbohydrate and fat rich foods, despite the knowledge that the absorption of these foods in the gastrointestinal tract is much less efficient compared to their younger years. It is here that the meal planner has a responsibility of substituting desirable things without seemingly interfering with established food habits. One has to study in detail the food habits of the old people in order to find out whether or not their meal planning is based on solid principles and what are the actual dietary errors (Sherwood, 1973). It is only after this intimate knowledge that suitable ways and means can be devised to introduce appropriate modifications in nutrition, while not disturbing the food habits of the individual in any significant manner.

In order to provide a balanced diet to the aged person, the meal planner should be conscious of the desirability of providing a variety of foods. Meat, poultry, eggs and fish are good sources of protein, fat, iron and vitamins, whereas dairy products are essential because of their richness in calcium as well as fat and vitamins. The importance of vegetables and fruits, especially citrus fruits for vitamin C, and dark green or yellow vegetables for Vitamin A, needs to be stressed. In most instances, the old people have been observed to have no fresh fruits and vegetables. This is not because these articles do not fit in with their food habits, but most often it is a result of changed circumstances, which have curtailed their mobility and economy so that they cannot afford to buy a balanced diet. The social circumstances tend to modify their availability of food and one may see old persons eating a lot of one food and ignoring the other. It is ironical that the income level of the old people goes down at a time when they need the extra money to buy protective foods to maintain themselves. For example, lean meats, fresh fruit and vegetables are always expensive and, ideally speaking, they are needed more by the old than the middle aged people. Jahnke described that the old folk, especially women, tend to consume a lot of fat and sweet things and in old men a preference for coffee as well as alcoholic drinks is seen (Jahnke, 1961). Old people seem to have a preference for refined foods.

One may outline certain principles, which may be applicable to a vast majority of the aged persons (Rao, 1973). It includes:

a. Intake of fewer calories in view of reduced physical activity and metabolism. Ideally, an aged person should try to maintain a weight pattern that existed in his or her middle twenties.

b. The intake of protein may be increased from the normally recommended 1.5 gms to 2.0 gms per kg body weight in order to maintain normal nitrogen balance. It may be desirable to have 20 to 25 percent of the calories from a protein source. On the other hand, the calories derived from fats should be reduced to approximately 20 percent of the total caloric intake. The food should provide enough *roughage* to prevent constipation.

c. Vitamin and mineral intake should be generous, particularly iron, calcium and vitamin C.

d. It is quite important that the aged should have a generous intake of water and fluids. It is recommended that the fluid intake should be equivalent to 6 or 7 glasses a day, so that the urinary output will be at least 1500 ml over a 24 hour period.

The basic principle of meal planning, however, is that the food should appeal to taste as well as smell, so that it is appetizing and attractive. Among the aged, not infrequently the sense of smell and taste are dulled.

Parosmia and anosmia, conditions characterized by loss of smell due to obstruction of nasal fossae or due to any disease in other parts of the nose, have been observed in a significant number of old people. In these conditions, the old person is aware of a persistent smell which could render the food offered to him quite monotonous, uninspiring and nonappetizing, thereby resulting in a loss of interest in food.

During the course of meal planning for the aged, adequate attention should also be paid to the dentition of the person concerned. Most of the old people use dentures for cosmetic purposes and are not able to use them well for chewing and crushing, and may tend to swallow the food. First of all, the food should not be very hard in consistency, but more important, the aged may need instruction and emphasis that they should not swallow their food without first masticating it sufficiently, thereby stimulating the flow of saliva and making use of salivary amylase, a necessary digestive enzyme.

NUTRITION NEEDS IN NORMAL HEALTH
Calories

The caloric requirements of old persons do not differ significantly from those of the middle aged. The caloric intake varies from person to person depending on the activity level. In very active person, a caloric intake of as high as 3,800 calories may not be excessive, whereas this high food intake may lead to obesity in a sedentary person. For the latter, a caloric intake of 2,000 may be enough. McGandy *et al.* described that in a group of men with sedentary work habits, the caloric intake ranged from 2,688 ± 584 cal/day at age 20 to 34. By the age of 75, the caloric intake went down to 2,093 ± 441 cal/day. Schematic conclusions about the daily caloric intake of old persons are not justified. The theoretical calculations of calorie requirements from metabolic tables may prove to be erroneous (Jahnke, 1961).

There are several factors which are important in determining the caloric requirements of aged persons. With advancing age, the basal metabolism slows down and the physical activity is also reduced to a great extent. A professional academician is likely to lead a sedentary life and in the old age should not need more than 2,000 calories, whereas a farmer of the same age, leading a very active life and indulging in great amounts of physical work, may consume 50 percent more calories (Gsell, 1956).

It is not merely the caloric needs that should be emphasized. It is more important in the old age that weight be maintained and the body be kept in good physical shape. The best index of determining the right amount is the maintenance of a particular weight level, which should be ideal for a person's height and age. Extra calories lead to weight gains and when taken over prolonged periods, result in obesity (Morgan, 1955). In these individuals, the rigid calorie control is a must, without falling into the trap of statistics of mortality and morbidity among the overweight. Even if the weight gain is slow, a constant addition of weight would lead to certain changes in the body conformation, which will be extremely deleterious in the advancing age. The Food and Agricultural Committee suggested that between ages 25 to 45, the caloric intake should be reduced by 3 percent from the caloric needs at the age of 25 years. Thereafter, between the ages of 45 to 65, a 7.5 percent decrease in caloric intake is recommended. The persons older than 65 may be well advised to reduce as much as 10 percent of their caloric needs at 25 years of age (FAO, 1957). Watkin (1968) described the consequences of slow increments in weight due to excessive caloric intake and accretion of body fat.

> Premature changes in the islets of Langerhans, accumulation of lipids in arterial walls, increased load on the heart and the incompletely known effects of subjecting certain enzyme systems to excessive metabolic loads increase the potential hazard of disease for all overeaters. Volunteers on low-calorie diets have demonstrated greater mechanical efficiencies than similarly trained subjects on high calorie regimens.

The results obtained from recent investigations have strongly emphasized that excessive intake of calories cuts down the life span by initiating certain disease processes, whereas restriction of calories and caloric intake in strict accordance to needs, helps prolong the life span. This has been amply demonstrated by a number of investigations on animals and is undoubtedly true of humans as well. Caloric restriction in early age helps to slow down the growth processes and, if the caloric restriction is not of a severe kind, it may help prolong life by reducing early mortality (Carlson and Hoelzel, 1947; Haleckvog and Chavapil, 1965). McCoy *et al.* investigated the experimental prolongation of the life span by feeding a well-balanced calorie restricted diet to rats. They not only succeeded in increasing the life span by more than double their normal expectancy, but also delayed sexual maturation for periods up to 1,000 days (longer than the normal life span) after which they resumed their normal growth and reproduction.

On the other hand, when the animals are given *ad libitum* diets, they become obese and their average life expectancy decreases significantly. If only we could prevent obesity in the advancing years by a combination of caloric restriction and moderate exercise, one could prolong his life expectancy by as much as four to five years (Mayer, 1962; Solomon and Shock 1919). In order to keep the body in good physical condition, the ideal thing to do is to combine reasonable caloric restriction with mild but regular exercise, e.g. walking is highly desirable for aged persons, as it will not only improve the muscle tone and the appetite, but also clear lipids from the blood.

Proteins

Although 65 gm/day is the average recommended figure of protein intake by an average sized elderly person, the actual protein requirement has not been satisfactorily determined. It is possible that with advancing age, larger quantities of essential amino acids may be needed. The studies of Ohlson *et al.* showed that an intake of 43 grams of protein was enough for a 50 to 75 year old woman weighing around 60 kg (0.88 grams protein per kg body weight per day) in order to maintain a positive nitrogen balance. Tuttle *et al.* (1957) conducted a series of experiments to prove that the aged person needed almost twice as much methionine and lysine compared to a young person in order to maintain nitrogen equilibrium.

On the other hand, a high protein diet will mean a much larger load on the kidneys because the excess protein has to be catabolized into urea and excreted through the kidneys. At the same time, it is well established that renal functions always deteriorate with age. The rate of protein synthesis is also slowed down (Chinn *et al.*, 1956). Some studies recommend the use of anabolic steroid hormones to stimulate protein synthesis, which also leads to improved nitrogen retention (Solomon and Shock, 1969).

In view of these facts, it is difficult to comment on the protein requirements of old people to everyone's satisfaction. Some studies do indicate that in ripe old age, the protein intake should be increased to as much as 1.5 to 2.0 gm/kg/ body weight (Kowitz *et al.*, 1953), although metabolic studies indicate that the elderly can maintain positive nitrogen balance on a diet containing 1 gm/kg/body weight content (Watkin *et al.*, 1953). Higher protein intake is recommended by some workers having based their conclusions that generous amounts of protein will have "specific effect, as it checks the tendency, common in old people, to accumulate fat" (Jahnke, 1961). They also argue that in the aged, there is a constant low level of serum albumin, which may be due to reduced protein synthesis by the liver. An effort should be made to give a diet which could provide all the essential amino acids in right proportions. Animal proteins may be preferred, but a wise selection and variety of vegetable proteins should be equally good in providing a good quality protein.

As a valuable source of high quality protein, the importance of milk in the diet of aged people may be rightly emphasized here. Since a majority of the old have lost their teeth, a liquid diet such as milk may go a long way in providing the basis of a good diet. The milk, in addition to proteins, is also a good source of dietary calcium, vitamin D, riboflavin and, to some extent, thiamin, ascorbic acid and iron. The intake of appropriate amounts of calcium is important as the years roll by. The development of osteoporosis with advancing age is a result of inadequate consumption of milk or other dairy products which creates a chronic shortage of dietary calcium intake. For those who cannot tolerate lactose, fermented milk products such as yogurt may be recommended (Boer, 1970).

It may be concluded that for practical purposes under conditions of average normal health, an aged person should not be considered different from a person in his middle years. The commonly recommended 1 gm/kg protein in the daily diet, provided it is of good quality, preferably derived from animal sources or by a judicious selection of vegetable sources, should be enough to meet the needs of the elderly person (Troll, 1971). The latter, however, could experience some sudden demands on his protein reserves by injury, disease or therapeutic measures, the incidence of which is likely to be more in old age than at any other time in life.

Carbohydrates

Carbohydrates provide the highest percentage of any nutrient in the diet of any age group. However, the calories derived from carbohydrates should be balanced with those

of fat and protein, which are equally essential. Excess carbohydrates, especially the refined ones (sugars) provide a
large amount of *empty calories* which may be harmful for
the elderly as it has been suggested that man's ability to
metabolize carbohydrates is reduced with advancing age.
The refined carbohydrates are a source of trouble to the
aged also because of the high incidence of diabetes among
them. The detailed investigations of Gordon revealed
that 20 percent of persons 65 to 74 years of age and 23
percent of those between 75 and 79 years show sugar in
the urine. The rising consumption of sugar and white flour
(refined carbohydrates) relates not only to diabetes but
also to the incidence of peptic ulcer, diverticular disease,
constipation, coronary heart disease, varicose veins, etc. (Taylor, 1972).

The level of carbohydrate intake may be regulated in
the vicinity of 55 to 60 percent of total calories in the diet.
Excess carbohydrates also play an important role in elevating
the level of serum cholesterol and serum triglycerides (Cohn
et al., 1962). As with fat absorption, the efficiency of absorption of carbohydrates is also diminished with the advancing
age and may be due to general inefficiency of the gastrointestinal tract. For example, in the elderly, the number of
absorbing cells is reduced. The efficiency of the mucosal
transport system is reduced and finally the blood supply to
the intestine may also be reduced due to arteriosclerosis
(Geokas and Haverback, 1969).

Another important effect of carbohydrates, especially
the refined ones, is their deleterious effect on the teeth. This
would result in a higher incidence of dental caries. The
problem of dental caries is not a very serious one in old age
because a high percentage of the aged do not have their
teeth. But if the harmful effects of excess sticky-type carbohydrates (candies, etc.) are stressed among the young and
middle aged, a larger number of old persons probably will
have their own teeth. There is no denying that the natural
teeth, even if somewhat worn, are better than new dentures.

Fats

The problem of quantity or quality of fat intake in the elderly is important because of its relationship to the problem of atherosclerosis. Some studies indicate that with advancing age, the ability to absorb fat decreases significantly and is probably due to inadequate production of pancreatic lipase or an impairment of some absorptive process in the intestinal mucosa or an abnormality in lipid metabolism (Becker *et al.*, 1950; Berkowitz *et al.*, 1959; Citi and Salvini, 1964).

The amount of desirable fat intake by elderly persons is indeed controversial in view of the fact that fat leads to elevated levels of cholesterol and coronary artery diseases are closely related to high cholesterol and lipoprotein levels in the blood (Watkin, 1968). From that point of view, the saturated fats must be reduced to a minimum possible level (*Nutrition Reviews,* 1967). It is recommended that fats should provide an average of 20 to 25 percent of the calories in the diet of the aged. This includes visible (added to the food) and invisible (bound with the food, such as meat and dairy products) fats.

In order to reduce the invisible fat in the diet, special emphasis should be placed on the consumption of skim milk, fish, poultry and lean meats. Sausages with as much as 50 percent fat should be avoided. It is wise therefore, to make the elderly aware of the harmful nature of excessive fat intake. Because of its richness in calories, it could easily lead to obesity. At the same time, forcing the aged to abandon their life-long food habits may not prove wise because such a compulsion to cut down fat or replace it with unsaturated fats may lead to the reduction in the intake of calories, proteins, vitamins and minerals as the palatability and satisfaction derived from fat-rich foods is diminished (Watkin, 1966).

Vitamins

In general, the vitamin needs of the old people do not

increase and they need not be given vitamin supplements if their dietary habits are based on sound principles. Most often problems arise due to their low vitamin intake for long periods of time (Melinghoff, 1959). It is possible that the elderly people overcook their food in order to help them in its mastication, as well as digestion, and a number of vitamins are destroyed in the process, especially vitamin C. Several studies have revealed that, in spite of dentures, a substantial proportion of aged persons does not use dentures while eating, and prefers to eat soft and somewhat overcooked foods. Commenting on the vitamin deficiencies among the elderly, Marks emphasized that it is time we take the vitamin deficiencies among this vulnerable section of our population seriously, because when clinical symptoms appear, the body is already yelling for help for survival. Before these symptoms appear, the aged person shows increasing ill health, loses body weight, appetite, and experiences malaise, insomnia and increased irritability. These are the complaints most often heard from elderly people, which, in reality, may be subclinical symptoms of vitamin deficiencies, curable simply by giving supplements. Marks added that:

> the clinical signs of a vitamin deficiency are the end result of a chain of reactions. The vitamins are taken in the food, absorbed from the intestinal tract, stored and utilized by the body cells. They are broken down or excreted and a balance is established between vitamin intake and vitamin loss. If vitamin loss exceeds intake, there is first a depletion of the vitamin stores, then a cellular metabolic change in consequence of the depleted coenzymes. Only after these metabolic changes have reached a critical level do the classical clinical signs appear. At a later stage still, anatomical changes in the tissues take place, some of which, e.g., keratomalacia, are irreversible (1969).

It may be worthwhile to give a systematic course of instruction to the elderly on their food needs, and ways and means to meet them under their changed circumstances. Special attention must be paid to make them aware of the losses, especially of vitamins, during the course of cooking or handling. For example, a milk bottle left in bright sunlight on the doorstep for a few hours by the milkman may lead to substantial losses of riboflavin (Marks, 1968). The general deficiency of B complex vitamins leads to a lack of general *vitality and vigor*. The chronic deficiency of thiamine is also observed in a great proportion of the old people. It results in loss of appetite, irritability and insomnia. When the symptoms are mild and the old person complains of cardiovascular complaints or absence of appetite, not too uncommonly, attention is not given to the deficiency of thiamine with the result that the situation keeps on deteriorating. When properly diagnosed, most symptoms disappear with vitamin supplements.

Marks (1969) emphasized that in most cases, doctors fail to look for and recognize the clinical symptoms and it may be due to erroneous thinking that vitamin deficiencies do not exist in the developed countries. Studies on a fairly large sample in the United States indicate that the average thiamine intake of elderly persons is around 0.7 mg, which is far lower than the recommended 13 mg (Brin *et al.*, 1964). Robinson recorded that out of 62 deaths from degenerative vascular disease, 12 cases (20%) showed clear evidence of beri beri.

Although not very common, polyneuritis among the aged results in great discomfort and pain. Large doses of thiamine lead to early relief of pain and muscular tenderness. Even a mild case of polyneuritis may cause so much distress as to immobilize an already frail patient. Wernicke's encephalopathy, especially among elderly alcoholics, may not be cured by giving supplements of thiamine, but the latter helps to a great extent in giving some relief, especially in ocular movements (Mayer, 1972). Greater thiamine needs have been indicated by several workers.

The deficiency of nicotinic acid is not by any means common among the aged but in some individuals, whose protein intake is very low and whose diets do not provide sufficient amounts of tryptophan, the niacin deficiency appears and can be helped to a great extent by large doses of niacin (Jelli He, 1940). Mayer described the progression of niacin deficiency in the elderly.

The onset is insidious and the earliest symptoms are vague (fatigue, irritability, depression, nervousness). Later, impairment of intellectual function supervenes, followed by stupor and coma. Associated with the clouding of consciousness are certain other neurologic signs, rigidity of the limbs, grasping and sucking reflexes, extensor plantar responses, exaggerated tendon reflexes, and sometimes polyneuritis and spinal cord lesions. Signs of classic pellagra (scaling, erythematous skin rash, glossitis, diarrhea) may or may not be present (1972).

Folic acid deficiency is not uncommon in aged people and is directly responsible for megaloblastic anemia. A direct correlation between low serum folate levels and certain brain disorders has been observed in a number of investigations, especially in old persons and in several cases, treatment with folic acid leads to a complete disappearance of the symptoms (Reynolds, 1967; Strachan and Henderson, 1967).

The requirements of vitamin B_{12} are not any different in old age as compared to middle age. In spite of some decrease of B_{12} in the serum, most of the aged persons get a sufficient quantity of this vitamin in their diets, irrespective of its quality. Some studies indicate that their retention of B_{12} when administered parenterally is better than the younger person (Watkin *et al.*, 1953). It is only during and after prolonged sickness that a deficiency of B_{12} may become evident (Theur, 1971).

In old people, the requirements of vitamins C and D, and calcium, are closely interlinked. It is not uncommon to observe aged persons complaining of backache, stiffness and skeletal deformities. Many investigators have observed a similarity in the symptoms characteristic of scurvy and senility. In both cases, the bones are rarefied, susceptible to fracture and defective in healing. Similar changes are observed in bones and tissues surrounding the teeth. In most cases, the capillary walls have become fragile. Large quantities of vitamin C are quite helpful. At the same time, it is essential that the old person be provided with adequate quantities of vitamin D and calcium in the diet. The amount of vitamin D derived from sunlight is generally small in old people as they are most often housebound. It is essential that the diet be supplemented with sufficient amounts.

The reasons for the prevalent vitamin C deficiency among the aged are the infrequent consumption of vegetables and fruits and the overcooking of vegetables, which destroys their vitamin C content. Taylor described that a survey of the elderly people on the lists of general practitioners revealed that 80 percent of them showed some degree of vitamin C deficiency, which manifests itself in the form of sublingual hemorrhages. Several studies have also indicated that there is a greater incidence of vitamin C deficiency among aged men than women (Brocklehurst *et al.,* 1968; Marks, 1968). Another interesting observation relates to higher incidence of vitamin C deficiency in the winter months as compared to summer (Andrews *et al.,* 1966; Chazan and Mistilis, 1963; Scobie, 1969).

Vitamin K deficiency in the elderly is very rare and will result only in very bizarre cases of a disease or bad eating habits when the dietary intake as well as synthesis by intestinal microflora will be insufficient. However, in certain diseases and therapy involving sulfa drugs and antibiotics, the internal sources of intestinal synthesis may be wiped out and result in inadequate synthesis of prothrombin, which may lead to "poor clotting and subsequent bleeding, purpura and poor wound healing" (Watkin, 1966).

Minerals

With the growing years, the mineral needs do not increase or decrease in any significant manner as compared to the younger years. Some comment on the desirability of caution with respect to certain minerals may be in order. Calcium is one of the most important minerals. There is a lot of stress laid in the literature on the calcium intake of older people. Some studies clearly indicate the desirability of higher calcium intake by the elderly.

Osteoporosis in old people is closely associated with the chronic deficit of calcium and vitamin D. Its presence is as common as 50 percent in the postmenopausal women and leads to progressive thinning and rarefaction of bone, making it more prone to fracture (Latham *et al.,* 1970; Smith and

Rizck, 1966). Gitman and Kamholtz found that in a group of 933 females, approximately 50 percent between the ages of 65 and 70 had osteoporosis. The incidence increased essentially linearly to 90 percent in women who are 90 or more years old. The incidence among old men is significantly lower for some reasons. Although lack of calcium seems to be the main reason for the onset of osteoporosis in old persons, some other factors may also play an important role. Special mention may be made of immobilization, castration and lesser availability of sex hormones such as estrogen (Morgan *et al.*, 1966; Saville, 1969). Gam *et al.* also showed that high calcium intake did not necessarily prevent the loss of bone density in old people (Gam *et al.*, 1967; Hegsted, 1967). A large number of elderly people can maintain calcium balance with a daily intake of 0.6 to 0.8 gm (Malus, 1958).

Is it not possible that calcium deficiency in old age may have been caused by some undefined metabolic defect associated with aging or the deficiency of some other mineral element (Watkins, 1950)? First of all, there is no calcium deficiency in the United States, where milk intake is quite high. Fluoride seems to have a beneficial effect. It becomes a part of the bone substance just as it does in dental enamel, replacing hydroxyl ions in the chemical composition of the bone and giving rise to a layer of bone crystal which may be less liable to resorption. A comparative study of two areas in North Dakota with differing amounts of fluoride in their water substantiated the claims that fluoride has a beneficial effect on the onset and incidence of osteoporosis (Bernstein *et al.*, 1966; Bernstein and Cohen, 1967; Hodge and Smith, 1968). Posner suggested that fluoride, by becoming a part of the bone mineral, makes a bigger and harder crystal from which calcium cannot be easily resorbed. Along with high intake of calcium, fluoride may help to reverse the alveolar bone loss in elderly people.

Iron, sodium and potassium are other minerals whose unsatisfactory intake by the aged person could cause metabolic problems. The serum iron level drops with advancing age and generally the recognizable anemia is due to iron deficiency. Adequate amounts of iron should be assured in the diet of the elderly. Watkin (1966) however, expressed that a resort to parenterally administered iron is usually unnecessary in terms of both inconvenience and expense, not to mention its potential carcinogenicity. The desirable iron intake is approximately 12 to 15 mg per day.

Regarding the sodium requirements, it must be emphasized that old people are prone to hypertension and water retention which should indicate a restricted intake of sodium chloride. In the industrialized societies of the West, it is difficult to estimate the amount of salt eaten because of its liberal use in all preserved foods such as canned foods, frozen foods, etc. It may be recommended that old people should, whenever possible, resort to eating fresh vegetables, fruits and meats. The desirable intake of salt is in the range of 5 to 7 gm per day (Melinghoff, 1959). Salt restriction is especially desirable if there is any indication or tendency of congestive heart failure, hypertension, cirrhosis of the liver and other conditions related to the retention of extracellular fluids.

The deficiency of potassium is quite rare in the middle aged people, as most of the green vegetables and fruits are quite rich in this mineral. Since the consumption of protective foods is greatly reduced in old age, special attention should be paid to seeing that their diets provide enough potassium. Several studies indicate that potassium deficiency in the elderly is caused by physicians who prescribe a number of drugs for certain ailments which deplete the cells of their potassium content, e.g. cortisone and related drugs (*Medical World News,* 1969). Taking laxatives causes the body to lose potassium, disorders interfering with absorption of food such as colitis or diarrhea create potassium lack, and occasionally drugs given for high blood pressure may disrupt the body's balance of potassium. It is speculated, with a certain amount of scientific evidence, that a crippling disease like muscular dystrophy may be a result of acute potassium deficiency.

It is difficult to comment on the desirability or undesirability of spices and seasonings and not much work has been done to investigate the effects on the gastrointestinal tract and digestibility in old people. Jahnke stated that

> seasoning is not only permissible in the diet of the old, but is also necessary, to enhance potability and toleration. We found that many old persons both like and tolerate piquant seasonings such as pepper and paprika, if used in moderation.

SOCIO-ECONOMIC, PSYCHOLOGICAL AND CULTURAL FACTORS AFFECTING THE NUTRITION OF THE AGED

It is the experience of many physicians, who look after the geriatric patients and aged persons capable of feeding themselves, that their dietary recommendations are not followed by them. Most often it is not because they do not respect the doctor's ideas of their need for the prescribed items, but they consider nutrition not as big a problem as their sociological and psychological hang-ups. No one who feels responsible for the care of the aged can divorce their psychological problems from the nutritional ones. Most common among the problems of the aged are concern for their families, for their belongings, preoccupation with religious ideas and concern for their future incomes, security, decreased social involvement and fear of desertion by their children.

Most often, those working with old people are fond of stressing these points, yet seldom do they do anything about it, and concern themselves with what they eat and what they should eat. Loneliness, eating alone, poor cooking facilities, lack of energy to go around and shop, and financial worries lead to depression that only old people can understand. Married old couples survive much better the vicissitudes of old age compared to isolated elderly persons, who could end up with a progressively deteriorating health on an ill-balanced monotonous diet. Physical inactivity leads to mental illness and lack of initiative and interest in life, which also may be accelerated by bereavements for dear and near ones.

A deeper analysis of the nutrition of the aged reveals

that there are certain factors, which are beyond their control, that determine their food intake and health care. The predominant ones are psychological and financial. It is common to see the old people showing disinterest in food because of their loneliness, which makes them psychologically lazy regarding the chores of meal preparation. Equally important are the financial factors which influence the nutrition of old people. It has been estimated that in the United States, 75 percent of the persons older than 65 years live on incomes which are significantly below their needs. The financial condition of old people in other countries is not much different. As a matter of fact, it is more on the dismal side. Under these circumstances, "one is tempted to glibly generalize that the most important deficiency afflicting many of the aged is not the deficiency of vitamins and minerals, but of money" (Burton, 1961).

Rao outlined some of the important factors which lead to an improper nutrition in old age:

1. Limited income may restrict the purchase of adequate amounts of the right kinds of food, proper cooking facilities, and refrigeration.

2. Loneliness, unhappiness and bereavement can lessen the appetite.

3. Reduced activity, increased fatigue and weakness, or living alone may affect the incentive for eating. Lonely men who are unused to cooking or women who used to cook for the family, lose interest in the process. Thus they tend to eat a poorly balanced diet consisting of foods which require little preparation.

4. Elderly persons living in urban areas are particularly prone to social isolation, which leads to mental and physical deterioration.

5. Many factors operate when support from family, friends or community is not available. Such deprivation often leads to apathy, depression and impairment of the appetite.

6. Food fads and fallacies and chronic alcoholism can pave the way for poor nutrition.

7. Chronic invalidism, of whatever origin, fosters lack of appetite and a poor nutritional status.

8. Poor dental health may be a serious factor in the poor eating habits of the elderly.

9. Mental disturbances, such as confusion or depression, significantly affect eating habits and the nutritional state.

10. In general, a combination of several of these factors makes the elderly especially vulnerable to malnutrition.

The culture of a particular country, region or community also has a profound effect on the nutrition and well-being of the aged. In some cultures, the old people are considered an asset to their family in terms of benefitting from their wide experience and baby sitting services, rather than any liability, and an honorable place is accorded to them. It is probably due to these cultural protections that, in most of the underdeveloped and developing countries, one does not come across any special government sponsored programs to help the old people at a time when they are incapable of agressively earning their means of subsistence. That does not imply that the governments in their countries are callous to the needs of their senior citizens. The cultural set-up in these countries seems to be potent enough to cause no special hardship to the subsistence of old people.

Let us take for example the Hindu cultural system, which divides a man's life into four parts, of a quarter of a century each. The first 25 years, according to this cultural tradition should be spent in growing and acquiring learning or trade in an unmarried state. The second 25 year period is meant for pursuing professions and procreation, whereas the third 25 year period is a transitional period in which the older person should prepare for retirement, give the leadership or head of the household status to his children and live under their patronage. In the last 25 year period, the man is expected to renounce the world and live a life of seclusion and devotion to God.

The impact of this cultural heritage has been quite strong over the society for thousands of years, until the last decade or so when the growing industrialization is forcing a change in the way of life of young as well as old people. The life expectancy in these countries is also very low and it is only a small fraction of the population that reaches the age of 70 or over because of the hardships suffered and the lack of good nutrition and material amenities throughout life. It is a truism to say that, in these cultures, the offsprings seem to develop a moral obligation towards the care of the older generation, because they always feel that they will reap the fruit by getting similar care from their own children. The children have, therefore, taken the role which is generally assumed by the government and the life insurance companies in the industrialized countries. Watkin has arrived at similar conclusions about the nutrition problems of the aged.

Technically underdeveloped societies have at present relatively fewer problems with the aged. High infant mortality rates of childhood and young adulthood, in the absence of adequate nutrition and systems for the distribution, availability and utilization of health services, result in only the genetically elite surviving into old age. The low level of concern about the aged also results from the fact that most technically underdeveloped societies are composed of extended families in which the genetically elite survivors to old age enjoy considerable honor, prestige and influence. However, in view of the drive towards industrialization and the improvement in nutrition and the delivery of the health services, more of the nonelite aged will be appearing on the scene with each passing year and as their numbers swell their burden on the extended family will increase. What has happened in technically advanced industrialized societies will undoubtedly recur in presently technically underdeveloped societies (1973).

While the scholarly conclusions of Watkins on the conditions of the old people in the underdeveloped countries seem valid, it seems that he has not paid adequate attention to the cultural influences on the *extended family system,* in those countries. Technical development or no technical development, it is doubtful if the extended family system in those countries would have survived for thousands of years without the moral bindings imposed by socio-cultural traditions. It is in these traditions that lies the future of the aged in all the poorer countries and, to some extent, the rich countries as well. Let us take for example the Hindu and the Chinese cultures. Even after the ancestors are dead, the younger generation voluntarily mourns their death once a year for a number of years and even offers food to the poor in their name or puts it on their grave. Reverence for the old age is culturally ingrained, which is reinforced by the feeling that the younger generations of today are the older generations of tomorrow. On the part of the older generation, as they grow older, they tend to give away the charge of running the household to the younger generation.

As mentioned earlier, the cultural traditions demand that as a man grows older than 50, he relegates his authority to his older son. By the time the man retires from active life and ceases to be an earning member, the older person has already relinquished his head-of-the-household status and takes over an advisory role. It is the author's contention that it is not the growing industrialization that is breaking the extended family system in those countries. The aged persons in most instances run into trouble when there is an evident breach of the cultural traditions on either side, such as the old man dominating the household and not relinquishing the head-of-the-household status to the younger generation, because as a result of contacts with the outside world, the younger generation is questioning the dominance of the older people.

The other reason for the somewhat strained relations between the young and the old generations in the underdeveloped countries is the evergrowing population, less productivity, unbearable increase in the cost of living, and static incomes. Suppose these countries had not gone through any industrialization; if the population growth had been as steep as it is at present; if the economics had been as stagnant as they are at present; and if the per capita productivity had been as low as at present—these strains between the young generation and the old generation would have appeared anyway.

In the industrialized advanced countries, the socio-cultural set-up is dominated by individualism. As the man grows, he is less worried in maintaining cordial relations with his children than with the life insurance company. Before he reaches retirement, an average person has been working for his income in old age either from his savings, life insurance, property, or the social security provided by the government. Children are not looked upon as an insurance for old age. This is not the place to discuss which is right and which is wrong. Both cultural set-ups have their own advantages and disadvantages. However, in the western cultural set-up, the biggest problem of the old is the psychological loneliness. As the children grow up, they go away to do their business of life. The old couple is left alone. Life becomes all the more lonely if one of the spouses dies. They do not have the energy to go around shopping for their material and nutritional needs, even if they have the money to buy them. Most of the old people have marginal economic resources and it is only a small percentage who have ample financial resources for their entire old age. This leaves us with the tradition that the children have no obligation to look after the physical, economic and psychological needs of their old parents. In this context, Sai posed a very interesting question.

> The present feeling that the old should be the care of the society alone is not only unattractive in humanitarian terms but it is likely, in the long run, to affect adversely the whole concept of family life. If one's children are going to leave one at a time of greatest need to be looked after by some bureaucratic institution called the state, what right have the children when they are young to demand that parents give them love and affection rather than simply assist the same bureaucratic state to look after them.

SOCIAL ISOLATION, SICKNESS AND OBESITY

In circumstances where husband and wife over the age of 65 are living together harmoniously, have their personal incomes (even though less than adequate), and are socially involved, the problem of caring for each other's health is generally not a problem. In most instances, the problem arises when an old person is either an isolate or a desolate. The former are men and women who are either widows or widowers who have lived long enough as single persons to be adapted to their state. There are more widows in this category who, having lost their husbands due to accidents, war or sickness, are living alone. Since they are quite used to taking care of the household and cooking, these widows are, in general, better able to take care of their health. The investigations of Lopata reveal that many widows live alone because they like it and their percentage is as high as 61 percent between the ages of 65 and 69.

The widowers in this category may be less efficient in taking care of their health because they are not trained to cook and take care of the household as women are, and may cross the threshhold of isolation into desolation. The fundamental difference between isolates and desolates is that, whereas the former are loners for most of their lives and like it that way, the desolates are forced by circumstances to loneliness and do not adjust to this way of life, and slowly and steadily find their way into hospitals, mental hospitals, nursing homes, retirement homes, and so forth. Most often, the desolates eat nutritionally unbalanced diets, which is a direct result of their social and psychological excommunication from the society. Troll expressed the view that the residential isolation may be less important than communicative isolation:

> One could live with other people but if one had no interaction with them, if one's presence were as meaningful to them as a piece of furniture pushed into a corner, one would be more effectively isolated than if one lived alone but talked on the phone daily with a friend on the other side of town, even if one saw that friend rarely face-to-face.

The common sickness of old age is generally a direct result of social isolation, disinterest in food due to loss of appetite, and decreased physical activity and certain pathological and psychosomatic processes. Due to a variety of reasons, the old persons are prone to conditions varying from a minor one such as constipation to serious conditions such as cardiovascular and respiratory disorders. Constipation is the most common ailment and is attributed to the reduction in muscle tone of the gastrointestinal tract as a result of decreased consumption of foods which provide roughage through the system. Fatty liver and cirrhosis of the liver are frequently observed in the aged. Similarly, the pancreas shows disorders of exocrine and endocrine secretion, which are a result of loss of functional pancreatic cells (Feldman, 1955). Similar atrophic changes are observed in the intestines which greatly affect the process of digestion of old people. The anatomical changes in the endocrine glands of old persons are similar to those that would be found in chronically ill or starved individuals of younger age (Goldzicher, 1956).

The old persons show more frequently problems of cardiovascular and respiratory systems. Atherosclerosis is a very common complication that would require a balanced and sensible nutrition pattern as a means of prevention or slowing down of the process. Hypertension and the presence of varicose veins, especially in the lower extremities, greatly reduce the activity level of the old, so much so that they do not get adequate exercise needed for maintaining muscular tone. Varicose veins greatly reduce the normal nutrition of the skin and subcutaneous tissue, so that healing of wounds or abrasions is a very slow process in the aged (Watkin, 1966; 1968). The respiratory problems of the aged are as crippling as are the cardiovascular disorders. Pulmonary tuberculosis and alveolar emphysema are the conditions found most commonly in the aged people and occasionally the condition is further complicated when another illness such as diabetes, mellitus, hepatic cirrhosis, cancer, alcoholism or chronic malnutrition is also present (Watkin, 1966).

The underlying reason for several of the ailments of old age is the persistence of overweight from their younger years. It has been estimated that between the ages of 30 and 60, the percentage of body fat increases from 28.7 to 44.6 percent in women and 30 to 32 percent in men (Norris *et al.*, 1963; Young *et al.*, 1963). An individual could be asking for trouble if the deposition of fat through advancing years is greater than the above figures (Schlenker *et al.*, 1973). Losing weight in old age results in sagging skin due to decreased elasticity, which prevents the skin from resuming its original contours (Solomon and Shock, 1969). The overweight elderly person succumbs to more diseases than his lighter counterpart. Even if one may not care about a few years' loss of life span due to obesity, one may have to look carefully into functional disabilities that the overweight old persons suffer which are not suffered by the leaner ones of the same age. Among the old people, obesity

often prevents ambulation and self-care in hemiplegia, arthritis and fractures of lower extremities . . . Physicians often are reluctant to institute a program of weight reduction for a very old patient who has done well in spite of excessive weight. One can certainly sympathize with the desire not to upset a physiologic and psychologic balance which seems to have endured, but it must be realized that weight reduction is commonly accompanied by improved ease of movement in any present (or potential) locomotor disability. A reduction in weight of not more than 10 kg may be sufficient to increase appreciably the rate and extent of ambulation and thus enhance the patient's enjoyment of life. Even in the absence of visible improvement in muscular strength, such a reduction in weight also lessens the probability of further locomotor disabilities consequent to arthritis, cardiovascular disorders, or accidents. Weight reduction in the aged is admittedly difficult. Activity is restricted, and thus a decrease in caloric intake may be the only variable available to create a deficit in the energy balance (Mayer, 1972).

Mention may also be made of the direct relationship between the heart diseases and the dietary fat among the old people. The intake of saturated fatty acids in larger quantities as may be the case in a predominantly meat diet, may increase the serum cholesterols at much higher levels in a sedentary old person than an active younger one. Although the protein requirements of the old are in no way different from those of the earlier years, one may be well advised to select alternate sources of protein to restrict the intake of large quantities of meat, which are rich in saturated fats and at the same time may not properly be utilized due to physical problems associated with dental health or digestion (Milne, 1972).

CONCLUSIONS

The food requirements of the elderly people are indeed hard to define as compared to food needs during the middle age. A large number of people over 65 (an age considered appropriate for retirement from active life) lead very active lives, are physically and psychologically quite strong and retain an active role in the community life. In some, the physiological changes due to aging are very prominent, whereas in others, such changes are hardly discernible. For example, an individual at the age of 80 may have renal function as good as a 50 year old. An assessment of nutritional requirements of the aged is strictly a personal evaluation of a subject's nutritional needs, food habits of the younger years and the type and degree of physiologic changes and how best some of the disabilities characteristic of old people can be minimized by a combination of good nutrition and social and psychological stimulation. Some of the chronic disabilities of the aged persons include osteoarthritis and rhumatoid arthritis.

According to several investigations, more than one-third of men and one-half of women at the age of 75 years or over show moderate to severe forms of these conditions. Even in the case of healthy individuals, the joints are not as mobile as one in the younger years (Barnett and Cobbold, 1968). Inadequate vision is another common disability among the aged which may have been due to slow physiological problems of the institutionalized aged. Walton observed that 53 percent of persons 80 years or older had vision around 20/50 and about 20 percent had less than 20/40 corrected visual acuity.

It may prove more effective to prepare the middle aged persons on the nutrition needs of the aged by making them accustomed to balanced diets and habituating them to the virtues and the substance of preventive nutrition. It is clear that sensible eating in the middle age and its continuation into advancing years is more useful than all the therapeutic measures taken in old age while having neglected nutrition in the middle age (Luhrs, 1973; Watkin and Mann, 1973).

It must be emphasized also that the society as well as the government has a moral obligation in taking care of the health needs of the aged persons. The government must make it easy for an old man to get medical help either free or at a price that he can afford, out of his old age pension or social security income. The physicians must develop a proper appreciation of the physical, mental, social and psychological problems of old age. They must not treat them like a spent bullet, and save time to devote to a young man to whom life may be more worthwhile. The aged person needs patience, care and help from his relatives, society and the country. The aged of today have paid taxes to the government all their lives and have given the best part of their years in the service of the society. It is a moral obligation, therefore, that the society and the government ensure free medical care to these senior citizens. This will ensure their right to live a long life and watch how the society in which they actively participated and helped shape is doing without them.

REFERENCES

Andrews, J., Brook, M., and Allen, M. A.: *Gerontol Clin, 8:*257, 1966.

Andrews, J., Letcher, M., and Brook, M.: *Br Med J, 2:*416, 1969.

Baker, S. P., Gaffney, G. W., Shock, N. W., and Landown, M. J.: *Geron, 14:* 37, 1950.

Barnett, C. H., and Cobbold, A. F.: *Ann Rheum Dis, 27:*175, 1968.

Beeker, G. H., Meyer, J., and Necheles, H.: *Gastroenterology, 14:*80, 1950.

Berkowitz, D., Sklaroff, D. M., and Likoff, W.: *J Am Geriat Soc, 1:*741, 1959.

Bernstein, D. S., Sadowski, N., Hegsted, D. M., Guri, C. D., and Stare, F. J.: *JAMA, 198:*499, 1966.

Bernstein, D. S., and Cohen, P. J.: *J Clin Endocrinol, 27:*197, 1967.

Birren, J. E.: In Birren, J. E., Imus, H. A., and Winole, W. (Eds.): *Process of Aging in the Nervous System.* Springfield, Thomas, 1959.

Birren, J. E.: *The Psychology of Aging.* Englewood Cliffs, Prentice Hall, 1964.

Boer, D.: *Soc Biol, 17:*163, 1970.

Brin, M., Schwartzberg, S. H., and Davies, D. A.: *J Am Geriat Soc, 12:*493, 1964.

Branfonbrener, M., Landown, M., and Schock, N. W.: *Circulation, 12:* 557, 1955.

Brocklehurst, J. C., Griffithes, L. L., Taylor, G. F., Marks, J., Scott, D. L., and Blackley, J.: *Gerontol Clin, 10:* 309, 1968.

Burton, B. T.: *Proc White House Conference on Aging.* January 9–12, 1961.

Carlson, A. J., and Hoelzel, F.: *J Nutr, 34:* 81, 1947.

Chalmas, J., Conorcher, W. D. H., Gardner, D. L., and Scott, P. I.: *J Bone Joint Surg, 49B:*403, 1967.

Chazan, J. A., and Mistilis, S. P.: *Am J Med, 34:*350, 1963.

Chinn, A. B., Lavik, P. S., and Cameron, D. B.: *J. Gerontol, 11:*151, 1956.

Citi, S. Z., and Salvini, L. J.: *Gerontology, 12:*123, 1964.

Cohn, C., Joseph, D., and Allweiss, M. D.: *Am J Clin Nutr, 11:*356, 1962.

Dublin, L. I.: *New Engl J Med, 248:*971, 1953.

Eisdorfer, C.: In *Symposium on Longitudinal Changes with Advancing Age.* San Francisco, Psych Assoc, 1968.

Evans, E., and Stock, A. L.: *Nutr Metab, 13:*21, 1971.

FAO. *2nd Committee on Calorie Requirements.* Rome, FAO, 1957.

Feldman, M.: *Geriatrics, 10:*373, 1955.

Fishbein, M., *J Am Geriat Soc, 21:*337, 1973.

Fisher, M. B., and Birren, J. E.: *J Psychol, 31:*490, 1947.

Fridenwald, J. S.: In Lansing, A. I. (Ed.): *Cowdry's Problems of Aging.* Baltimore, Williams and Wilkins, 1952.

Gam, S. M., Rohmann, C. A., and Wagner, B.: *Fed Proc, 26:* 1729, 1967.

Geokas, M. C., and Haverback, B. J.: *Am J Surg, 117:* 881, 1969.

Gitman, L., and Kamholtz, T.: *J Gerontol, 20:* 32, 1965.

Goldzicher, M.: *Geriatrics, 1:* 226, 1956.

Gordon, T.: *Natl Center Health Statistics,* PHS Publ. #1000, Series 11, No. 2. Washington, U.S. Govt. Printing Press, 1964.

Gregarman, R. I., Gaffney, G. W., and Shock, J. W.: *J Clin Invest, 41:* 2065, 1962.

Gsell, D.: *Gerontologia, 2:* 321, 1956.

Haleckvog, E., and Chavapil, M.: *Gerontologia (Basel), 11:* 96, 1965.

Hayflick, L.: *Am J Med Sci, 265:* 432, 1973.

Hegsted, D. M.: *J Am Diet Assoc, 50:* 105, 1967.

Hodge, H. C., and Smith, F. A.: *Am Rev Phenom Col, 8:* 395, 1968.

Jahnke, K.: In Brock, J. F. (Ed.) : *Recent Advances in Human Nutrition.* Boston, Little, 1961.

Jelliffe, N., Bowman, K. M., Rosenblume, L. A., and Fein, H. D.: *JAMA, 114:* 307, 1940.

Kallstrom, B., and Nylof, R.: *Acta Psychiatr Scand, 45:* 137, 1969.

Kowitz, W. B., Ackermann, P. G., Khein, T., and Toro, G.: *Geriatrics, 8:* 63, 1953.

Latham, M. C., McGandy, R. P., McCann, M. D., and Stare, F. J.: *Nutrition Scope Manual.* Kalamazoo, Upjohn, 1970.

Lopata, H.: *Living Arrangements of American Urban Widows.* Paper presented before Gerontological Society, Toronto, 1970.

Luhrs, C. E.: *Am J Clin Nutr, 26:* 1150, 1973.

Malus, O. J.: *Calcium Requirement and Adaptation in Adult Men.* Oslo, Oslo University Press, 1958.

Marks, J.: *The Vitamins in Health and Disease.* London, Churchill, 1968.

Marks, J.: *Royal Society Health Journal, 89:* 289, 1969.

Mayer, J.: *Postgrad Med, 32:* 394, 1962.

Mayer, J.: *Human Nutrition.* Springfield, Thomas, 1972.

McCoy, C. H., Pope, F., and Lunsford, W.: *Bull NY Acad Med, 32:* 91, 1956.

McGandy, R. B., Barrows, C. H., Sparias, A., Meredith, A., Store, J. L., and Norris, A. H.: *J Gerontol, 21:* 581, 1966.

Medical World News, October 6, 1969.

Melinghoff, K.: *Dtsch Med Wochenschr, 84:* 1138, 1959.

Milne, H.: *Can Hosp, 49:* 40, 1972.

Morgan, A. F.: *Calif Health, 13:* 65, 1955.

Morgan, D. G., Wales, M. D., Preloertaft, C. N., and Fourman, P.: *Lancet, 1:* 772, 1966.

Norris, A. H., Shock, N. W., and Wayman, I. H.: *J Appl Physiol, 5:* 589, 1953.

Norris, A. H., Lundy, T., and Shock, N. W.: *Ann NY Acad Sci, 110:* 623, 1963.

Nutrition Reviews, 25: 130, 1967.

Ohlson, M. A., Brewer, W. D., Cederquist, S. C., Brown, E. G., and Robergs, P. H.: *J Am Diet Assoc, 24:* 744, 1948.

O'Leary, J. L.: In Lansing, A. I. (Ed.) : *Cowdry's Problems of Aging.*

Baltimore, Williams and Wilkins, 1952.

Posner, A. S.: *Fed Proc, 26:* 1717, 1967.

Rao, D. B.: *J Am Geriatr Soc, 21:* 362, 1973.

Reynolds, E. H.: *J Psychiatr, 113:* 681, 1967.

Riley, M., and Foner, A.: *Aging and Society, An Inventory of Research Findings.* New York, Russel Sage Foundation, 1968, vol. 1.

Robinson, J. J.: *South Med J, 53:* 1446, 1960.

Rothschild, D.: *Geriatrics, 2:* 155, 1947.

Rudd, T. N.: *J Am Geriatr Soc, 21:* 342, 1973.

Sai, F. T.: *Proc R Soc Med, 66:* 123, 1973.

Saville, P. D.: *J Am Geriatr Soc, 17:* 155, 1969.

Schlenker, E. D., Feurig, J. S., Stone, L. H., Ohlson, M. A., and Mickelsen, O.: *Am J Clin Nutr, 26:* 1111, 1973.

Scobie, B. A.: *New Zealand Med J, 70:* 398, 1969.

Sherwood, S.: *Am J Clin Nutr, 26:* 1108, 1973.

Shock, N. E.: In *Annual Rev Physiol at V E Hall.* Palo Alto, Annual Reviews, Inc., *97,* 1961.

Shock, N. W.: *Sci Am, 206:* 100, 1962.

Shock, N. W., Watkin, D. M., Yiengst, M. U., Norris, A. H., Gaffney, G. W., Gregerman, R. I., and Falsone, J. A.: *J Gerontol, 18,* 1963.

Smith, R. W., and Rizek, J.: *Clin Orthop, 45:* 31, 1966.

Solomon, N., and Shock, N. W.: *South Med J, 62:* 1523, 1969.

Strachan, R. W., and Henderson, J. G.: *Q J Med, 36:* 189, 1967.

Taylor, G. F.: *Community Health, 3:* 244, 1972.

Theur, R. C.: *J Dairy Sci, 54:* 627, 1971.

Troll, L. E.: *J Am Diet Assoc, 59:* 456, 1971.

Tuttle, S. G., Swendsird, M. E., Mulcare, D., Griffith, W. H., and Bassett, S. H.: *Metabolism, 6:* 566, 1957.

Tuttle, S. G., Bassett, S. H., Griffith, W. H., Mulcare, D. B., and Swendsird, M. E.: *Am J Clin Nutr, 16:* 229, 1965.

Walton, W. G.: *Am J Optom, 44:* 319, 1967.

Watkin, D. M., Long, C. A., Chow, B. F., and Shock, N. W.: *J Nutr, 50:* 341, 1953.

Watkin, D. M.: *Mammalian Protein Metabolism, 2:* 247, 1964.

Watkin, D. M.: In Beaton, G. H., and McHenry, E. W. (Eds.) : *Nutrition.* New York, Acad Pr, 1966, vol. III.

Watkin, D. M.: In Wohl and Goodhart (Eds.) : *Modern Nutrition in Health and Disease.* Philadelphia, Lea and Febiger, 1968.

Watkin, D. M.: In Rechcigl (Ed.) : *World Rev Nutr Diet,* 1973, vol. 16.

Watkin, D. M. and Mann, G. V.: *Am J Clin Nutr, 26:* 1159, 1973.

Weiss, A. D.: In Birren, J. E. (Ed.) : *Handbook of Aging and the Individual.* Chicago, Chicago U Pr, 1959.

Williams, S. R.: *Nutrition and Diet Therapy.* St. Louis, Mosley, 1969.

Young, C. M., Blardin, J., Tennusion, R., and Fryer, J. H.: *Ann NY Acad Sci, 110:* 623, 1963.

CHAPTER VI

OBESITY AND MALNUTRITION—
CAUSES AND EFFECTS

OBESITY

IN THE PRESENT AGE, science and technology in the western world have created a degree of affluence in material goods as well as food that most everyone can afford to eat big meals three times a day. The psychology of food as a source of sensual pleasure was created in those days of the ancient and medieval periods of human history when there was a general scarcity of food all the year round and periodically food became almost unattainable. In those days, whenever extra food became available, it was an occasion for celebration and overeating. Somehow this psychology in which food was regarded as a reward and as a primary agenda in meetings, social gatherings, parties, celebrations, etc., has persisted to the extent that, in most instances, the sensual pleasure of eating a lot of food becomes an obsession. The social and cultural acceptability of alcohol has helped ingestion of large quantities of calories in celebrations and has come to be accepted as normal.

If this psychology is stretched to other situations, a resort to food when one is happy or when one is sad becomes a part of one's life. In childhood, parents use choice foods as rewards and the child learns to get comfort from food when it is not forthcoming from his parents or guardians. Some mothers, being consciously unable to provide love, try to substitute for love by giving a lot of food to the child.

To some parents, it is easier to give their children pocket money to spend on sweets than to communicate love. . . The unhappy or neglected child may withdraw into himself in his inability to relate to others, and seek solace in food. Increasing obesity leads to disinclination to join his fellows in play, resulting in further withdrawal and more eating. The observation has been made that even before the development of obesity, such children are clumsy and awkward. They adopt sedentary habits and their interests are often artistic rather than athletic (Jones, 1972).

PREVALENCE OF OBESITY AND APPRAISAL OF THE PROBLEM

If obesity is defined as a form of *malnutrition* (imbalanced diet), its widespread occurrence is a problem of as much gravity as the prevalent undernutrition due to lack of body building proteins and calories for energy. Broadly speaking, undernutrition is a grave problem facing the underdeveloped and developing poor countries, and obesity has an equally grave prognosis for the industrialized, richer countries of the world (JAMA, 1970). One only needs to consult the statistical records prepared by the insurance companies to get an insight into a correlation between extra weight, mortality and morbidity. These records tend to substantiate the remarks of Plato that the human is endowed with a body and a soul; when one does not function well, neither does the other (Hutton, 1971). As many as 30 percent of young males and 20 percent of young females are obese. Significant still, its prevalence is approximately 50 percent in both sexes from age forty upwards (Anderson, 1972). It is safe to say that obesity is the most prevalent metabolic disorder of the Twentieth Century.

The National Center for Health Statistics discussed the weight, height and body dimensions of the adult population and showed an increasing trend toward extra fat deposition in the United States' populations. It is probable that this trend is attributable to the modern living habits, abundance of labor-saving conveniences, and easy availability of abundant food to eat. A closer examination further reveals that women tend to be obese after the delivery of their first baby;

whereas, men tend to add weight between the ages of 25 to 40. It is very likely that the pattern of food consumption in childhood and adolescence, when extra food can be consumed because of the demands of growth, is not changed in middle age, in spite of the fact that the tempo of physical activity decreases, resulting in extra deposition of fat. The Metropolitan Life Insurance Company considers 29 percent of 40 to 49 year old men to be 10 to 19 percent or more overweight. For women in the same age groups, the figures are 19 and 40 percent, respectively. The incidence of overweight in persons 50 to 59 years old is even higher. These numbers indicate that the majority of middle aged Americans are obese (Mayer, 1969). The Chicago Tribune of October 27, 1970, called obesity an epidemic in the United States, and commented that if the money spent for policing marijuana were spent on obesity, much more could be accomplished.

Contrary to the old belief that it is the affluent who are obese, a careful evaluation reveals that the reverse may be true, especially in the technologically advanced countries. In the poorer countries, where there are chronic shortages of food, a majority of the obese may come from a relatively well-to-do class engaged in business or professions involving little physical activity. In some cultures, a higher social status is given to those who weigh more, probably because it reflects prosperity and success. A class survey of the prevalence of obesity in India showed that this is primarily a condition of the affluent. The lower classes probably cannot afford to buy enough food to eat, much less to overeat (Berry, 1971). In the industrial societies where food is in abundance, especially the carbohydrate-rich beverages, this may not hold true. Based on a study of 3,344 obese children, Stunkard *et al.* (1972) showed that obesity is more prevalent in the lower class girls than those of the upper class, and nine times as prevalent by age six.

A similarly significant difference in boys is also evident. Knowing that obese children grow into obese adults (the odds against an obese child becoming a normal weight adult are more than four to one at age twelve, rising to twenty-eight to one if weight has not been reduced by the end of adolescence) (Stunkard and Burt, 1967), the problem of obesity among the lower classes becomes a social problem of great magnitude and must be taken up on an urgent basis. The poor eat more and unsensibly because they are probably compensating for the hard realities of their life. The upper classes are obese probably because of the opulence and instant availability of all kinds of attractive foods as well as conveniences which greatly reduce their physical activity levels. With increasing upward mobility from the lower classes to the middle class, the women have tended to move from obese to the thin category, while men move from obese to the *normal* category (Goldblatt *et al.,* 1965). In the southern part of the United States, obesity is more common among white males as compared to black males who earn their living mostly by hard physical labor. On the other hand Mayer theorizes that obesity is more prevalent among black females as compared to white females because of the employment of the former as housemaids, in which capacity they are closer to the kitchen and the food. At the same time, a white female has social pressures of maintaining a figure, which are absent in the case of the black female (Mayer, 1972).

The word *obese* is a very ambiguous term that has come to be used in a very unspecific manner. A person must not be labelled obese without a comprehensive assessment of his health. Weight may not be a good index of fatness; along with it is needed a thorough assessment of other important factors such as sex, age, body type, state of health, skin fold thickness, etc. Every individual is unique in certain respects including his body structure and weight. A person who has been labelled as overweight by the standards of some tables actually may have more skeletal or muscle mass and may not be obese at all.

On the other hand, a person with a small skeleton may fall in the normal range of the weights recommended by those tables but still may be obese because of excessive proportion of adipose tissue or fat. Obesity may, therefore, be defined as an excessive accumulation of triglyceride fat in the adipose tissue storage of the body. This is mainly the result of energy imbalance caused by intake greater than utilization. Physical inactivity and lower basal metabolism as one grows older are probably the reasons for smaller utilization of the available calories while, at the same time, maintaining or increasing the level of food intake. In an obese person, "fat is in a dynamic metabolic state, storing excess calories not metabolized immediately after ingestion in the form of triglyceride, and releasing free fatty acids when these are required for energy (Anderson, 1972).

This is not to say that the weight and body measurements are in any way useless—they do provide guidelines for a more detailed examination. If the weight pattern conforms to certain standards, one may not worry unnecessarily about obesity. The ideal general rule of thumb is: for women, beginning with a height of five feet, use one hundred pounds and add five pounds for every inch over five feet; for men, beginning at five feet, use 110 pounds and add five pounds for every inch over five feet (Williams, 1969). More than body measurements, the assessment of tissue composition is important. This can be done by measuring specific gravity or weight of tissue per unit volume, that is, of lean tissue and excess fat (Widdowson, 1961). Figure 5 gives a comparative picture of the fat content of the obese, normal, and lean person (Jokl, 1964).

The fat content of the individual is indeed the most reliable index of the extent of obesity. An examination of the body measurements would reveal that in individuals with normal health, the chest circumference will be larger by a few inches, but if the abdominal circumference is equal to or exceeds the chest measurements, this is an indication of deposition of fat. Measurement of skinfold thickness has been often used to get a fair idea of the subcutaneous fat. Table XI represents the minimum triceps skin fold thickness in males and females of various ages indicating obesity (Latham *et al.*, 1970; Mayer, 1972; Root, 1972).

In obese persons, most of the extra fat is deposited subcutaneously. If a pinch of fat reveals skin thickness larger

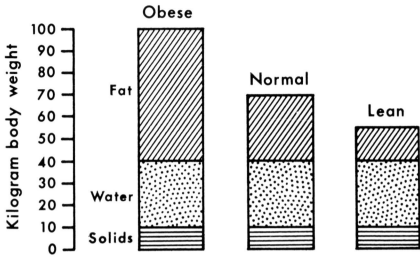

Figure 5. A comparative picture of the fat content of the obese, normal and lean person.

than an inch, it indicates excess fat and an obese state. Based on thousands of measurements of the skin fold with the help of accurate calipers, Redaksie calculated that lean men and women have a skin fold thickness of 1.5 and 2.0 cm respectively, compared with 1.5 to 2.0 cm in men and 2.0 to 2.5 cm in women in cases of mild obesity; 2.0 to 2.5 cm in men and 2.5 to 3.0 cm in women in moderate obesity, and 2.5 cm and over in men and 3.0 cm and over in women in cases of severe obesity. These figures could serve as a general guideline for the measurement of obesity (Redaksie, 1969). Besides measurements of fat deposits by calipers, obesity may also be appraised by estimating the body electrolyte count (Forbes *et al.,* 1967). A number of researchers have used, besides the anthropometric measurements, the skeletal measurements, basal oxygen consumption, and creatinine excretion, etc., to assess the ratio of body fat to lean mass. Soft tissue X-ray technique would be another precise way to visualize the fat pads.

It is an established fact that the majority of fat people eat more than their physiological needs. This tendency in most

TABLE XI

OBESITY STANDARDS FOR
CAUCASIAN AMERICANS
*(minimum triceps skinfold thickness
in millimeters indicating obesity)*

Age (years)	Skinfold measurements	
	Males	Females
5	12	14
6	12	15
7	13	16
8	14	17
9	15	18
10	16	20
11	17	21
12	18	22
13	18	23
14	17	23
15	16	24
16	15	25
17	14	26
18	15	27
19	15	27
20	16	28
21	17	28
22	18	28
23	18	28
24	19	28
25	20	29
26	20	29
27	21	29
28	22	29
29	23	29
30–50	23	30

From: J. Mayer, *Human Nutrition* (Springfield, Thomas, 1972).
C. C. Seltzer and J. Mayer, *Postgrad Med, 88:* 2, 1965.

instances starts in childhood and it is during this period that the body goes through the adaptive phenomenon of taking care of excessive amounts of calories that remain unutilized due either to too much intake or physical inactivity or both. In a normal growth pattern,

fat increases steadily for the first nine months of life. At this time a plateau is reached and thereafter a slight increment occurs until approximately age seven, when fat once again increases. A final spurt of deposition of adipose tissue occurs during adolescence. In females the early fat loss is less, as is the development of lean body mass; hence the average female finishes as an adult with a greater amount of body fat (Falkner, 1966; Knittle, 1972).

In children who are physically inactive and do not utilize the ingested calories, the pattern of fat deposition undergoes a drastic change right from the young age. In these subjects, the number of adipose cells increases in number as well as size. Biopsy studies show that there is a threefold increase in the number of adipose cells in the subcutaneous tissues in obese persons as compared to lean ones (Hirsch *et al.,* 1966). Considering that the adipose cells are greatly increased in size as well, an obese person has provided for himself a lot of space to store the extra fat (Hirsch and Knittle, 1970).

In most instances, it is during childhood when this anatomical and physiological adaptation takes place, and a number of studies point in that direction. For example, 80 percent of those who are obese as children remain so during their adult life (Asher, 1966; Knittle, 1972). Recent studies at New York's Mount Sinai Hospital have shown that the foundation of chronic obesity is laid in early childhood; as early as six weeks of age (*Nutr Review,* 1970). In response to abundant availability of food which cannot be utilized, children develop excessive numbers of fat-containing cells, which become a part of the body, never to disappear. In times of food shortages these fat cells shrink, to become prominent again as soon as extra food is available. Obese five and six-year-old children (with 30 percent or more weight than the ideal for height and age) have more fat cells than normal adults, and these cells continue to increase in number along with the general body growth (*Newsweek,* 1970). The studies of Drs. Knittle and Hirsch of Rockefeller University showed that obese rats, when put on a restricted diet, did not show any permanent effects on their obesity. As soon as the diet ended, they regained all their weight.

In the childhood period, too, there is a pattern of the onset of obesity that is interesting. Among the 100 obese children selected randomly, at least 45 of them were obese before the age of six (Robertson and Lowry, 1964). If a child is heavier than normal for his age in the early part of infancy, his physiological adaptation for storing extra fat in increased numbers of adipose cells is all the more perfect and becomes a part of his existence. The children whose shoulder and hip girdles are wide for their heights—that is, the so-called stocky type—are particularly prone to obesity. Asher showed that children who are obese at six months of age continue to be so, and at the age of five those children are on the average 4.2 kg heavier than those who weighed in the average range at six months of age.

These observations have tended to confirm Mossberg's hypothesis that there are two critical periods in childhood at which times the weight pattern has a direct relationship with the onset of obesity in adulthood. The first one is between birth and four years, with another between seven and eleven years (Mossberg, 1948). The first one appears to be determined by the feeding pattern established by the mother, whereas during the second period the child expresses his own eating habits, which are likely to continue into adult life. Those who have established for themselves as a large number of adipose cells during the critical periods of development are likely to retain their obesity, whereas those babies who have not resorted to developing an extra number of adipose cells outgrow their *baby fat*.

OBESITY, PHYSICAL INACTIVITY AND EXERCISE

It is an unfortunate truth that there is no direct relationship between physical activity and the appetite. No doubt very active persons have large appetites and they consume large quantities of food, but when these active persons become inactive, they do not lose appetite in the same proportion. It is as if the *appetite-stat* has been physiologically set at a certain level. A person generally maintains that level, irrespective of changes in the load of physical work. That is the reason for slow and steady accumulation of excess fat in the sedentary middle aged persons who have no other physiological abnormality whatsoever. In certain cases, the food intake actually increases in spite of lesser exercise. As the age goes by, if constant attention is not paid to physical exercise, the active tissue is slowly and steadily replaced by fat (Gubner, 1973).

In other words, one does not have to increase weight per se to increase the percentage of fat in the body. The fat content of inactive older people is significantly higher than an active person of the same age or the same weight. A somewhat overweight athlete cannot, therefore, be put in the same category as a relatively inactive person of the same weight with respect to proneness to disease processes. Based on a number of studies, it may not be incorrect to advise that a male should try to maintain his weight at the age of 25 and the female her weight at age 21 or 22. In most instances, unless extraordinary athletic activity is pursued, the extra weight accumulated after these ages is in the form of fat deposition. "If *homo laborans* becomes *homo sedentarium* rather than *homo sportius,* obesity will be an automatic consequence for many of our citizens (Mayer, 1972).

A better understanding of calorie intake and calorie expenditure can be brought about if one is aware of the calorie consumption with a particular amount of work, which should help an adult person to realize the extent of his calorie requirements, after the requirements of growth have ceased. A 160 pound man, as an example, uses 350 calories an hour when he walks at the rate of 4 miles an hour. He uses 300 calories an hour when he plays golf, and 500 calories or more an hour in a game of tennis (Mayer, 1972). Generally, the activity level of persons decreases with marriage. It is not always easy to find partners who will be equally interested in sports and the responsibilities of a married life warrant more time out for work and less for sports or exercise.

The obese, overweight and fat people are generally lethargic and tend to save energy at every step of their lives, and this pattern of inactivity may be the chief villain in the onset and persistence of obesity. According to Bruch it reflects a deepseated apprehension of their inability to master any athletic skills. Jokl described that fat people do not make a single unnecessary step. Whenever possible, they will sit down and control the environment from their big chairs (Bruch, 1957). It is their inhibition of activity that represents a more fundamental disturbance than overeating (Jokl, 1964). Stunkard and Chirico compared the spontaneous walking activity of nonobese and obese women. The mean walking distance which an obese woman covered came to around 2.0 miles per day compared to 4.9 miles per day covered by a nonobese woman. Measuring on the basis of locomotor activity, one has to walk 35 miles to lose one pound. An obese woman will gain an extra pound every 12 days, just because of lessened walking activity compared to the nonobese, keeping the food intake constant in both cases. A large number of obese fuss that they eat a lot less than the average and yet they gain weight. Some investigators also tend to confirm this (Weng *et al.*, 1956); that the obese eat fewer calories. It is the lack of exercise and physical inactivity that is at the root of their continuing obesity.

The obese can lose fat if they exercise regularly and if they undergo a sustained program of intense physical training, which could profoundly affect their physique and character (Jokl, 1964). To emphasize the importance of exercise, Jokl described a case of a 15 year old boy, 5 feet 5¾ inches tall and weighing 209 pounds. For a period of 10 months, 3 hours per day were devoted to exercise and recreation without any specific dietary or medical measures. During this period, he lost 55 pounds. He must have lost more fat because a differential analysis of the body changes due to training revealed that he had gained at least 15 pounds of active body tissue resulting in a remarkable reorganization of his body. At the end of the training period, the boy's measurements and weight were within the normal range for his skeletal frame (Jokl, 1964).

SOCIO-MEDICAL ASPECTS OF OBESITY

Obesity is a complex social as well as a medical problem. In the latter category, a number of cardiovascular, digestive and endocrine abnormalities result from obesity, which may prove fatal in a large section of the obese population. The mortality rates among men who are about 10 percent over-weight are approximately one-fifth higher than the normal. In those people who are 20 or more percent overweight, the mortality rate is about one-third higher. Among the common conditions that obesity contributes to are hypertension, congestive heart failure, varicose veins, rupture of inter-vertebral discs, osteoarthritis and many other varieties of bone and joint diseases (Mayer, 1972). Excessive amounts of fat increase the probability of hepatic disease, whenever it causes actual fatty infiltration of the liver. No one would say that obesity causes these conditions, but it is as good as a direct implication when the overweight increases their incidence many-fold in obese people. Some of the metabolic disorders associated with obesity have been discussed in detail in the next section.

At this stage it may be sufficient to say that an obese per-son is a medical liability, who has reduced his life expec-tancy in general. Those obese persons who reduce their weight to normal range and stay reduced increase their life expectancy and reduce their liability to the above-mentioned diseases as compared to those who do not lose weight or go through a cycle of losing and gaining. If an obese person is involved in an accident, his chances of recovery through operation are significantly less than a person of average weight, because even in a simple surgical operation, an obese person has much higher chances of extra complications. The anesthesiologist especially experiences much more difficulty in taking care of an obese patient, and it is always recom-mended to lose extra weight before a surgical operation (Mayer, 1959).

More than a medical problem, obesity is a social problem of great magnitude. Intimately intertwined with social problems and social attitudes are the psychological and en-vironmental factors which not only perpetuate obesity, but also are detrimental to its prevention. Obesity, bad as it is for the individual, has been stigmatized by the society. The obese go through so much physical, emotional and social pressures that a majority spend most of their energy coping with discrimination, rather than curing their condition. As mentioned elsewhere, the medical profession does not accord to obesity any serious attention, and since their success in controlling the condition is slight, they tend to blame the patient for his being "weak-willed, ugly, and awkward" (Maddox and Liederman 1969). Little do we realize that society is to a great extent responsible for instilling into obese persons a sense of inferiority which results in such personality traits as "withdrawal, passivity, expectation of rejection, and extraordinary concern with self-image" (Kalisch, 1972). Day after day, an obese person finds himself discriminated against in privileges, opportunities and status that the leaner persons get without struggling for them. These discriminations become so ingrained in the minds of obese persons that even if they are able to reduce their weight to the normal range, they are not able to revise the self-concept and eradicate the self-hate and feelings of inadequacy. The result is often that the obese person is unable to retain his weight loss, because in order to gain emotional stability, he finds himself sliding slowly under the security-providing umbrella of food.

In general, the obese are often hostile, frustrated and depressed people. Weight reduction without taking care of the underlying emotional problems may prove to be an incomplete method of understanding these problems. Various studies have shown that the obese individuals respond to their environment in a manner quite differently than people of normal weight. The fat adolescent is often uncommunicative and withdrawn; the theory of being *fat and happy* is contrary to his true emotional state (Editorial, 1970). It has been said that inside every fat woman is an unhappy thin woman. It may be worthwhile to try to liberate this thin woman with a minimum of inconvenience and expense. A study of mental illness in lower class normal, obese and hyperobese women revealed that the obese and hyperobese ate when anxious and depressed, even though they lacked hunger and appetite (Holland *et al.,* 1970). Systematic observations reveal that obese people are more easily stimulated for food by external stimuli of taste, smell or sight as compared to the normal people (Rosenstock, 1969).

A survey of dieters for weight-reduction purposes revealed that women are more concerned about their extra weight and are more likely to do something about it compared to men who come in the same degree of obesity (Duyer and Mayer, 1970). Women worry about overweight for its aesthetic disadvantages. However, since men reduce their weight for health reasons, they have a bigger incentive to do the same thing and do so successfully compared to women.

Since overeating is used to compensate for the less desirable circumstances and emotional upsets, it may be a beneficial factor in a certain sense. Eating may provide certain solutions to emotional problems with the result that the suicide rate among the obese is much lower than the nonobese population. Also, there are certain cultural and environmental factors which predispose the members of a society to becoming obese or overweight. Hard physical work in certain cultures is not a favorable thing to do, and a white collar job is preferable to a blue collar job. In a country like the United States, physical hard work is not frowned upon, but cultural food habits in combination with opulence of food tends to make a meal concentrated in calories. Stunkard *et al.* believed that the *obese* tend to overeat in the evenings (Stunkard and Burt, 1967). With advancing urbanization, the facilities for exercise proportionately decrease. In some cases, certain physiological situations (e.g. iron deficiency) or psychological traumas also decrease the activity level of the individuals, leading to underutilization of calories.

Often a question is asked as to whether there is any positive relationship between giving up smoking and unnecessary weight gain. People who give up cigarettes seem to put on some extra weight. It is, however, probable that in an effort to give up smoking, they start eating candies or snacks more often in order to keep themselves away from the cigarettes. It is these additional calories that add to the weight. It is also possible that smoking reduces appetite by inhibiting hunger contractions. The smoker may be eating less food, but once smoking has been given up, he may return to his pre-smoking food levels. Brozek conducted a study of changes in body weight in normal men who stopped smoking cigarettes. He found that smokers who cease to smoke do gain weight, although it is not obvious that such a weight gain is a permanent part of the body (Brozek, 1956). Faced with a choice between smoking, which is positively dangerous to health, or obesity, which may be equally hazardous, the dilemma is very real and unpleasant. A Public Health Service Report on smoking and health suggests that the reduced mortality of ex-smokers, directly attributable to cessation of smoking, more than offsets possible increases in mortality due to a weight gain of five to ten pounds (Smoking and Health, 1964).

METABOLIC DISORDERS ASSOCIATED WITH OBESITY

The main reason for the onset of obesity is an imbalance of the caloric intake. Due to physical inactivity and/or excessive food intake, the level of energy utilization is a lot less, with the result that the extra calories must be deposited in the body in the form of fat. However, it is recognized that certain metabolic factors can play an equally important role in its perpetuation, especially the derangement of glucose and fat metabolism, endocrine disorders or some disorder of the hypothalamic centers which control satiety and appetite. Gordon pointed out that there are at least twenty-seven metabolic differences between the obese and the nonobese individuals. This would indicate that obesity is not merely a matter of simple gluttony. It could be anything from the consumption of extra calories to the involvement of the pituitary-hypothalamic area (Gordon, 1970). The reader is referred to a couple of excellent review articles on metabolic aspects of obesity by Gordon and Sassoon. These reviews have tried to answer some of the most important questions: Are obese people metabolically different from normal ones?; and are there time factors in pattern of food consumption that lead to obesity? Is the metabolic abnormality genetic or acquired? Are the obese simply uncontrollable gluttons, or are they helpless at the hands of their changed metabolism? Is the compulsive eater under the spell of numerous complex nervous pathways that connect the hypothalamus with other areas of the brain, having a profound influence on the emotional state of the individual?

The defect in glucose metabolism results in decrease of glucose tolerance, and in these subjects, plasma insulin is also increased. These abnormalities of glucose and insulin metabolism may or may not be accompanied by any other clinical complications such as diabetes. It is not clear at this stage whether, in the obese patients, these metabolic abnormalities precede or follow the development of obesity. However, it is evident that when the abnormalities of carbohydrate metabolism are present, the adipose depots are enlarged and, when these depots are reduced, the functioning of carbohydrate metabolism is significantly improved (Salans *et al.*, 1968). The carbohydrate metabolism regulates food intake, mediated through the rate of passage of glucose into the glucoreceptor cells of the ventromedial hypothalamic area, the seat of *satiety* center (Young, 1973).

On the other hand, if the dorsomedial meleus of the hypothalamus is disturbed, say by creating a lesion in the area, enormous amounts of food are eaten by the patient, which may be attributed to a relief of emotional disturbances. The patient may be completely free of all inhibitions related to the realities of his life and develop an abnormal appetite for food. It has been found that some patients with lesions in the dorsomedial hypothalamus gained as much as 100 pounds. An obese person shows low level of glucose utilization and high level of glucose formation. Like the hibernating animals who grow fat before their hibernating act, the obese person is primed for a period of starvation. The fat effectively wraps up the lean tissues in a physical as well as thermal blanket, as it has been shown that the skin temperature of an obese person is 2° F higher than the lean one. The problem with human obesity is that the person is not going to hibernate and is likely to continue to gorge himself on food, thereby converting one of his assets (better chances of surviving in a shipwreck or arctic life) into a liability which promotes metabolic disorders that are hazardous to his health and longevity.

In obese persons, fat metabolism may also be altered, and show itself in high blood levels of free fatty acids. It is possible that the high plasma free fatty acids may cause the tissue insensitivity to insulin in the obese and could stimulate the pancreas to greater insulin secretion (Jones, 1972).

Obesity affects the adrenal function adversely. At least in 30 to 60 percent of obese persons, increased adrenal cortical function has been found. It is not clear, however, how it may be related to the development or maintenance of the obese state (Schteingart and Conn, 1965).

That obesity has a profound effect on the secretion of growth hormone has been demonstrated by several workers (Beck *et al.,* 1964; Copinschi *et al.,* 1967). In volunteers in whom obesity was induced experimentally, the growth hormone secretion was quite abnormal and the level of hormone returned to normal only after weight loss (Ball *et al.,* 1970b). Although several workers have established a correlation between the growth hormone levels and the degree of weight loss, it may be that growth hormone secretion is irreversibly impaired (El-Khodary *et al.,* 1970), and that altered levels of the growth hormone may be a primary phenomenon in obesity (Root, 1972). Following physical exercise, the growth hormone concentration may (Shwarz *et al.,* 1969) or may not (Glick, 1969) increase in the obese patients. The female patients, however, respond better than males in this respect (Root, 1972).

Experimental evidence indicates that damage to the noradrenergic system of the brain leads to overeating and obesity. In laboratory animals the destruction of noradrenergic terminals is achieved by destroying at midbrain levels a fiber system supplying the hypothalamus.

The metabolic consequences of obesity are much more serious than is generally recognized. Obesity is associated with at least a transitory abnormality of almost every body function. The first and foremost consequence is the problem of supplying oxygenated blood to the extra tissue. Respiratory problems in obese people are much more common than in people of normal weight and musculature (Bortz, 1969). Cardiovascular problems always compete with respiratory irregularities for first place in metabolic dysfunctions in obese people. The latter show more hypertension and greater risk of heart ailments or even heart failure. An effective loss of weight and maintenance of weight could be very important in the prevention of circulatory disorders. Obesity also increases the risk of skin ulcers and other skin disorders, especially among those who already have varicose veins.

Several attempts have been made to correlate obesity and hypertension. Studies have revealed that hypercholesterolemia and hypertension develop independently of obesity, although one may accelerate the onset of the other. In several studies in the United States, a correlation between obesity and hypertension has become quite apparent. In the general population, one fifth to one third of all people who have hypertension are also overweight. A survey of 22,000 U.S. Army officers revealed that, after the age of 45, hypertension among overweight persons was two-and-one-half times more than their average-sized colleagues (Mayer, 1969). In most instances, a significant loss in weight simultaneously lowers the blood pressure as well. It could be that since obesity increases oxygen consumption and increases cardiac output and work for the left ventricle, a decrease of adipose tissue could greatly relieve the cardiac load, which should, in turn, lower the blood pressure. In a group of 194 obese patients who lost more than ten pounds, the average blood pressure fell from 154/96 to 133/86. Among a group of 62 patients with a systolic pressure of 200 mm mercury or more, blood pressure in 22 patients who had a substantial weight loss fell from 219/119 to 176/108 (Mayer, 1969).

There is some evidence that excessive fat stores in men, especially on the upper part of the thighs, may lead to folds of adipose tissue around the scrotum, which may in turn lead to infertility.

The problem of hyperinsulinism associated with obesity has not been satisfactorily answered. So far the condition has been viewed as a compensatory adjustment of the pancreatic beta cell to the antagonism of peripheral tissues to insulin (Merimee, 1971). Hyperinsulinism may be a result of increased ingestion of carbohydrates (Kolkhoff *et al.*, 1971), as patients generally reduce insulin secretion on a low carbohydrate diet or a consequence of the insulin antagonism associated with obesity (Grey and Kipnis, 1971). Hypothyroidism is also believed to be associated with obesity, although there is no conclusive proof of the same. Two forms of obesity that are certainly associated with metabolic disorders of the body are obesity associated with diabetes mellitus and obesity accompanying Cushing's syndrome, or adrenocortical hyperfunction. In the former, there is a positive relationship between overweight or excessive amount of adipose tissue and the development of the disease. A common observation shows that a vast majority of the people having diabetes are grossly obese as well. As the disease appears and advances, these obese people do not lose weight. Gordon explained the metabolic implications of both these disorders, and it may be worthwhile to reproduce them here.

There must be some connection between the hormonal and metabolic derangements of the diabetic state and the deposition of excess weight. Many such diabetics are clearly guilty of excessive overeating and marked underactivity so that the deposition of excess weight is easily understood, but this is not true of all diabetics, and the question still remains, why should diabetics be more susceptible to obesity than the general population? In the present state of our knowledge, it seems like a good possibility that the excessive production of insulin in this form of diabetes may in some way account for the progressive accretion of excess adipose tissue. But, when the phenomenon is studied in detail, it appears that the *hyperinsulinism* of adult onset, noninsulin-dependent diabetes is more a consequence than it is a cause of obesity. In Cushing's disease, it is recognized that the excessive production and release by the adrenal cortex of adrenocortical steroids of the cortisol type impose upon the total metabolism a marked resistance to the physiological action of insulin. This, in turn, places a stress upon the beta cell mechanism of the pancreas, and excessive amounts of insulin are produced. Since insulin is a powerful lipogenic agent, it would appear that obesity is then a secondary metabolic consequence of adrenocortical hyperfunction; but despite this, from the thermo-dynamic standpoint, it is still necessary to account for the excess weight in terms of a positive caloric balance.

The genetic inheritance of obesity has not been proven and probably there is no genetic basis of obesity. Common observations, however, suggest an indirect hereditary relationship. Obese parents produce children who turn out to be obese as well. When one parent is obese, the possibility of obesity in the children is about 40 percent, but when both parents are obese, the possibility of obesity in the children rises to about 80 percent. It is difficult to say finally whether this is a familial occurrence or simply an extension of the eating habits of the family. It is possible that profession and social status, generation after generation, have a profound effect on not only the level of physical activity, but on the eating habits as well. Mayer believes that it is probably the intervention of genetic and environmental factors which determines the onset of obesity in individuals or groups of individuals (1972). The full implications of genetic inheritance of obesity have still to be worked out, but at this stage of our knowledge it may be likened to a metabolic abnormality in the same category as hereditary hyperglycemia (Ingelfinger *et al.,* 1966; Mayer, 1960).

MANAGEMENT OF OBESITY

For the purpose of treatment, it is necessary that the prevalence of obesity be rationally estimated. People who are overweight by 5, 10 or 15 percent of their desired weight do not run a great risk of morbidity due to cardiovascular complications unless they keep increasing steadily. Maximum attention needs to be focused on those who are at least 25 to 40 percent overweight. It is in these heavy individuals that one begins to see enough of a difference in the mortality and morbidity rates to be worrisome.

Obesity is a relatively simpler disease as compared to other morbid conditions. This is probably one of the main reasons that the success rate is one of the lowest. We have psychologically accepted its presence in society, and most physicians find it uninteresting, unrewarding, and quite unglamorous. Dr. Glenn rightly remarked that a physician will spend whatever time may be needed to correct an acute condition, even if it is not very serious, but he often fails to spare time to instruct a patient on a chronic condition such as obesity, which may take twenty years off the patient's life expectancy (Mayer, 1973).

So far, there is no fool-proof treatment of obesity because of the complexity of the problem. Lecturing the patient and instilling in him a feeling of guilt could not only be unhelpful, but damaging as well. Whenever there is a case of repeated failure to reduce weight or to maintain reduced weight, the doctor may be well-advised to help the patient by psychological persuasion to accept his obesity (*Medical Letter*, 1971). It is believed that the best results are obtained when the following criteria are adequately satisfied: 1) the patient has a genuine desire to lose weight; 2) an explanation of how the condition has arisen and how it is to be treated is described to and understood by the patient; 3) stress is laid on dietary reduction based on his established food habits rather than excessive restriction or substitution of a diet unfamiliar to the tastes of the patient; and 4) there is frequent contact between the patient and the physician, and, if possible, the dietician (Anderson, 1972).

At the same time, it must be recognized that there are a complex series of metabolic, psychologic, socio-economic and genetic factors involved in the onset of obesity affecting the whole personality as well as outlook of an individual. The state of obesity cannot be cured unless all the factors involved are properly taken care of and the individual is adjusted to his new role and outlook on life in order to stay on the slimmer side (Young, 1973). At best, the situation at the present time is confused. All kinds of approaches have been mentioned in the literature and tried with varying results. A combination of diet therapy and psychological approach appears to be, by far, the best. However, in both areas, the confusion is as great as the problem of obesity itself. Let us discuss the diet first.

Diet Therapy

There is no such thing as a diet for the obese or a diet for reducing one pound a week, or two pounds a week. There are certain principles that can be followed in recommending a diet for reducing, but there is no diet which can be recommended for everybody. Prescribing a diet for obesity is a tailor-made individual operation, which should be adapted to the magnitude of obesity, the patient's level of physical activity, psychological and emotional state, the degree of motivation and, above all, the tastes of the individual. That is why there is no such thing as the "American Medical Association's Diet" for weight reduction. Mayer has rightly emphasized that all an obese person needs to understand as well as appreciate is the *portion* sizes. He should continue to eat the same food to which he is accustomed. There is no need to change to any special diet, if the patient eats smaller portions of all the things that he normally eats. If he previously ate an *average* sized potato, with an *average* sized meat serving, all he has to do is to select half the size of potato with half of his usual serving of meat. For adding bulk, one may add some extra salad.

It is worthwhile to educate the patient to count the caloric content of various foods and various portion sizes so that in his bid for reducing, it may be easier for him to count a deficit of approximately 500 calories per day, while understanding the concept of a balanced diet which should contain about 15 percent protein, 30 percent fat, and 55 percent carbohydrates, with refined sugar reduced to the minimum level. "The downward calorie adjustment of existing food habits by reducing portion size is an easy way to place the patient on a diet acceptable to him in terms of economics and style of eating" (Mayer, 1972). Hutton suggested to his patients that they keep a scratch pad and write every item of food before they put it into their mouths. This will help the patient get a realistic idea of his daily food intake, as well as help the doctor to guide the patient in his dietary schedule.

This is probably the only way, not only to reduce sensibly, but to maintain the weight loss. The goal of maintaining a reduced weight is as important as losing the initial weight. Drastic reducing may not only hurt physiologically, but the patients may tend to regain once the psychological pressure of reducing is lifted. The commerciogenic obesity-reducing diets may have a balanced composition in terms of nutrition, but since they do not cater to the individual likes and dislikes of the person, they cannot be eaten over a prolonged period of time. If and when the patient reverts to his original pattern of eating, he quickly starts regaining the weight. For similar reasons, some of the *crash* diets, made from unusual mixtures of food, have been unsuccessful (Stillman and Baker, 1968). First of all, such foods do not represent culturally-based food patterns of any patient and are not liable to be followed for a long time. Secondly, once the patient is off this diet and back to his regular diet, the sheer pleasure of eating his favorite foods could lead to overindulgence, resulting in weight rebound. Fad food can never become a permanent part of one's menu; hence, there is a desirability of having a food plan which is based on the eating habits of the individual (Williams, 1969).

It seems extremely important to re-emphasize that an obese person must be aware of the crash reducing diets. One can make a long list of such diets which have been commercially advertised with all their merits. Popular magazines thrive on promoting such things as the "sweet-tooth diet, the lollipop diet, the whipped cream diet, the champagne diet, the grape diet, the operant-conditioning diet, the stone age meat diet, and the working man's diet" (*Medical World News*, 1973). The extreme examples are macrobiotic diets which may be the cause of scurvy, or total fasting without medical supervision, and the patient may find himself in the next world due to unexpected heart failure. The crash diets must be avoided simply because they are *crash* diets. Any *crash* way of losing weight is bound to be a *crash*. One does not gain weight in a *crash* manner, and one must not lose it that way. The ideal thing is to lose approximately one pound, or even half a pound, per week. One pound is equivalent to about 3,500 calories, so a meagre 250 calories less per day should bring about a reduction of half a pound a week, or approximately twenty-five pounds over a year's time. I would rather have an overweight person reduce at this rate on a continuing basis, provided he does so by adjusting the calorie value of his regular meals.

The human is not strictly a biochemical engine. We eat for pleasure, and eating is probably one of the most satisfying pleasures. No attempt at reducing is likely to be successful for a lifetime if it is at the cost of the pleasure and satisfaction that food gives. No wonder 85 percent of all the dieters do not stay at their reduced level of weight for more than two years! They generally return to their reducing diet, giving it one more try, and end up in the same manner, hurting their bodies instead of helping them. As Dr. White put it, "There is some evidence that obese individuals who lose weight and gain it back have a gradual increase in their blood cholesterol and blood lipid levels; and the next time they lose weight and gain it back, these levels are even higher. It must be tough on the psyche" (*Medical World News*, 1973).

A sensible well-balanced diet, deficient in calories, therefore, remains the most important treatment for a weight reduction program. An obese person must eat enough quantities of foods to which he is accustomed according to his cultural pattern, except that he must be made calorie conscious and vigilant about the deficiencies of protein, vitamins or minerals. A calorically reduced diet, which could at the same time be balanced in other nutrients and still be the favorite food of the patient, could reduce two or more pounds on a monthly basis without much inconvenience. Such a dietary pattern over a prolonged period of time could not only reduce sufficiently, but may be a sufficient incentive for the patient to continue on that pattern for maintenance to safeguard reversal to the obese state. The characteristics of a good diet are well described by Young; that diet should satisfy all nutrient needs except calories; should be adapted as closely as possible to the tastes and habits of the patient for whom it is intended; should protect the patient from between meal hunger insofar as possible and leave him with a sense of wellbeing and minimum of fatigue; should be easy for the patient to obtain at home or away from home, without feeling different; and should be such that it can be followed over a period of time and retain eating habits so that with suitable caloric addition it may become a pattern for lifetime eating.

Schauf (1973) recommended the following regimen, which takes into account the quality and quantity of food and the frequency of ingestion.

1. Eat at least three meals per day.
2. Eat animal protein (eggs, meat, fish, fowl or cheese) at each meal (3–4 ounces per serving of meat or fish).
3. Limit carbohydrates to between 15 and 25 grams per meal.
4. Restrict sugar containing and caffeine containing foods to breakfast.
5. Do not eat carbohydrates between meals.
6. Ensure an adequate water intake.
7. Use polyunsaturated oils (e.g. corn, safflower, soybean, peanut, and olive oils).
8. Finish each meal feeling nourished and alert, but never full.

Some differences of opinion exist about the advisability of giving artificial sweeteners as a substitute for sugar and the restriction of salt. Both should be left to the discretion of the physician. Artificial sweeteners may help to make certain foods more palatable. Salt restriction may be advisable because it helps the patient in three ways. Low salt diet prevents the water retention, which is often observed as the patient loses weight. A low salt diet is often not very tasty and it is likely that the overweight person may successfully overcome the temptation to overeat. A low salt diet can also help as a preventive measure to curb the tendency of heart disease, which is not uncommon among the obese persons (Mayer, 1972). However, it is difficult for most people to adhere for a long time to a low salt diet because food is eaten for taste and a low salt diet should be recommended only for those to whom a heart attack has already given a warning.

A special mention may be made of a *reducing diet* that has evoked more controversy than anything else like this in the field. It is called *Dr. Atkins' Diet*, which he propounded in his book, "Diet Revolution" (Atkins, 1972b). Dr. Atkins' whole philosophy of a reducing diet is based on the hypothesis that since most of the overweight or obese people have a disturbed carbohydrate metabolism and their physiology cannot handle this the way an active lean person does; the carbohydrate must be pronounced the main villain and must be excluded. Dr. Atkins believes that if carbohydrates are eliminated from the diet, there is no need to count calories. If the patient wants to, he can go ahead and eat as many as 4,000 calories per day and still lose weight. As Atkins explained:

> My diet cuts out carbohydrates altogether at first, then keeps them down permanently. My patients lose weight whether they eat more or less than usual. Most people eat less, but it's only because the diet so completely satisfies their hunger, they find they just can't eat as much as they used to. But some have lost thirty, forty or one hundred pounds while consuming 2,000 to 3,000 calories a day—or even more. The most permanently effective treatment for overweight is the removal of all carbohydrates from the diet. By carbohydrates, I don't mean just bread and pastry, but all foods with carbohydrate content—including such things as apples, raisins, carrots, catsup and yogurt with fruit. One reason why this diet works is that when you take away carbohydrates, you take away hunger. Proteins and fats have satiety value, but carbohydrates actually provoke hunger by stimulating the insulin release that sends blood sugar plummeting down (Atkins, 1972a).

According to that author, overeating pattern in the obese is not due to any psychological disturbance, as is generally believed. Most of them eat larger quantities because of the abnormal pattern of carbohydrate metabolism which makes them feel an elevated degree of hunger.

Since carbohydrates, as a ready source of energy, are seldom stored for more than two days, their nonavailability in the diet puts the body in a state of ketosis because the excessive fat is being utilized in order to provide energy and, in the process, large quantities of ketones (carbon particles released as by-products of burning fat) are released. In other words, the body "converts from a carbohydrate-burning engine to a fat-burning engine" (Atkins, 1972b). Dr. Atkins' regimen recommends that, during the first week of treatment, carbohydrates should be eliminated altogether from the diet, which puts his metabolic engine to a fat burning engine or in a state of ketosis. From then, small quantities of carbohydrates may be added to the diet so long as one's body remains a fat burning engine. While fat is being summoned as a source of energy, the pituitary gland releases the fat mobilizing hormone. The mechanism of action of this hormone on weight reduction has not been adequately explained by Dr. Atkins, except that he has provided data that his male patients lose an average of 15 to 20 pounds and female patients, 10 to 15 pounds during their first month of his diet therapy program. Along with the diet is highly recommended an optimum dosage of vitamins and minerals. For example, it is recommended to have daily as much as 800 units of vitamin E, 1,000 mg of vitamin C, and double the minimum requirements of the full spectrum of the vitamin B complex. This diet has been violently attacked in a sixteen-page monograph by the American Medical Association Council of Foods and Nutrition, and the same degree of disapproval has been accorded by the Medical Society of the County of New York.

There is nothing new about the desirability of reducing carbohydrates for the purpose of reducing weight. It has always been considered desirable to have a low caloric, low carbohydrate, low fat diet. A 1,000 calorie diet with carbohydrates restricted to the level of 30 to 50 gms is considered drastic reducing, but nonetheless acceptable; but what about a diet which forbids carbohydrates yet sanctions the unlimited intake of fats? When protein-rich and fat-rich steaks are recommended in unlimited quantities, the intake of saturated fats and cholesterols could be significantly high. "In individuals who respond to such a diet with an elevation of plasma lipids and an exaggerated alimentary hyperlipemia, the risk of coronary artery disease and other clinical manifestations of atherosclerosis may well be increased—particularly if the diet is maintained over a prolonged period." (*Medical World News*, 1973) . Before this *revolutionary* diet is recommended to the *overweight* population of the world (the numbers do run into hundreds of millions of people) , it should go through a thorough examination of the long-term effects of continued ketosis.

The people who are prone to gall bladder related diseases may find their gall bladders damaged beyond repair. It is quite possible that Dr. Atkins has come out with an unconventional approach that may solve this grave human problem, but since neither Dr. Atkins nor anybody else can explain the full implications of prolonged ketosis, its wholesale use by thousands of individuals may be premature. A high fat diet generally raises cholesterol levels but Dr. Atkins says that, among his patients who have cut down carbohydrates, the cholesterol level goes down; however, he cannot explain why. We must understand the long-term effects of continued ketosis as well as the full implications and mechanisms of a low carbohydrate, high fat diet before it is recommended for widespread use.

There is yet another diet, which is gaining recognition among the weight reducing enthusiasts. It is based on a regular intake of cider vinegar, lecithin, kelp, and vitamin B_6, besides reduced caloric intake. It is believed that the cider vinegar from apples is rich in potassium; the lecithin is a natural diuretic and to some extent a cholesterol reducer; kelp is rich in iodine helping to tone up the metabolic system and vitamin B_6 helps to set up a body balance of sodium and potassium, which regulates body fluids and avoids unnecessary water retention (Crenshaw, 1974) . The diet needs elaborate scientific examination before any opinion is expressed about it.

Clinical Approach
A variety of methods for reducing obesity are practiced.

These include specifically formulated diets, drugs, hormones, hypnosis, psychotherapy, behavior therapy, etc. Every approach has its merits, demerits and assumptions. For example, behavior therapy is based on the assumption that excess eating is due to special behavior patterns that can be unlearned. So far, there is little evidence that this is more effective than other types of individual or group psychotherapy (*Medical Letter*, 1971). That new methods keep coming up regularly indicates the relative failure of the existing approaches in promoting sustained weight loss among obese patients.

The clinical approach mainly consists of using certain categories of drugs or surgical procedures. For example, diuretics, anorexigenic agents, thyroid preparations, or other drugs have been used to obtain a sustained weight loss. The use of diuretics in excessively obese patients who have clear indications of water retention may be good, but an indiscriminate use of them is inadvisable. The weight loss may be solely due to sodium and water excretion, while the amount of adipose tissue may not be diminished. Prolonged use of diuretics could be a cause of real damage; however, some patients with idiopathic edema may have it for a number of days. Hutton believes that the diuretics are better taken at bedtime (Hutton, 1971).

Anorexigenic agents as appetite suppressants have also been tried in an effort at quick reduction of obesity (Wohl, 1968). These include such habit-forming drugs as amphetamines. It is believed that these drugs act by stimulating the satiety-controlling centers such as the ventromedial nucleus of the hypothalamus (JAMA, 1963). The amphetamine preparations depress the appetite and decrease the amount of food eaten at a meal. There may be some metabolic merit in their use, and some studies indicate that four to six weeks' use may have helped to reduce obesity, but we do not yet understand the exact mode of action of these drugs on the nervous system and the manifestations of side effects, which are occasionally as bad as restlessness, irritability, insomnia, etc. Cardiac patients or people with some complications of hypertension may especially be hurt by the use of amphetamines (Mayer, 1972). Even if these drugs are useful for a short term, they should not be recommended because their long-term effects could be quite hazardous. It is important that whenever used, the patient must be under the continued supervision of a qualified physician. Knittle strongly emphasized that

> the use of drugs such as amphetamines is of little value in the long range treatment of obesity and should be assiduously avoided. This is especially true in children and adolescents who are exposed to a drug-oriented society. The introduction of yet another medically approved drug creates the risk of subsequent harm from misuse.

Thyroid preparations have also been prescribed to reduce obesity, whether or not the patient is in a hypothyroid state. This prescription is made with the belief that the obese patients are hypometabolic. Mayer believes that the administration of thyroid hormone is in part self-defeating as it depresses endogenous thyroid secretion, the depression being very slow to reverse (1965). Extra thyroid extracts could induce a hyperthyroid state which could increase appetite and also have undesirable side effects such as tachycardia, palpitation, nervousness and insomnia, creating an unpleasant and potentially dangerous situation (Mayer, 1965).

Biguanides also have an insignificant role in the treatment of obesity. However, phenoformin and metaformin have been reported to induce weight loss in some obese nondiabetic persons (Roginsky and Sandler, 1968). The biguanides cause a reduction in the gastrointestinal absorption of carbohydrates and reduces the tendency of hyperinsulinism often present in the obese (Czyzyk, 1969).

> Results using these drugs are not consistently good, but a trial of one or the other is recommended, particularly in those who are diabetic or who have a family history of diabetes. Metaformin is usefully given in the form of glucophage, 850 mg twice daily, and phenoformin as the dibotin sustained-release capsule, 50 mg twice daily. In each case, the drugs should be given with or after meals to minimize gastric irritation (Anderson, 1972).

Triiodothyroxine is another drug that has been used in the 1950's and early 1960's, along with caloric restriction, as a treatment of obesity. Reports indicate that this drug does not cause thyrotoxic side effects up to a certain dosage. It is believed that triiodothyroxine "enhances the lipolytic effect of epinephrine on adipose tissue and increases the glomerular filtration rate and renal blood flow of obese patients."

Other drugs used are human chorionic gonadotropins— marked as Antuitrin-S, APL and Folutein. Hutton described the regimen followed by the late Dr. A. W. Simeons:

> In general, the program consists of injections of 125 to 250 units daily or three times weekly depending on circumstances. Simeons gave 125 units daily six times weekly until forty injections had been given. He then stopped the injections for six weeks, during which time the patient was not expected to lose any more weight. If more weight needed to be lost, a second series was begun at that time.

Mention may be made of the bulk-producing agents such as methyl cellulose, which have been recommended to add bulk to the restricted quantity of food for the treatment of obesity. They may produce a temporary feeling of satiety, but they have not proven successful because most men do not eat for bulk but for energy (Anderson, 1972). Dietary dilution studies in rats and men have proven the same point (Teitelbaun and Epstein, 1962).

It is hard to decide whether or not to resort to fasting as a method of reducing weight. Bloom, who used fasting as an introduction to the treatment of obesity, and several other workers (Ball *et al.*, 1970a; Bloom, 1959) found that the major portion of the weight loss during a period of starvation is not fat, but water and protein. It is not clear at this time why the obese are unable to accelerate fat loss in response to such drastic measures as fasting (*JAMA*, 1970).

Surgical operation is another approach which would not be recommended as a weight reduction plan, although in cases of severe intractable obesity, surgery has been used. Jejunocoli shunts, bypassing the small intestine, have been successfully used, but most of these patients develop malabsorption syndromes along with other side effects, such as megaloblastic anemia, iron deficiency and impaired vitamin B_{12} absorption. It is believed that short-circuiting of the small intestine lacks a sound physiological basis and can be accompanied by undesirable physiological as well as psychological sequelae (Wohl, 1968).

For the purpose of controlling the metabolic disorders produced as a result of obesity or vice versa, Gordon proposed to use the following scheme of things which are purely speculative as well as hypothetical; however, they are worth considering in view of the increasing prevalence of obesity in our society.

1. Increased energy expenditure in the form of physical exercise should be prescribed. Not only the exercise itself would drain off large quantities of reserve fuel through total oxidation to carbon dioxide and water, but the large amount of wasted heat generated by exercise would increase the energy cost of such activity.

2. By means of some hypothetical drug, the lipolysis-fatty acid esterification cycle could be *speeded up* so that more energy could be wasted and dissipated as heat.

3. The alternate pathway principle of the fatty acid syntheses-oxidation cycle could be stimulated by some means unknown at present, with the further loss of substantial amounts of energy as heat.

4. The glycerophosphate shuttle could be accelerated to produce wasted energy as heat. At present this may be accomplished by the use of a low-protein diet and the additional *induction* of the dehydrogenase enzyme with thyroid hormone. Exposure to cold environmental temperature and injection of catecholamine drugs (epinephrine, norepinephrine) will also achieve this result.

5. Uncouple oxidative phosphorylation by some pharmacological means. Hopefully drugs of the dinitrophenol type may be found that would also be safe therapeutic agents to use.

6. Find some method to increase the urinary loss of partially metabolized foodstuffs, perhaps through injection of fat-mobilizing agents.

7. Suppress the appetite center in the hypothalamus or stimulate the satiety center. The effect should be accomplished through pharmacological manipulation. But regardless of method, the intake of energy-containing foodstuff should be curtailed.

Psychological Factors

Obesity is not a typical illness that should respond to

clinical treatment. It requires a very deep understanding on the part of the therapist and psychological confidence on the part of the patient, the degree of which will determine the cooperation and motivation that could be expected of him.

Psychological disturbances of children and adults often lead to certain abnormal behavior, and overeating is one of them. To some obese people, eating is an escape from the worries, frustrations and disappointments of their life, and they resort to it at the slightest psychological disturbance, as if eating will compensate for the hard realities of their life. Overeating, therefore, may be considered as a substitute gratification for a depressing situation. Such a trend of running to food at a time of emotional stress generally has its roots in the early years of life. Very few children with balanced personalities and belonging to secure, loving, well-adjusted homes eat themselves to obesity. A balanced child devotes more attention to play and exploring his environment than to keeping himself busy eating. On the other hand,

> if home offers a child little security, he may make food a substitute for the love and sense of security he craves and needs. An obese child is an unhappy child; overeating is his weapon against failure and disappointment. The abnormal eating habits developed by such a child may persist into adult life, and combined with physical indolence, lead to obesity in maturity (Wohl, 1968).

That overeating or developing an addiction for food is a sign of emotional instability and is a response to stress situations has been pointed out by a number of prominent psychologists. According to these studies, overeating which results in obesity is a symptom of emotional illness, depression, and inability to face the realities of life, and is sought after as an outlet for frustrations. A psychiatric study of obesity in women revealed that most fat girls come from less than happy family situations, and sexual maladjustment may be a reason for some adolescent girls to be obese. "A fat figure may be a defense for individuals wishing to avoid contact with the opposite sex or secretly desiring to have physical attributes of the other sex" (McWilliams, 1967). Among children dur-

ing their growing years, normal psychological struggles are
not positively supported by the child's environment, and the
child feels insecure and emotionally unstable (Bruch, 1957).

Bruch (1961) believes that the obese literally do not
know when they are physiologically hungry. She believes
that this lack of knowledge about the sensation of hunger
stems from their early childhood, when they were not taught
to differentiate between hunger, fear, anger and anxiety,
because with all these emotions, they tended to eat. Such a
tendency persists in the adult life when they label every
form of arousal as hunger (Bruch, 1961). The extensive
studies of Schachter also point out that the obese are relatively insensitive to variations in the physiological correlates
to food deprivation, but highly sensitive to environmental,
which explains better why the obese lose significant weight
in a controlled environment such as a hospital ward, but
fail to maintain it and return to the original weight upon
their return to normal living in an environment full of hopes
as well as fears, anxieties as well as tensions (Schachter,
1968).

A study of anxiety and depression in obese dieters reveals
that more of the obese than the nonobese tend to be poor,
single, divorced, separated or widowed. Obesity in such
cases is caused by lack of self-control, self-pity or serious
abnormalities of personality (Hutton, 1971). Such people,
who are psychologically depressed by virtue of their circumstances, will go through an extra stress and strain when put
on a restricted diet in order to treat their obesity. Such a
procedure in an emotionally unstable person may turn out
to create more neurotic symptoms as well as pronounced
depression or psychosis. This may be especially true when
eating has been used by the patient as an escape or defense
against his psychological disturbances or the depressive
environment in which he lives.

Psychological analysis could go a long way in allaying
fears which are indirectly responsible for obesity. A resolution of anxieties and stressful conditions, which result in overeating, could decrease considerably the caloric intake. By

not blaming the patient and by not expecting him to be a hero of strong will, the psychologist may put things in the right perspective for the patient and may develop in him the movitation to steadily achieve a reduction in weight, or to at least maintain it. A more favorable psychological approach can be created by group therapy. Mass discipline is always the best discipline, and in most instances, it is the lack of motivation that stands in the way of following successfully a weight reduction program. When a group of people is involved, an exchange of views among the patients helps to increase the motivation of an individual.

It must be emphasized that the obese are acutely aware of the attitudes of the society towards their figures and the kind of labels such as gluttonous, self-indulgent, weak-willed, with which they are viewed. This kind of awareness often causes psychological taxing which further reduces one's ability to reduce weight by a voluntary plan of food restriction. A number of prominent psychologists have noted that the uneven distribution of food intake by the obese reflects a state of depression that the obese take the shelter of food when hurt psychologically. If society expects the obese to reduce, then something needs to be expected from the nonobese in order to help the obese to conform to the desirable norms. The nonobese will help by describing the overweight as jovial, cheerful and easygoing, rather than snubbing them as being lethargic, lazy and weak-willed. Obesity cannot be cured by blaming the person. We do not ridicule any other congenital condition because we have learned to associate other such conditions as states of sickness and, therefore, in need of our sympathy and support. Maybe we should apply some psychological readjustment towards the obese, and call their condition a complex medical problem. An obese person, more than anybody else, needs comfort rather than ridicule. This could help him in overcoming some of the serious psychological problems associated with reducing and staying reduced thereafter.

We must realize that when an obese person is put on a reducing diet, he faces the hard prospect of overcoming the physiological as well as psychological difficulties that made him obese in the first place, i.e. being hungry a large part of the time. Reducing by those whose obesity is of metabolic origin is all the more painful in terms of psychological and physiological stress. They may go into a negative balance or may lose the valuable proteins along with the fat. Mayer described that

> even in those persons in whom metabolic factors are not primary in the etiology of obesity, burning of body fat does not fulfill satiety requirements to the same extent as does food. This may explain why so many fat patients react to dieting as though they were starving. They show an acute craving for all sorts of food, even some which they do not usually like. They are constantly in a state of extreme tension; they feel dizzy and are sleepless at night, and in some extreme cases, they may show an almost complete disintegration of their personality (1972).

PREVENTION IS BETTER THAN CURE

Obesity is one of those conditions where prevention is likely to be more successful than the cure, as the treatment of established obesity is often unsuccessful or disappointing. When an obese person loses weight, only a slight degree of carlessness about food intake prompts the regaining of the lost weight. It is believed that the practice of frequent weight gains and losses by unmotivated dieters may be more harmful than the maintenance of a steady weight at a higher level. The fluctuations in weight patterns may subject the body to more atherogenic stress than a stable, though excessive, weight. The elevation of serum cholesterol levels, which accompany every incidence of weight gain, may increase the risk of coronary heart disease, because with decrease in weight, the cholesterol levels may not decrease. It appears that regaining the lost weight is much more efficient than the first weight gain. This could be the most compelling argument in favor of prevention of obesity. This is especially true in childhood, when its seeds are sown in the form of increased numbers and sizes of adipose cells and before other irreversible physiological changes take place. In the prevention program, it is the fatty component of the food and, later,

the fatty part of the body that are the most desirable to curtail. Such a reduction of fat may make all the difference in
the prevention of certain diseases associated with obesity
and which affect the mortality rate among the obese people.

At a time when prevention is most desirable, i.e. the early
years of life, the obese state is generally considered a state
of good health. Most parents are happier to see healthy,
plump and good-looking children who continue to consume
large quantities of food. The parents are proud to see their
children growing bigger and bigger, year after year. It is
as though they get the feeling of being competent parents
when their child outgrows the neighbor's child in body build
and the size of clothes. A fat child has been socially considered as a healthy child and, to a great extent, a beautiful
one, too. It is interesting that one can hear the mother of
those very obese children fussing about their lack of appetite! These children may be among those who do not feel
hunger until they begin to eat, but then have difficulty in
stopping (Knittle, 1972). The most dangerous is the *clean
plate syndrome,* which in simple language would mean that
the mother insists that the child finish everything that was
put on the plate. Imagine if this tendency continues to adult
life! Parents must be made to understand that a child of
six months does not look prettier if he is as large as a normal
one-year-old, nor is he likely to be more intelligent. Instead,
overfeeding is putting more stress on his cardiovascular
system. Obesity during early childhood may delay motor
development so that a two year old obese child may not be
able to learn to walk, which, in turn, could have severe consequences of exploration of environment so necessary for a
child of this age (*Br Med J,* 1970).

In feeding the child, an individualized approach has to
be followed. It is unwise to generalize that a child of this
weight should get a diet containing that many calories. The
reason for such nutritional differentiation is the individual
activity levels that are characteristic of every child. Even
at very early stages of infancy, some children spend long
periods crying and kicking, whereas others quietly sleep

most of the time. The energy requirements of these kinds of children are different. Giving extra food to a sleeping-type of baby will not only make him obese, but may further reduce his level of activity.

A very potent factor in the prevention of obesity is the deeper involvement of the pediatrician. If a pediatrician makes it a routine procedure to explain the nutritional requirements of the child and the pattern of child growth to the parents, it will not only help the baby, but may indirectly influence the eating patterns of the adults in the family as well (McWilliams, 1967). It is only the pediatrician who can loosen the stranglehold of the age-old dictum that "a fat baby is a healthy baby." Instead, it should be that a "lean and active baby is a healthy baby." Parents must not underestimate the food needs of the baby, as is done in the overpopulated countries of the East, but at the same time, there is no need to exaggerate the nutritional needs of the baby, just because he is growing. It has been estimated that only 8 to 10 percent of the total calories are consumed for the growth of new tissue (Widdowson, 1961). The bulk of the calories in children are consumed by physical activity and basal metabolism. Since the level of physical activity varies from child to child, there is no need to equate the food requirements of two children. A lean and active child is likely to consume many more calories than a fat child who is more likely to play sitting at one place. It is interesting that the basal metabolism accounts for 45 percent of the total calories; 9 percent of the calories are found in the feces; 8 percent are used for growth; and 38 percent are available for physical activity (Mayer, 1968). A fat child does not make use of this large chunk of calories, and hence, tends to accumulate it in the form of fat.

It is difficult to determine at this stage whether inactivity leads to obesity or obesity leads to inactivity. The reasons for inactivity could be genetic, or due to other metabolic disturbances discussed elsewhere. Because of the fact that we do not have a satisfactory answer to this extremely important question, a great caution is needed to enforce a drastic curtailment of calories in our anxiety to prevent obesity. It is possible that an overweight child is simply endowed with a heavy skeleton, larger muscle mass, or a combination of heavier bony mass, unusual amount of muscle and large quantities of adipose tissue. It is essential that an overweight child be thoroughly examined for his fat content or total body fat. Mayer has rightly emphasized that:

> if the fat baby does not have a larger-than-normal intake, great caution must be used in cutting down on how much he eats. First, there is a risk of diminishing growth rather than fat accumulation. Second, it may well be that any curtailment of a moderate intake will cause hunger and with it a great increase in crying, muscle tone and (rage) activity, which will magnify the size of the calorie consumption to a level much above that anticipated and again compromise growth. Although decreasing excessive fatness in babies is probably very useful, the *dieting* prescription should be determined with caution and accompanied by frequent checks on the maintenance of growth in length, health, and a reasonably happy disposition (Mayer, 1972).

This puts a great responsibility on the parents to help the children develop dietary habits which prevent overweight. At this point, two things become apparent: one, the dietary habits of the parents and their physical state; and two, the nutritional knowledge of the parents and how well they use this knowledge for the guidance of their children. A study of obesity, social class and mental illness points out that people's preoccupation with foods results from limited opportunities for recreational pursuits, excessive use of habitual foods which are generally high in carbohydrates or fats, and, above all, lack of knowledge or education as to what to purchase and the importance of keeping one's weight within the normal limits (Moore *et al.,* 1962). Acquisition of new hobbies or recreational interests will help to prevent the boredom that often leads to overeating.

An important criteria of prevention of obesity is an inducement for children to greater activity and harder play, especially in the case of children with bigger skeletal size and musculature (Seltzer and Mayer, 1965). Starting from a very short period of exercise, the amount of exercise should be increased on a regular basis. A program of regular exercise will not only result in burning of extra calories, but will improve muscle tone, flexibility of the joints, and physical, mental and social fitness (Wohl, 1968). In certain obese people who find it extremely hard to lower significantly their calorie intake, exercise can help them in caloric expenditure. Calculating a weight loss based on moderate exercise such as walking one mile a day (one has to walk thirty-five miles to lose one pound), one could lose ten pounds in a year, provided the caloric intake is constant.

This is not the place to discuss the use of health clubs and modern conveniences of exercise. They have their own useful role to play. However, it is generally true that few people visit them regularly over a period of several years. An obese person is motivated for some time, and will visit such a place until, in a few days or weeks, he reduces somewhat and then loses motivation. Planning for the type of exercise that is done, not out of necessity, but out of pleasure, is always preferable. A husband and wife can develop walking habits which, in addition to the needed exercise, give some time for mutual discussions that may, in turn, lead to better communication. A badminton court in the backyard, mowing the lawn and doing things around the house can be fun as well as provide the needed exercise.

CONCLUDING THOUGHTS

It is evident that obesity is a very complex problem. There is no single factor that leads to it and there is no single cure which can treat it. Every obese person must be treated as an individual case with his individual problem and a tailor-made regimen of dieting. Psychotherapy and other remedial measures may be equally important in helping him to reduce as well as to learn to live with his new diet and physical size.

Greatest stress needs to be placed on the prevention program, in view of the high degree of prevalence. The seeds of obesity are sown soon after birth of the baby in the form of a dietary regimen, unless genetically inherited. The pediatrician needs to play a key role in regulating the dietary intake of the infants and in educating the mother on the meaning of sound nutrition of the baby. The baby reacts to excess quantities of food by making extra fat cells in which to store it. These extra fat cells stay with the individual for the whole life. The concept of food as a reward for good behavior needs to be changed. In the same way, it is desirable to check at an early age the desire to eat whenever psychologically hurt or upset. A lot needs to be learned about the eating habits of the children under different types of stimuli such as hunger, happiness, pain, disturbance, deprivation, insecurity or even ready availability of everything as soon as desired. Education of the parents in the art of infant feeding is a must, but we have to go deeper into the problems of the mechanism of the inception of obesity in childhood because it is in the early life that, in most instances, the seeds of obesity are sown.

The treatment of obesity must not be viewed from a short-range program of reducing and leaving him alone. The whole approach, by the very nature of the condition, has to be based on a life-long pattern. The diet regimen must be a simple modification of the eating patterns which an individual is accustomed to for his whole past life and which are likely to continue. A person may stick to an unfamiliar schedule for a few years with the best of will-power and motivation, but he is likely to revert back to foods which have always given him the satisfaction, pleasure and satiety. The reducing regimen must conform to his cultural and individual tastes of food, otherwise an obese person will never be able to extricate himself from a vicious cycle of weight loss followed by weight gain.

Weight loss by drastic reduction of calories or fasting may be harmful in the long run. The whole approach should be a slow reversal of the process. Nobody becomes obese in a short time of one year and nobody should be expected to lose it all in one year. Varying from person to person, it may be better to reduce constantly in the same proportion as the patient gained. This will give him ample time for readjusting himself to a somewhat thinner state and the way of life that will accompany it. Obesity in most instances is a result of physical inactivity. Reducing should be accompanied by a slow, steady increase in physical activity. As explained by Knittle, "weight loss should be monitored in terms of body composition rather than total body weight. Indeed the maintenance of a constant weight with an increasing ratio of lean body mass to body fat with normal linear growth is a desirable result."

MALNUTRITION
THE VULNERABLE GROUPS

Although not many starve to death in the present day world, there are millions who are chronically undernourished and malnourished. Besides pockets of mass poverty in Africa, South America, and elsewhere, the Asian continent is the most overcrowded, technologically backward and unable to afford a decent level of nutrition for its vast populations. It has been estimated that 0.5 to 7 percent of children below five years of age in these countries are malnourished, and about three million of them die every year due directly or indirectly to malnutrition (Miladi, 1971).

In the year 1975, 329 million children below 15 years of age out of a total of about 815 million will not receive adequate diets if the present disparity in per capita food production between the developed and developing countries remains. As the trend goes, there is a no reason to believe that the present status is going to change (Cravioto and DeLicardie, 1973; May and Lemm, 1969). Malnutrition, whether it is caused by lesser quantities of protein, carbohydrates, vitamins or minerals, leaves a person debilitated and prone to various kinds of diseases (Gopalan and Srikantia, 1973; McLaren, 1973), and incapable of putting in his best. A worker who is undernourished is not likely to be as productive as a worker who is well-nourished. When a whole community is undernourished, it has an adverse effect on the economic development of the community. Production lags and so does the availability of food. To put it in a simpler manner, "malnutrition roadblocks human progress and socio-economic and cultural development" (Paarlberg, 1973).

In most of the underdeveloped and developing countries which are overpopulated and are unable to produce sufficient foods, the average per capita caloric consumption is less than 2,000, which is woefully inadequate. It must be added here that, when a national average falls less than 2,000 calories, there will always be a substantial population which gets a lot less than that amount. At that calorie level, coupled with insufficient quantities of protein, vitamins and minerals, the poorer sections of the society will lead a very lethargic and unproductive existence. Consider for a moment the fate of malnourished children born to malnourished parents. After two decades this generation of inadeequately nourished individuals is supposed to enter the public, cultural and social life of their nation. What will be the values of this generation? How will they rule the destinies of their country? What kind of society and government will they have with its impact on the international scene? White warned that

> malnutrition as a deterrent to social progress should not be taken lightly. Malnutrition can be involved directly or indirectly in the initiation and perpetuation of a disheartened, listless segment of a population, thus producing considerable drag on society. Social development requires involvement, and it is difficult to become involved after the world has passed one by (White, 1971).

For details, the reader is referred to the author's earlier book on *Malnutrition and Retarded Human Development*.

Whereas there is no evidence that the adult population suffers from any mental impairment under the influence of malnutrition, a good deal of scientific data exist which clearly underline the dangers to a baby in its prenatal and postnatal life, if it fails to get adequate nutrition during this critical period of its development. We must, therefore, recognize a vulnerable group, which should be given priority in feeding and special attention be given to their nutritional needs. These vulnerable groups are the pregnant and lactating mother and the baby in its preschool years. In a number of traditional societies, there is absolutely no concept of the extra food needs of the pregnant or lactating mother, or that of the baby in its infancy. Only proper guidance in nutrition can break the hold of these misinformed and dangerous concepts in the underdeveloped countries. It must be recognized that the diet and general health of the mother before and during pregnancy has a profound influence on the health and well-being of the baby.

Studies on animals are producing precise evidence as to the mechanisms underlying the deleterious effects of poor maternal nutrition on the physical and physiological growth of the fetus. There is a direct relationship between the fetal growth and the maternal diet. A significant percentage of mothers whose growth has been stunted because of their nutrition, shows abnormal pelvic shapes conducive to disordered pregnancy and delivery. Baird noted during a study of 13,000 deliveries that fetal mortality rates were more than twice as high in women five feet one inch tall or less as compared to those five feet four inches tall or more. Thomson also studied more than 26,000 births and concluded, "It is evident that whatever the nature of the delivery, the fetus of the short woman has less vitality and is less likely to be well grown and to survive than that of a tall woman."

During the early stages of pregnancy the requirements of the fetus can be met from the nutritional reserves of the mother. But if the latter does not get adequate quantities of nutrients from her diet, during the later part of pregnancy the host-parasite relationship between the mother and the fetus is likely to be strained to the detriment of both. This is especially true of the third trimester of fetal growth. It is during this period that 70 percent of the birth weight and 93 percent of the fat are acquired (Brock, 1972). A woman whose dietary intake is defective or does not have nutritional reserves accumulated in her tissues from the preconceptional period, will have low plasma amino nitrogen and very small quantities of amino acids to make available to the fetus with the result that the latter is adversely affected.

Small, low birth weight babies are often born to mothers who have been undernourished in their periods of childhood, adolescence and during pregnancy. The low birth weight babies are either *preterm,* born before 37 weeks' gestation, or *small for date,* born at full term. It is the latter group that has suffered fetal growth retardation that is our major concern because, whereas the *preterm* may make up their losses by better diet in their early postnatal life, the full term retarded infant may have his growth trajectory altered to the extent that the *catch up* may not be possible. Although birth weight is not a conclusive index of physical and mental retardation, it is a very adequate parameter for assessing the damage and chances of the survival of the baby (Habicht, *et al.,* 1973).

> WHO figures show that of every 1,000 infants born live and weighing 1,000 gm or less, 912 will die shortly after birth. Of the 1,000 babies between 1,000 gm and 1,500 gm, 512 will quickly die, while in the group between 1,500 gm and 2,000 gm, 180 will not survive. And, of 1,000 weighing between 2,000 gm and 2,500 gm, 41 will die soon after birth. In the group between 2,500 gm to 3,000 gm, only nine of 1,000 will soon succumb. The best chances for life are found in the group over 3,000 gm where just four of every 1,000 will die (Symposium, 1972).

Several investigations have indicated that it is most desirable that the female is very healthy in her adolescent life so as to nurture a healthy fetus, but it is of utmost importance that she be given a richer diet during the last trimester of her pregnancy. This may be illustrated better by two studies. In the first study conducted in England, the Indian and Pakistani immigrants took full advantage of the maternal and child welfare facilities along with their British counterparts. These women were very well fed during their entire gestation period. The death rates between 1 and 11 months were similar in the two groups under study. But it is surprising that the neonatal death rate among the immigrant group was 2.4 times greater than the British group. The investigators concluded that the preconceptional nutritional status of the immigrant mothers was poorer as compared to that of the British girls. The former went through greater stress of pregnancy, encountered more clinical problems, and the birth weight was generally lower. After the babies survived their neonatal period, both groups took equally good care of them (Akyroyd and Hussain, 1967). A study in India included pregnant mothers of lower socio-economic groups. A random sample from this group was admitted to the nutrition ward of the hospital during the last four weeks of gestation. During this period they were given 85 gms of protein and a diet containing over 2,500 calories along with full rest. The mean birth weight of the babies in this group was over 2,900 gms compared to 2,000 gms in the control group not admitted to the hospital (Venkatachalam, 1962).

Occasionally, the mother may hurt the baby during *in utero* growth and development not because of any serious problems of nutrition, but because of her way of life. A working mother with extra responsibilities of running a home or caring for other children may overexert herself and develop hypertension. This is especially true of those career women who try to work on their jobs until the last day. The social practice of giving up to three months' paid pregnancy leave is very useful and is practiced in a number of countries. At a recent symposium in New York, Dr. Minkowski, a prominent French scientist, told of how China has eliminated the problem of hypertension during pregnancy. "A pregnant woman's blood pressure is measured every week, no matter how remote the factory, town or commune in which she lives. If her blood pressure ever reaches 130/90, she is put to bed for a month, order of The Chairman Mao."

Genetic endowment is important to a great extent in determining the ultimate size of the offspring but may not be as big a contributing factor as the level of maternal nutrition when it comes to the growth of the fetus (Graenwald, 1968). There also exists a definite relationship between the quality of the mother's diet during pregnancy, particularly with respect to its protein content, and the length of the baby at birth. Protein supply in the diet appears more important than the number of calories in the maternal food as a determiner of the length of the baby (DeSilva and Baptist, 1969). However, the height of the mother, which directly or indirectly influences the shape of the pelvis, may have the same influence. It is believed that rounded or long oval pelvis is functionally superior for childbearing and is more common in well-off, well-grown, taller women.

The mother's diet has a profound effect on the pattern of development of the fetal tissues. If she fails to provide adequately, not only does the overall body growth rate decrease, but most of the fetal tissues are affected as well. It is interesting to note, however, that all organs of the body of a malnourished fetus are not affected in the same proportion. The brain gets the maximum priority over the available nutrients, especially during the last trimester. The next in line are the heart and lungs; the pancreas and kidneys are also affected, but the liver and spleen in these malnourished infants are disproportionately small. The number of parenchymal cells in the liver, spleen, and pancreas are greatly reduced (Naeye, 1966). These infants also show disturbance in carbohydrate metabolism which manifests itself at a later stage in mental dysfunction. Basic research indicates that fetal malnutrition impairs cell replication *in utero* which largely depends on protein synthesis. Because of their small size and limited storage of subcutaneous fats, the malnourished infants show a limited ability to conserve body heat. They also show low serum total protein (albumin and immunoglobulin) levels at birth with the result that they are more predisposed to catch common infections and less able to combat them.

The intrauterine growth retardation not only affects the organs grossly, but also the metabolic patterns of the individual cells. Recent investigations from our laboratory and others have pointed to reduced activity of certain energy generating enzymes in the cells of different organs. These observations point out a slowing down of metabolic processes (Manocha and Olkowski, 1972; 1973). It is hoped that more insight will be developed soon as to the mechanisms by which malnutrition affects the metabolic processes.

Although it is not the rule, some of the infants who suffer intrauterine growth retardation, show abnormalities in their cytogenetical make-up. For example, the fetuses which show evidence of Down's and Turner's syndromes, also fail to thrive and their chances of *in utero* or postnatal survival are greatly reduced. The abnormalities of the chromosomes lead to prenatal and postnatal growth retardation (Chen and Falek, 1974). The loss of the short arm of the X-chromosome is directly related to such stunting of growth and leads to dwarfism and other characteristic features of Turner's syndrome (Reisman, 1970).

A note on breast feeding may not be inappropriate here due to its importance. Here also, the preconceptional health of the mother is of extreme importance. It appears that undernutrition in childhood and adolescence impairs the development of mammary tissues with the result that a malnourished woman may not be able to lactate adequately. Her child may suffer adversely in its early postnatal life (Jelliffe, 1972; 1973). After the baby is born breast feeding is the best thing to do anywhere in the world. The milk is sterile (uncontaminated by disease carrying germs), cheap and readily available at the time of need. Recent studies in biochemistry, immunology and psychology have proven the superiority of human breast milk over animal milk (cow's or buffalo's) for the health and well-being of the infant. Strangely, in the poorer countries, the practice of breast feeding is declining which is aggravating the already bad situation (Donoso, 1971; Jelliffe, 1971).

Breast feeding in certain conditions may run into problems to the detriment of the child's health. A malnourished mother may be unable to produce quantitatively as well as qualitatively adequate milk to promote satisfactory growth of the baby. A baby whose growth has already been retarded while being inside the body of such a weak mother now suffers during its critical early period of life which most certainly will affect its physical and mental development. In most of the poor developing countries, the results of artificial feeding are generally disastrous for the baby. The milk is expensive and the family may not afford to buy enough quantities. In the absence of refrigeration facilities, pure uncontaminated water and the necessary knowledge required in artificial feeding, the baby is likely to be the victim of recurrent infections and diarrhea. Studies from many places indicate a disastrous decline in breast feeding, especially among the inhabitants of poorer urban and periurban areas which are growing so rapidly in all the developing countries (Jelliffe, 1972). It is indeed unfortunate!

MALNUTRITION AND MENTAL IMPAIRMENT

The peak period of brain growth, which occurs during the last 15 weeks, coincides with the period of maximum growth of the fetus on the whole. During this period the nutritional demands of the growing fetus are greatly enhanced and if the mother fails to meet those demands, the satisfactory growth of the brain is likely to be adversely affected. Maternal malnutrition may therefore interfere with fetal neuronal development. The growth of human brain involves enormous proliferation of neurons, extension of axons and dendrites, and the process of myelination. All these processes involve a large amount of protein synthesis. During its peak growth period, synthesis of proteins and lipoproteins make up to 90 percent of the dry weight of the brain (Cowley and Griesel, 1966).

It has been estimated that protein substances increase more than 2,000 times during the process of maturation of a neuroblast into an anterior horn cell. If this figure is magnified for the entire brain the latter at the time of birth is gaining weight at a rate of 1 to 2 mg/minute. A generous supply of nutrition is, therefore, essential for the mother, who in turn must obtain it from her dietary source. Whereas a marginal supply of nutrients to the mother from her dietary source may be enough to sustain the fetus in its early stages of pregnancy, the needs of the rapidly growing infant during the last trimester are indeed considerable and may outstrip maternal supplies if no serious attempt is made by the mother to increase significantly her nutrient intake during this period. If the mother fails to provide the needed nutrients, the results are disastrous for the baby because it is likely to change the composition of the brain (Roeder and Chow, 1972). The deficiency of essential nutrients affects the intellect by directly modifying the growth and biochemical maturation of the brain. Dobbing (1968) and Manocha (1972) have suggested a direct damage to the structure of the brain in humans and monkeys during their period of fastest growth, which occurs at about the time of birth. Those newborn babies who succumb to malnutrition soon after birth show a marked reduction in their brain cellularity (Winick and Rosso, 1969). Some of the survivors in this group are left permanently with a smaller cellular endowment (Winick, 1970). Such anatomical damage manifests itself in irreversible functional impairment (Monckeberg, 1969). Both animal and human studies suggest that various regions of the brain have once in a life opportunity to grow properly and during this period (late Prenatal and less than two years of Postnatal life), even mild to moderate malnutrition may produce irreversible damage. It is quite probable that satisfactory brain development during this period is a prerequisite for satisfactory subsequent bodily growth (Winick, 1972; Dobbing, 1973, 1974; Dobbing and Sands, 1973). It may be remembered that by the time a child is three years old, 80 percent of his brain development has been completed compared to only 20 percent of his body development. Under these conditions, malnutrition that affects the growth of the baby is likely to affect the brain development as well (Livingston, 1971; Widdowson, 1972). Scott produced structural and functional lesions of the central nervous system of young rats by specific amino acid deficiencies in the diet (Scott, 1964). To prove a similar point, Flexner *et al.*, showed that inhibition of protein synthesis by puromycin causes loss of memory in mice (Flexner *et al.*, 1962).

Electroencephalographic (EEG) abnormalities are a good index of functional impairment, which most likely reflects anatomical damage (Stoch and Smythe, 1963). If the degree of malnutrition suffered in its intrauterine life, because of the mother's inability to provide the nutrients is severe enough, the EEG abnormalities may never become normal even if the child is apparently physically rehabilitated in his later life.

Hypoglycemia of the neonate whose growth has been retarded in its intrauterine life, may also be responsible for damage to the brain. The hypoglycemic infants show a deficiency of hepatic glycogen. This will adversely affect the brain of a newborn baby which has very little stored glycogen and is totally dependent on blood glucose for its energy requirements (Naeye, 1966). With respect to the direct involvement of the nervous system during the episode of severe malnutrition, one may reasonably conclude that malnourished babies do exhibit a profound ability for catch up growth including physical size, brain growth or head circumference, but there is a critical period during intrauterine and neonatal life during which malnutrition may cause irreversible damage to the brain and adversely affect learning ability.

It is indeed a very difficult proposition to assess the damage to the mental development or intellectual functioning of the infant caused by *in utero* malnutrition of the fetus due to inadequate supply of nutrients by the mother. At the time of birth, those infants who die can be useful subjects for investigating the anatomic damage to the nervous system. But the assessment of intellectual functioning of the survivors has to wait until the organism's cognitive and neurointegrative competence can be judged and compared to their healthy counterparts. This must, therefore, take into account the most important part of early postnatal life. Since the mother is mainly responsible for feeding the baby during this period, the mother's own nutritional state in relation to the mental development of the baby may be of extreme importance here. It must be stated, however, that during this period, the environmental influences also come into play. Unfortunately, infants who are malnourished in their fetal life belong to parents who belong to the lowest socio-economic groups and are steeped in poverty, illiteracy and technical backwardness. A child belonging to them is not only malnourished, and prone to catching common infections because of the unsanitary dwelling in which he lives, but also experiences retardation in language, personal, social and psychological behavior because of the cultural impoverishment of the parents (Barnes, 1972; Craviota and DeLicardie, 1968; Monckeberg, 1968, 1972; Scrimshaw, 1968; Cheek *et al.,* 1972; Vahlquist, 1972).

Malnutrition at an early age results in loss of learning time which interferes with learning during the critical periods of development. If a child spends most of his time thinking about food, he will have no mental inclination or ability to focus his attention on learning (Kallen, 1971). For example, such a child, when he looks at a busy road, does not have the energy to quickly observe and grasp what is going on. This changes the very course of growth of the child and results in abnormalities that manifest themselves in changes in personality and motivation. Such a person in his adult life develops such a low level of aspiration that he is simply unwilling to attempt difficult tasks (Kallen, 1973). This is because his inherent capabilities have been retarded by malnutrition in the early years of his life (Sulzer *et al.,* 1973). A certain degree of apathy appears in the child which could have the effect of diminishing the parents' responsiveness to him. As Craviito and DeLicardie put it,

Apathy can provoke apathy and so contribute to a cumulative pattern of reduced adult-child interaction. If this occurs it can have consequences for stimulation, for learning, for maturation, and for interpersonal relations, the end result being significant backwardness in performance on later more complex learning tasks.

There is, therefore, a genuine concern in the overpopulated countries for the children of low socio-economic groups because of an increasing association of bad nutrition, social, cultural and economic poverty with depressed levels of intellect and increased rates of school failure. Most of the retardation observed in the malnourished children is the result of the twin impact of bad nutrition and poor environment (Chandrasekhra, 1972). Not only are the adolescent girls and pregnant mothers woefully undernourished but they also have inherited a particular pattern of child care, social values and depressed motivation that heavily contributes to a lowered intellectual level and poor academic performance in their children. It is the infant who has suffered some degree of damage to the developing nervous system during the *in utero* existence that suffers most of the consequences of poor nutrition and poor environment in its postnatal life. If we take birth weight as an index of *in utero* retardation, the effects of maternal nutrition on the mental and intellectual development of the baby become evident at once. There are several reports of the inability of such apparently rehabilitated children to learn a language as well as their matched controls. In some cases the experimental children are more retarded in their perceptual and abstract ability than their memory and verbal ability.

It may be worthwhile to summarize the findings of a few pertinent investigations which indicate the effects of early malnutrition on intellectual performance. Cabak and Najdanvic studied the effects of undernutrition in early life on the physical and mental development of 36 Serbian children who were hospitalized for severe malnutrition between 4 and 24 months of age. After complete rehabilitation they were studied between 7 and 14 years of age. It was found that their mean I.Q. level was 88 as compared to an average of 93 in children of unskilled Serbian workers. Fifty percent of these children showed an I.Q. below 90 and six children in the group scored less than 70. This difference is quite significant because in the general population the children of the same age and socio-economic condition, 32 percent of them showed an I.Q. score over 110. Kagan believes that during the period of 12 to 18 months, some important cognitive changes occur in the child's mental development. It is likely that malnutrition at this critical age vitally affects the cognitive development of the child.

An Indonesian study of Liang *et al.* in a group of children who were malnourished between the ages of two and four years, also showed signs of vitamin A deficiency, revealing that after rehabilitation these children lagged significantly in their I.Q. levels; and the authors concluded that if the nutritional status of a child in the preschool years is known in detail, the intellectual development and physical development can be predicted with a high degree of accuracy. An Indian longitudinal study on kwashiorkor and mental development on a group of children malnourished between 18 and 36 months, along with their matched controls, revealed significant differences between groups not only in intelligence but also in the level of intersensory adequacy (Champakan *et al.*, 1968). The maximum difference was observed in children who were malnourished at a younger age.

To the list of these studies may be added a very detailed investigation in Mexico by a team of very prominent workers in this field (Cravioto *et al.*, 1969). The children in this study suffer from malnutrition before their 30th month. Along with their controls, a number of tests including the Wechsler intelligence scale, recognition of geometric forms, analysis of forms, and auditory-visual integrative ability were administered. It was concluded that "it is not only general environmental deprivation but also factors which are closely related to the event of early severe malnutrition that are contributing to a further depression of intellectual performance and learning" (Cravioto and DeLicardie, 1973). There is also a strong correlation between the height of the children and their I.Q. The detailed investigation of Klein *et al.* showed that the children who were tall for their age performed better on the I.Q. tests than those who were short for their age.

A low birth weight of around 1,500 gm would be quite a critical factor in putting the neonates to a permanent intellectual disadvantage. Warkany studied 22 such children for a prolonged period of time and found only five of them within the normal range of intelligence. Lubchenko studied a large number of ten year old children who were born with a birth weight of around 1,500 gm. Twenty-five children out of his sample showed abnormalities in their electroencephalograms, 35 children appeared to have normal intelligence but twenty out of these had problems in their progress at school. Drillien studied a sample of 112 babies whose birth weights were 1,360 gm or less. Those babies showed obvious signs of physical and mental handicaps. Of the 66 children in this group at school age, only six showed an I.Q. above 100 and the majority of them showed significantly retarded mental development and abnormal behavior. A long term British study conducted on 17,000 babies indicates that a birth weight two pounds below the normal translates itself into a six month lag in learning skill at school age (Butler, 1973). The differences are most apparent in neurointegrative competence and auditory-visual integration.

It may be reasonably concluded that children who suffer severe episodes of malnutrition in their early life suffer severe handicaps in their adult life, fail to learn the substance of human culture and do not acquire the skill necessary for competing in this aggressively competitive world. Cravioto and DeLicardie suggested that

> survival from severe malnutrition may constitute the event that starts a developmental path characterized by psychological defective functioning, school failure and subsequent subnormal adaptive functioning. . . . Such survivors are themselves more at risk of being the victims of their poor socio-economic environment, being less effective than otherwise would be the case in their social adaptations. In turn, they will choose mates of similar characteristics and may rear children under conditions and in a fashion fatally programmed to produce a new generation of malnourished individuals (1973).

Birch weighed the pros and cons of the effect of malnutrition on learning and intelligence and stated that the

> simplest hypothesis would be that malnutrition directly affects intellect by producing central nervous system damage. However, it may also con-

tribute to intellectual inadequacies as a consequence of the child's loss in learning time when ill, of the influences of hospitalization, and of prolonged reduced responsiveness after recovery.

In our present state of knowledge this is probably the most acceptable hypothesis on the effect of malnutrition on the intellectual performance of the human organism. In the same context, it may also be worthwhile to quote the beautiful summary presented by Ricciuti, which represents a very balanced conclusion derived out of many hundred scientific investigations over the last decade.

First, there is reasonably good evidence that protein-calorie malnutrition occurring in the first year of life, which is severe enough to markedly impair physical growth and to require hospitalization and treatment, may have adverse effects on the child's mental development, perhaps even to the extent of producing in some instances borderline or more severe mental retardation which does not appear to be readily remediable under conditions of nutritional rehabilitation. Severe malnutrition beginning in the second year of life or later, often taking the form of kwashiorkor, appears to produce adverse effects on mental development which are not as severe and seem to be more amenable to treatment. In both instances, however, it is not entirely clear whether the condition of postnatal malnutrition is the sole or even the principal determinant of impaired intellectual functioning, nor do we fully understand how its influences are mediated.

Secondly, when we consider the chronic, moderate-to-mild protein-calorie malnutrition which appears to be endemic in many economically disadvantaged populations, then the evidence as to effects on intellectual and learning functions attributable to malnutrition as such, independently of the concomitant influences of social and environmental factors, is very weak and unclear indeed, and we need considerable further research on this question before it can be satisfactorily answered. It's reasonable to assume, however, in the light of our present knowledge of child development, that the effects of moderate or mild malnutrition on intellectual development and school learning are probably minimal, in comparison with the influences attributable to other major environmental, experiential, and genetic determinants of mental development.

THE INTERRELATIONSHIP BETWEEN NUTRITION AND ENVIRONMENT

In human situations, it is always extremely difficult to

isolate the effects produced by bad nutrition from those for which the quality of the surrounding environment can be held responsible. It is rare to find malnourished children who are not also culturally and socially deprived. Invariably the malnourished children come from poor backgrounds, low socio-economic conditions and a deprived atmosphere. The nutritional deprivation goes side by side with emotional deprivation and helps to make a complex situation in which significant retardation is the end result (Cobos and Guevara, 1973). Malnutrition in combination with poor environment predisposes a child to a period of behavioral unresponsiveness. A strange sense of apathy and indifference towards the surroundings dominates the behavioral pattern of the child, with the result that he wastes a certain period of his life in which he would lose a great deal of learning. The child does not have the motivation to interact with the environment and the environment itself is so poor as to provide no stimulating experience. This produces in him marked degree of retardation in language, adaptive personal, social and psychological behavior. Malnutrition has a catalyzing or accelerating effect. The apathy provoked by a dull environment, which does not allow a healthy interaction of physical, biological and social factors, provokes more apathy and results in reduced adult-child interaction. If this trend continues the child shows significant developmental lags and the psychologists then pronounce the child mentally retarded and significantly backward in intellectual performance (Manocha, 1972).

A study of the factors conditioning malnutrition in widely separate geographical regions of the earth reveals that there is a particular setting (cultural, economic or social) under which malnutrition generally thrives. This setting generally involves illiteracy, low income, low cultural level, low intellectual performance, bad sanitary conditions and deep-rooted cultural or racial prejudices (Monckeberg, 1970). It is futile to fight malnutrition in these areas without a deep insight into this complex socio-economic religio-cultural setting. A malnourished child may respond posi-

tively to a better diet if his environment continues to be
"culturally and economically destitute or, in other words,
devoid of stimuli. The child will remain in intellectual
jeopardy. This reasoning can be applied to the individual
family as well as to the community" (White, 1971). Similar sentiments were expressed by Dr. Lowe before a U.S.
Senate committee on nutrition and human needs. "When
malnutrition is coupled with the constellation of adverse
environmental factors that are characteristic of life in poverty, it is clear that intellectual growth will be jeopardized."

In a practical sense, the dietary and environmental influences are so intertwined that it is difficult to assess or dis-
tinguish the effects of one from the other. We do not find
malnourished children in the well-to-do families, who not
only give good nutrition but also provide a stimulating environment for a fuller growth. That a stimulating environment greatly helps has been shown by a controlled study
of 30 babies in Lebanon aged 2.5 to 16 months. These babies
were hospitalized for marasmus for a period of four months.
During this period half the group was housed in a colorful
ward with pictures, music, toys, caretakers to play, sing,
handle the babies as well as the nursing care. The other
half of the group were housed in the conventional ward.
The clinical and nutritional care of both groups was exactly
similar. Yet the stimulated group with better envirionments
showed faster recovery and greater scores in the mental
development scale (Elias, 1971; Yatkin and McLaren, 1970).
Enrichment of environment definitely helps to accelerate
the mental development of the babies (Karras *et al.*, 1970).

A person who greatly influences the immediate environment of the child and who greatly determines the course of
emotional and behavioral development of the child is the
mother. The mother, with her tender touch, imparts a sense
of security and emotional stability from the earliest period
of infancy. Under normal circumstances, the child, from
this secure citadel, explores his environment with confidence
and is able to move about with a sense of dignity and be-
longingness. An illiterate mother who does not question

the centuries-old traditional methods of child care, fails to provide that security. An educated mother, receptive to new ideas of child raising, often exerts a positive socializing influence. Even in the absence of toys and books, the mother may encourage the child to play with kitchen utensils or other articles and provide a varied and interestingly stimulating experience. Such a mother, by constant attention and talking, can greatly help in language development and other facets of the child's personality.

In some of the developing countries, the socio-economic and cultural conditions for certain communities or groups are such that malnutrition is a life-long process and probably has been there for generations, with consequent physiological adaptations. In such communities, a combination of poor diets and poor environments produces conditions that are quite ideal for retarded development, physical as well as mental. A child subjected to dietary abuse and poor environment cannot realize his full genetic stature. The apathy introduced by poor environment affects the sensory responsiveness, which affects the chemical environment of the nervous system and the emotional state of the individual. We cannot minimize or underestimate the role played by environment on the physical and mental growth of the child. A number of studies have shown that, even when a child is getting adequate nutrition, his physical and mental growth may be retarded if his environments are poor.

As it is with nutrition, there is a critical period of life when emotional disturbance could prove more detrimental to a child's mental development. During this critical period the poor environment predisposes a child to emotional deprivation and affects his mental development. It has been observed that children admitted to orphanages (which often fail to provide security and stimulating environment) at the age of one year or less are more emotionally disturbed and show lower performance at a later age than those who are admitted at the age of three or four or older, in spite of the same dietary pattern in both groups (Rajalakshmi and Ramakrishnan, 1972).

It may be concluded that the chances of mental retardation because of bad nutrition in the critical period of growth are indeed great. However, the poor environment in certain sections of society also acts to modify the growth and development of the central nervous system because the general apathy resulting from lack of energy causes the individual to lose the motivation to learn from his daily experiences. The lasting behavioral deficits are generally a result of interaction of nutrition with impoverished environments. It is safe to presume that the poor socio-economic conditions set the stage of malnutrition, which determines the intersensory development and the physical stature of the individual. A combination of poor food and poor environment affects not only the all-round development of the child, but the future of the human species as well.

CONCLUDING THOUGHTS

From the above account of malnutrition in relation to the growth and development of the baby, it is evident that the undernutrition of the mammalian organism during early development can affect the body size and induce various kinds of abnormalities in metabolism and functional capabilities. These effects may persist long after an adequate supply of nutrients becomes available and may even be transferred on to the next generation. More and more scientific evidence is accumulating that there is a close association between protein-calorie malnutrition early in life (intrauterine and early postnatal) and subsequent retardation in intellectual development. Recently, Dobbing (1974) stressed the adverse effects of malnutrition during the first 18 months of life on the mental development of the baby, in the belief that a prenatally malnourished child has some chances of rehabilitation if he does not suffer any more nutritional insults in the postnatal period; but if the episode of malnutrition continues, the degree of mental impairment may be severe enough to cause learning impairment of a permanent nature. However, the contributing part played by poor environment should not be ignored, for it is rare to find malnourished children who are not also culturally and socially deprived. A combination of chronic undernutrition, widespread infection, and psycho-environmental deprivation result in a situation in which the undernourished and malnourished children not only fail to achieve their physical growth potential but suffer functionally as well.

Improved nutrition of the mother can increase the infant's birth weight and chances of survival, as well as improve its learning abilities (Chow, 1973). A well nourished and well grown woman will meet most of the requirements of the growing fetus from her tissue reserves. A poorly nourished woman, on the other hand, will have scanty tissue reserves. In the event of super-imposition of undernutrition during gestation, she may not be able to provide for the growing fetus. Poor levels of maternal nutrition before and during pregnancy lead to smaller birth weight, decreased chances of survival, and learning impairment. These deleterious traits may be passed on to the next generation as recent studies on rats have indicated. Learning deficiencies produced by protein deprivation of the mother are observed in her grandchildren even though the first generation offspring are reared on a normal rat diet (Zamenhof *et al.*, 1968). The intergenerational effects of mother's nutrition upon mental development need to be strongly emphasized. Poor health of the mother when she was a girl results in a woman who has a high level of reproductive risk. The child that she produces lags in neuro-integrative ability and has below normal I.Q. If this child happens to be a female, it is not hard to imagine the risks involved as she matures through childhood and adolescence on a poor diet and environment, and in turn becomes a mother. Birch, based on the evidence so far produced by scientific investigations, stated that "one can reasonably construct a chain of consequences starting from the malnutrition of the mother when she was a child, to her stunting, to her reduced efficiency as a reproducer, to intrauterine and perinatal risk to the child, and to his subsequent reduction in functional adaptive capacity." It is important, therefore, that we recognize the importance of nutrition of the female during her childhood, adolescence and pregnancy if we are to secure the health and wellbeing of the next generation.

While it is true that environment has its own role to play, there is a period of rapid growth in which the level of nutrition has the maximum effect. This period extends from mid-gestation to the first 6 to 9 months of postnatal life. Prior to birth, it is the mother's nutritional supply that determines growth. After birth, in most instances, it is the mother's lactating ability which determines it. In this critical period of rapid growth, the baby depends almost completely on the mother.

The learning potential of a child is most likely determined by the brain composition at birth and during the first few months of life when the child depends on the mother for growth, development, and cellular differentiation. Studies have indicated that a child born to a severely malnourished mother may catch up to a great extent in physical growth with adequate diet, but the impairment of the nervous system may be irreversible and leave the individual permanently damaged with respect to intellectual functioning. Some recent studies have, however, indicated that if a timely action is taken "some retarded developmental characteristics are remediable through treatment beginning in the preschool years" (Sulzer *et al.*, 1973). It is believed that malnutrition in the early postnatal period interferes with the otherwise explosive increase in dendritic complexity and the establishment of synoptic connections which are extremely important to the development of brain function (Dobbing, 1974).

While we are convinced of the deleterious effects of malnutrition which are further aggravated by unsanitary, overcrowded, unstimulating environment, we must not lose time in taking remedial measures. Besides making a concerted effort to increase the total food output, we have to pay adequate attention to the uncontrolled growth of population as well as the care of the vulnerable sections of our society, especially the female. The malnourished female children of today are the mothers of the next two decades. A drastic curtailment of population in the future and adequate attention to those who are already born is the only way out of the prevailing situation of generation-to-generation transfer of ignorance, poverty and malnutrition. This situation has grave consequences for the human species and needs to be tackled now without further delay. We need to implement our goals for a planned growth of population, which can be fed adequately (Chandrasekhra, 1972). The prevalent malnutrition is to a great extent due to a losing battle that is being fought every day between the available food and the ever-increasing number of mouths that lay claim to that food. Slater rightly remarked, "Because there are too many of us, a man does his neighbors more harm than good, just by staying alive. As numbers increase this will become a more self-evident factor in our lives."

While it is absolutely essential to narrow the gap between food supply and demand, it will, nevertheless, be most profitable to try to educate the mother and the housewife in the principles of simple nutrition. As the gatekeeper of the family's nutrition, she must be educated as to her own extra needs during pregnancy and lactation and the importance of food for her baby during the first few years of life. Studies have shown that there is a positive correlation between the nutrition level of the children and intelligence or education of the mother, as also a correlation between the nutritional states of children and their intelligence (Monckeberg, 1969). In other words, education of the mother is of paramount importance. It is also the mother who needs to be educated in the principles of family planning in order to space her children over her reproductive period. A combination of nutrition education and principles of family planning may go a long way in correcting the present state of affairs.

In developing countries deep-rooted cultural influences often prevent the mothers and children from using food that may otherwise be consumed to their benefit. A number of examples can be cited where protein rich foods are available but are withheld from the child because of certain cultural prejudices to those foods (Manocha, 1972). For example, in Malaya, fish is not given to children because it is believed to produce worms. In some other parts, young mothers are discouraged from eating eggs because they are believed to cause debility. Milk and fish must not be consumed with the same meal for fear of getting leprosy or leukoderma. Brain must be avoided because it is likely to cause premature graying and baldness. The eating of goat tongue by children and young women may make them talkative. Eating goat legs leads to the underdevelopment of the knee and ankle joints, and pig's stomach eaten by young women will darken their complexion. In Bangladesh, a pregnant or lactating mother is put on a dry diet and is not allowed to have fluids. In Indochina, nursing mothers are advised to take less food than required. In certain cultures, milk is rejected with revulsion because it is regarded as an animal mucous discharge. In India, infants are maintained on insufficient breast milk while supplementary foods are withheld up to one year of age in the belief that they cannot be digested. Such cultural taboos need to be cleared if maximum utilization of the available food is to be made (Manocha, 1972). Scientists can play an important role in not only discrediting these beliefs, but also in leading the way in society's need to develop priorities for the usage of available food. The educators and scientists of a nation need to get out of their ivory towers in the institutions and universities and join adult education programs designed to interpret scientific findings to the masses (Manocha, 1973). It is only the joint efforts of educators, social scientists, nutritionists and other health related personnel working in or through a health delivery system, that can make a dent in the solution of this grave human problem (Vitale, 1973).

REFERENCES

Obesity

Ahlskog, J. E., and Hoebel, B. C.: *Science, 182:* 166, 1973.
Anderson, J.: *Br Med J, 1:* 560, 1972.
Asher, P.: *Arch Dis Child, 41:* 672, 1966.
Atkins, R. C.: *Woman's Day,* p. 52, Sept., 1972a.
Atkins, R. C.: *Dr. Aktins Diet Revolution.* New York, McKay, 1972b.
Ball, M. F., Canary, J. J., and Kyle, L. H.: *Arch Intern Med, 125:* 162, 1970.

Ball, M. F., El-Khodary, A. Z., Aldridge, C., and Canary, J. J.: *Clin Res, 18:* 354, 1970.

Beck, J. C., Ganda, A., Hamick, M. A., Morgen, R. O., Rubinstein, D., and McGarry, E. E.: *Metabolism, 13:* 1108, 1964.

Berry, J. N.: *Ind J Med Res, 59:* 585, 1971.

Bloom, W. L.: *Metabolism, 8:* 214, 1959.

Bortz, W. M.: *Ann Intern Med, 71:* 833, 1969.

Br Med J: The overweight child, *2:* 64, April, 1970.

Brozek, J.: *Body Measurements and Human Nutrition.* Detroit, Wayne U Pr, 1956.

Bruch, H.: *The Importance of Overweight.* New York, Norton, 1957.

Bruch, H.: *Psychiatr Qu, 35:* 458, 1961.

Chicago Tribune, October 27, 1970.

Copinschi, G., Wegienka, L. C., Hane, S., and Forsham, P. H.: *Metabolism, 16:* 485, 1967.

Crenshaw, M. N.: *Family Circle,* January, 1974.

Czyzyk, A.: *Acta Diabetologica latina, 6:* 636, 1969.

Dwyer, J. T., and Mayer, J. J.: *J Am Diet Assoc, 56:* 510, 1970.

Editorial: *J Iowa Med Soc, 60:* 910, 1970.

El-Khodary, A. Z., Ball, M. F., Krop, J. M., and Canary, J. J.: *Proc 52nd Meeting Endocrinol Soc,* abst. *#157,* 1970.

Eid, E. E.: *Br Med J, 2:* 74, 1970.

Falkner, F.: In Falkner, F. (Ed.): *Human Development.* Philadelphia, Saunders, 1966.

Forbes, G. B., Gallup, J., and Hursk, J. B.: *Science, 133:* 101, 1967.

Glick, S. M.: In Ganary, W. F., and Marteni, L. (Eds.): *Frontiers in Neuroendocrinology.* New York, Oxford U Pr, 1969.

Goldblatt, P. B., Moore, M. E., and Stunkard, A. J.: *JAMA, 192:* 1039, 1965.

Gordon, E. S.: In Levine, R., and Luft, R. (Eds.): *Advances in Metabolic Disorder.* New York, Acad Pr, 1970.

Grey, N., and Kipnis, D. M.: *N Engl J Med, 285:* 827, 1971.

Gubner, R. S.: *S Afr Med J, 47:* 868, 1973.

Hirsch, J., Knittle, J. L., and Salans, L. B.: *J Clin Invest, 45:* 1023, 1966.

Hirsch, J., and Knittle, J. L.: *Fed Proc Symp, 29:* 1516, 1970.

Holland, J., Masling, J., and Copley, D.: *Psychosom Med, 32:* 351, 1970.

Hutton, J. H.: *Ill Med J, 140:* 137, 1971.

Ingelfinger, F. J., Relman, A., and Finland, M. (Eds.): *Controversy in Internal Medicine.* Philadelphia, Saunders, 1966.

JAMA Council on Drugs: *JAMA, 186:* 62, 1963.

JAMA, 211: 492, 1970.

Jokl, E.: *Nutrition, Exercise and Body Composition.* Springfield, Thomas, 1964.

Jones, H. E.: *Practitioner, 208:* 212, 1972.

Kalisch, B. J.: *Am J Nurs, 72:* 1124, 1972.

Kolkhoff, R. K., Kim, H. J., and Cerletty, J.: *Diabetes, 20:* 83, 1971.

Knittle, J. L.: *J. Pediatrics, 81:* 1048, 1972.

Landano, J. M., Gallagher, T. F., and Bray, G. A.: *Metabolism, 81:* 986, 1969.

Latham, M. C., McGandy, R. P., McCann, M. D., and Stare, F. J.: *Nutritionscope Manual.* Kalamazoo, Upjohn, 1970.

Maddox, G. L., and Liederman, V.: *J Med Educ, 44:* 214, 1969.

Mayer, J.: *Postgrad Med, 25:* 4, 1959.

Mayer, J.: *Am J Clin Nutr, 8:* 712, 1960.

Mayer, J.: *Postgrad Med, 38:* 3, 1965.

Mayer, J.: *Postgrad Med, 44:* 4, 1968.

Mayer, J.: *Postgrad Med, 46:* 253, 1969.

Mayer, J.: *Human Nutrition.* Springfield, Thomas, 1972.

Mayer, J.: *Medical World News,* April 27, 1973.

McWilliams, M.: *Nutrition for the Growing Years.* New York, Wiley, 1967.

Medical Letter, 13: 61, 1971.

Medical World News, April 27, 1973.

Merimee, T. J.: *N Engl J Med, 285:* 856, 1971.

Moore, M. E., Stunkard, A., and Srole, L.: *JAMA, 181:* 926, 1962.

Newsweek, October 19, 1970.

Mossberg, H. O.: *Acta Paediatr,* [Suppl] *35:* 2, 1948.

Nutr Review, 28: 184, 1970.

Redaksie, V. D.: *S Afr Med J, 43:* 1273, 1969.

Robertson, A. F., and Lowry, G. H.: *Mich Med, 63:* 629, 1964.

Robertson, E. C.: In Beaton and McHenry, E. W. (Eds.) : *Nutrition.* New York, Acad Pr, 1966, Vol. III.

Roginsky, M. S., and Sandler, J.: *Ann NY Acad Sci, 148:* 892, 1968.

Root, A. W.: *Human Pituitary Growth Hormone.* Springfield, Thomas, 1972.

Rosenstock, I. M.: *Am J Public Health, 59:* 1992, 1969.

Salans, L. B., Knittle, J. L., and Hirsch, J.: *J Clin Invest, 47:* 153, 1968.

Sassoon, H. F.: *Am J Clin Nutr, 26:* 776, 1973.

Schachter, S.: *Science, 161:* 751, 1968.

Schauf, G. E.: *J Am Geriatr Soc, 21:* 346, 1973.

Schteingart, D., and Conn, J.: *Ann NY Acad Sci, 131:* 388, 1965.

Shwarz, F., TerHarr, D. J., Van Riet, H. G., and Thijssen, J. H. H.: *Metabolism, 18:* 1013, 1969.

Seltzer, C. C., and Mayer, J.: *Postgrad Med, 38:* 2, 1965.

Smoking and Health. *Publ Hlth Serv Bull #1103,* Washington, D.C., 1964.

Stillman, I. M., and Baker, S. S.: *The Doctor's Quick Weight Loss Diet.* New York, Dell, 1968.

Stunkard, A. J., and Burt, V.: *Am J Psychiatry, 123:* 1443, 1967.

Stunkard, A. J., and Chirico, A. M.: *N Engl J Med, 263:* 935, 1960.

Stunkard, A., d'Aquili, E., Fox, S., and Filias, R. D. L.: *JAMA, 221:* 579, 1972.

Teitelbaum, P., and Epstein, A. N.: *Psychol Rev, 69:* 74, 1962.

Weng, L., Heseltine, M., and Bain, K.: *Hospital, 30:* 64, 1956; *30:* 74, 1956.
Widdowson, E. M.: *Proc Nutr Soc, 20:* 83, 1961.
Williams, S. R.: *Nutrition and Diet Therapy.* St. Louis, Mosby, 1969.
Wohl, M. G.: In Wohl and Goodhart (Eds.) : *Modern Nutrition in Health and Disease.* Philadelphia, Lea and Febiger, 1968.
Young, C. M.: *World Rev Nutr Diet,* 1973, Vol. *16.*

Malnutrition

Akyroyd, W. R., and Hussain, M. A.: *Br Med J, 1:* 42, 1967.
Baird, D.: *J Pediatr, 65:* 909, 1964.
Barnes, R. H.: Conference: *Early Nutritional and Environmental Influences upon Behavioral Development.* Seattle, Dec. 6–7, 1971.
Birch, H. G.: *Am J Public Health, 62:* 773, 1972.
Brock, J. F.: *S Afr Med J, 47:* 1109, 1972.
Butler, N.: *Medical World News,* Jan. 5, 1973.
Cabak, U., and Najdanvic, R.: *Arch Dis Child, 40:* 532, 1965.
Champakan, S., Srikantia, S. G., and Gopalan, C.: *Am J Clin Nutr, 21:* 844, 1968.
Chandrasekhra, S.: In *Infant Mortality, Population Growth and Family Planning In India.* London, George Allen & Unwin, Ltd., 1972.
Cheek, D. B., Holt, A. B., and Mellits, E. D.: PAHO Pub #251, 1972.
Chen, A. T. L. and Falek, A.: *Humangenetik, 21:* 13, 1974.
Chow, B. F.: *Nutr Rep Int, 7:* 247, 1973.
Cobos, F., and Guevara, L.: In Kallen, D. J. (Ed.) : *Nutrition, Development and Social Behavior.* Washington, DHEW Publication #242, 1973.
Cowley, J. J., and Griesel, R. D.: *Brain Behav, 14:* 506, 1966.
Cravioto, J., and DeLicardie, E. R.: In Scrimshaw, N. S., and Gordon, J. (Eds.) : *Malnutrition, Learning and Behavior.* Cambridge, MIT Press, 1968.
Cravioto, J., and DeLicardie, E. R.: In *Food, Nutrition and Health. World Rev Nutr Diet,* 1973, Vol. 16.
Cravioto, J., Pinero, C., Arroyo, M., and Alcalde, E.: *The Symposium Swedish Nutr Foundation.* Uppsala, Almiquist and Wiksells, 1969.
DeSilva, G. C., and Baptist, N. G.: In *Tropical Nutritional Disorders of Infants and Children.* Springfield, Thomas, 1969.
Dobbing, J.: In Scrimshaw, N., and Gordon, J. (Eds.) : *Malnutrition, Learning and Behavior.* Cambridge, MIT Press, 1968.
Dobbing, J.: *Nutr Rep Int, 1:* 401, 1973.
Dobbing, J.: *Pediatrics, 53:* 2, 1974.
Dobbing, J. and Sands: *J Arch Dis Child, 48:* 757, 1973.
Donoso, A.: *Proc Sixth Symp Nutrition and Health.* Am U Beirut, 1971.
Drillien, C. M.: *The Growth and Development of the Prematurely Born Infant.* Baltimore, Williams and Wilkins, 1964.
Elias, M. F.: Personal communication, 1971.

Flexner, L. B., Stellar, E., De La Haba, G., and Roberts, P. B.: *J Neurochem,* 5: 595, 1962.

Gopalan, C., and Srikantia, S. G.: *Food, Nutrition and Health. World Rev Nutr Diet,* 1973, Vol. 16.

Graenwald, P.: *Public Health Rep, 83:* 867, 1968.

Habicht, J., Yarborough, C., Lechtig, A., and Klein, R. E.: *Nutr Rep Int, 1:* 533, 1973.

Jelliffe, D. B.: *Food Tech, 25:* 55, 1971.

Jelliffe, D. B.: *UNICEF News, 71:* 6, 1972.

Jelliffe, D. B.: *Food, Nutrition and Health. World Rev Nutr Diet,* 1973, Vol. 16.

Kagan, J.: *Nutrition, Development and Social Behavior.* Washington, DHEW Publ. #242, 1973.

Kallen, D. J.: *JAMA, 215:* 94, 1971.

Kallen, D. J.: *Nutrition, Development and Social Behavior.* Washington, DHEW Publ. #242, 1973.

Karras, M. B., Teska, J. A., Hodges, A. S., and Badger, E. D.: *Child Dev, 41:* 925, 1970.

Klein, R. E., Hibicht, J., and Yarborough, C.: *Nutrition, Development and Social Behavior.* Washington, DHEW Publ. #242, 1973.

Liang, P. H., Hie, T. T., Jan, O. H., and Giok, L. T.: *Am J Clin Nutr, 20:* 1290, 1967.

Livingston, S. K.: *J Nutr Ed, 3:* 18, 1971.

Lowe, C.: Interim report, *U.S. Senate Committee on Nutrition and Human Needs.* August, 1969.

Lubchenko, L. O., Horner, F. A., and Reed, L. H.: *Am J Dis Child, 106:* 101, 1963.

Manocha, S. L.: *Malnutrition and Retarded Human Development.* Springfield, Thomas, 1972.

Manocha, S. L.: *Everyday Science, 18:* 1, 1973.

Manocha, S. L., and Olkowski, Z.: *Histochem J, 4:* 531, 1972.

Manocha, S. L., and Olkowski, Z.: *Histochem J, 5:* 105, 1973.

May, J. M., and Lemm, H. J.: *JAMA, 207:* 2401, 1969.

McLaren, D. S.: *Food, Nutrition and Health. World Rev Nutr Diet,* 1973, Vol. 16.

Miladi, S.: *Proc Sixth Symposium Nutrition and Health.* Am U Beirut, 1971.

Minkowski, A.: *Symposium on Nutrition and Fetal Development.* March of Dimes, Nov. 13–14, New York, 1972.

Monckeberg, F.: In Scrimshaw, N. S., and Gordon, J. (Eds.): *Malnutrition, Learning and Behavior.* Cambridge, MIT Press, 1968.

Monckeberg, F.: Paper presented at *Conference Nutrition and Human Development,* East Lansing, 1969.

Monckeberg, F.: In Gyorgy, P., and Kline, O. L. (Eds.): *Malnutrition is a Problem of Ecology.* Basel: S. Karger, 1970.

Monckeberg, F.: PAHO Pub #251, 1972.

Naeye, R. L.: *Am J Obstet Gynecol, 95:* 276, 1966.

Paarlberg, J. D.: *Food, Nutrition and Health. World Rev Nutr Diet,* 1973, Vol. 16.

Rajalakshmi, R., and Ramakrishnan, C. V.: *World Rev Nutr Diet,* 1972, Vol. 15.

Reisman, L. E.: *Pediatr Clin N Am, 17:* 101, 1970.

Ricciuti, H. N.: In Kallen, D. J. (Ed.) : *Nutrition, Development and Social Behavior.* Washington, DHEW Publ. #242, 1973.

Roeder, L. M., and Chow, B. F.: *Am J Clin Nutr, 25:* 812, 1972.

Scrimshaw, N. S.: In Scrimshaw, N. S., and Gordon, J. (Eds.) : *Malnutrition, Learning and Behavior.* Cambridge, MIT Press, 1968.

Scott, E. B.: *J Exp Mol Path, 3:* 610, 1964.

Slater, E.: In Cox, P. R., and Peel, J. (Eds.) : *Population and Pollution.* New York, Acad Pr, 1972.

Stoch, M. B., and Smythe, P. M.: *Arch Dis Child, 38:* 546, 1963.

Sulzer, J. L., Hansche, W. J., and Koenig, F.: *Nutrition, Development and Social Behavior.* Washington, DHEW Publ. #242, 1973.

Symposium, *Nutrition and Fetal Development.* March of Dimes, Nov. 13–14, New York, 1972.

Thomson, A. M.: *Br J Nutr, 13:* 509, 1959.

Vahlquist, B.: *Acta Ped A Scient Hung, 13:* 309, 1972.

Venkatachalam, P. S.: *Bull WHO, 26:* 193, 1962.

Vitale, J. J.: In Kallen, D. J. (Ed.) : *Nutrition, Development and Social Behavior.* Washington, DHEW Publ. #242, 1973.

Warkany, J., Cravioto, J., and Stephen, J. M. L.: *Adv Protein Chem, 15:* 131, 1960.

White, P. L.: *JAMA, 215:* 110, 1971.

Widdowson, E. M.: *Bibl Nutr Diet, 17:* 5, 1972.

Winick, M.: *Med Clin N Am, 54:* 1413, 1970.

Winick, M.: PAHO Pub #251, 1972.

Winick, M., and Rosso, P.: *Pediatr Res, 3:* 781, 1969.

Yatkin, U. S., and McLaren, D. C.: *J Mental Def Res, 14:* 25, 1970.

Zamenhof, S., Van Marthens, E., and Margolis, F. L.: *Science, 160:* 322, 1968.

APPENDICES

APPENDIX I

1973 World Population Data Sheet—Population Reference Bureau, Inc.
POPULATION INFORMATION FOR 163 COUNTRIES

Region or Country	Population Estimates Mid-1973 (millions) [2]	Birth Rate [3]	Death Rate [3]	Annual Rate of Population Growth (percent) [4]	Number of Years to Double Population [5]	Population Projections to 1985 (millions) [2]	Infant Mortality Rate [5]	Population under 15 Years (percent) [6]	Population over 64 Years (percent) [6]	Life Expectancy at Birth [7] M F	Per Capita Gross National Product (US $) [8]
WORLD	3,860 [9]	33	13	2.0	35	4,933 [9]	—	37	5	—	—
AFRICA	374	46	21	2.5	28	530	—	44	3	—	—
NORTHERN AFRICA	95	44	17	2.7	26	140	—	45	3	—	—
Algeria	15.5	50	17	3.3	21	23.9	86	47	1	—51—	300
Egypt	36.9	37	16	2.1	33	52.3	118	43	1	—53—	210
Libya	2.1	46	16	3.1	23	3.1	—	44	5	—52—	1,770
Morocco [10]	17.4	50	16	3.4	21	26.2	149	46	1	—51—	230
Sudan	17.4	49	18	3.1	23	26.0	121	47	—	—48—	120
Tunisia	5.6	38	16	2.2	32	8.3	120	46	1	—52—	250
WESTERN AFRICA	110	49	24	2.5	28	155	—	45	2	—	—
Cape Verde Islands [11]	0.3	39	14	2.5	28	0.3	121	42	1	—	160
Dahomey	2.9	51	26	2.6	27	4.1	149	46	1	—39—	90
Gambia	0.4	42	23	1.9	37	0.5	125	38	1	—41—	120
Ghana [10]	9.9	47	18	2.9	24	14.9	156	45	1	—46—	310
Guinea	4.2	47	25	2.3	30	5.7	216	44	7	—	120
Ivory Coast	4.6	46	23	2.4	29	6.4	159	43	1	—41—	310
Liberia	1.2	50	23	2.7	26	1.6	137	37	1	—37—	240
Mali	5.5	50	27	2.3	30	7.6	190	49	1	—	70
Mauritania	1.3	44	23	2.1	33	1.7	187	—	—	—37—	140
Niger	4.2	52	23	2.9	24	6.2	200	45	1	—41—	90
Nigeria	59.6	50	25	2.6	27	84.7	—	43	1	—37—	120

Region or Country	Population Estimates Mid-1973 (millions) [2]	Birth Rate [3]	Death Rate [3]	Annual Rate of Population Growth (percent) [4]	Number of Years to Double Population [5]	Population Projections to 1985 (millions) [2]	Infant Mortality Rate [5]	Population under 15 Years (percent) [6]	Population over 64 Years (percent) [6]	Life Expectancy at Birth [7] M	F	Per Capita Gross National Product (US $) [8]
Portuguese Guinea [11]	0.6	41	30	1.1	63	0.7	—	37	L	-34-	—	250
Senegal	4.2	46	22	2.4	29	5.8	—	42	L	-41-	—	230
Sierra Leone	2.8	45	22	2.3	30	3.9	136	37	5	-41-	—	190
Togo [10]	2.0	51	26	2.5	28	2.8	163	48	L	—		140
Upper Volta	5.7	49	29	2.0	35	7.7	182	42	L	—		60
EASTERN AFRICA	106	47	22	2.5	28	149	—	45	3	—		—
Burundi	3.9	48	25	2.3	30	5.3	150	47	L	—		60
Comoro Islands [11]	0.3	—	—	—	—	0.4	—	44	L	—		140
Ethiopia	26.8	46	25	2.1	33	35.7	—	44	L	-39-	—	80
Kenya [10]	12.0	48	18	3.0	23	17.9	—	46	L	-48-	—	150
Malagasy Republic	7.5	46	25	2.1	33	10.8	102	46	L	-38-	—	130
Malawi	4.8	49	25	2.5	28	6.8	120	44	L	-39-	—	80
Mauritius	0.9	25	8	1.7	41	1.2	65	42	L	59	62	240
Mozambique [11]	8.2	43	23	2.1	33	11.1	—	42	L	-41-	—	240
Reunion [11]	0.5	30	8	2.2	32	0.7	58	46	L	—		800
Rhodesia	5.6	48	14	3.4	21	8.6	122	48	L	-51-	—	280
Rwanda	3.9	52	23	2.9	24	5.7	133	—	—	-41-	—	60
Somalia	3.0	46	24	2.2	32	4.2	190	—	—	-39-	—	70
Tanzania	14.3	47	22	2.6	27	20.3	162	44	L	-41-	—	100
Uganda [10]	9.3	43	18	2.6	27	13.1	160	46	L	-48-	—	130
Zambia [10]	4.7	50	21	2.9	24	7.0	159	46	L	-44-	—	400
MIDDLE AFRICA	38	44	24	2.1	33	52	—	42	3	—		—
Angola [11]	6.1	50	30	2.1	33	8.1	192	42	L	-34-	—	300
Cameroon	6.2	43	23	2.0	35	8.4	137	39	L	-41-	—	180

Central African Republic	1.6	46	25	2.1	33	2.2	190	42	L	—	140
Chad	4.0	48	25	2.3	30	5.5	160	46	L	—	80
Congo (People's Rep. of)	1.0	44	23	2.1	33	1.4	180	42	L	—41—	300
Equatorial Guinea	0.3	35	22	1.4	50	0.4	—	35	L	—41—	210
Gabon	0.5	33	25	0.8	87	0.6	229	36	7	—	630
Zaire (Dem. Rep. Congo)	18.7	44	23	2.1	33	25.8	115	42	L	—	90
SOUTHERN AFRICA	25	41	18	2.4	29	34	—	40	4	—	—
Botswana	0.7	44	23	2.2	32	0.9	175	43	L	—41—	110
Lesotho	1.1	39	21	1.8	39	1.4	181	43	5	—44—	90
South Africa [10]	21.7	41	17	2.4	29	29.7	138	40	L	—49—	760
Namibia (Southwest Africa) [11]	0.7	44	25	2.0	35	0.9	—	40	5	—39—	}
Swaziland	0.5	52	24	2.8	25	0.7	168	47	L	—41—	180
ASIA	2,204	37	14	2.3	30	2,874	—	40	4	—	—
SOUTHWEST ASIA	84	44	16	2.8	25	121	—	43	4	—	550
Bahrain	0.2	50	19	3.1	23	0.3	—	44	L	—	950
Cyprus	0.6	23	8	0.9	77	0.7	26	33	7	—	—
Gaza [11]	0.5	44	8	3.6	19	0.8	—	50	L	—	—
Iraq	10.8	49	15	3.4	21	16.7	104	48	5	—52—	320
Israel	3.1	28	7	2.4	29	4.0	23	33	7	70 73	1,960
Jordan	2.6	48	16	3.3	21	3.9	115	47	L	—53—	250
Kuwait [12]	0.9	43	7	9.8	7	2.4	39	38	L	—64—	3,760
Lebanon	3.1	—	—	—	23	4.3	—	—	—	—	590
Oman	0.7	50	19	3.1	23	1.1	—	—	L	—	350
Qatar	0.1	50	19	3.1	23	0.1	—	—	L	—	1,730
Saudi Arabia	8.4	50	23	2.8	25	12.2	—	47	L	—42—	440
Syria	6.8	48	15	3.3	21	10.5	—	42	L	—53—	290
Turkey	38.6	40	15	2.5	28	52.8	119	42	L	—54—	310
United Arab Emirates	0.1	50	19	3.1	23	0.2	—	32	L	—	2,390
Yemen Arab Republic	6.2	50	23	2.8	25	9.1	—	—	—	—42—	80
Yemen, People's Republic of	1.4	50	21	2.9	24	2.0	—	—	—	—42—	120
MIDDLE SOUTH ASIA	828	44	17	2.6	27	1,137	—	43	3	—	—
Afghanistan	18.3	51	27	2.4	29	25.0	—	45	L	—38—	80

Region or Country	Population Estimates Mid-1973 (millions) [2]	Birth Rate [3]	Death Rate [3]	Annual Rate of Population Growth (percent) [4]	Number of Years to Double Population [5]	Population Projections to 1985 (millions) [2]	Infant Mortality Rate [3]	Population under 15 Years (percent) [6]	Population over 64 Years (percent) [6]	Life Expectancy at Birth [7] M F	Per Capita Gross National Product (US $) [8]
Bangladesh [13]	83.4	—	—	—	—	123.3	—	—	—	—	—
Bhutan	0.9	—	—	2.2	32	1.2	139	42	L	—	70
India [10]	600.4	42	17	2.5	28	807.6	—	46	L	—	110
Iran	31.1	45	17	2.8	25	45.0	—	44	L	—50—	380
Maldive Islands	0.1	46	23	2.3	31	0.1	—	40	L	—	100
Nepal	12.0	45	23	2.2	32	15.8	142	45	L	—41—	80
Pakistan [13]	68.3	51	18	3.3	21	100.9	—	40	L	—	100
Sikkim	0.2	48	29	1.9	37	0.3	—	41	L	—	80
Sri Lanka (Ceylon)	13.5	30	8	2.2	32	17.7	48	—	L	—62—	110
SOUTHEAST ASIA	313	43	15	2.8	25	434	—	44	3	—	—
Burma	29.8	40	17	2.3	30	39.2	—	40	L	—48—	80
Indonesia	132.5	47	19	2.9	24	183.8	125	44	L	—48—	
Irian, West [11]	1.0	—	—	—	—	1.3	—	—	—	—	80
Khmer Republic (Cambodia)	7.8	45	16	3.0	23	11.3	127	44	L	—	130
Laos	3.2	42	17	2.5	28	4.4	—	—	—	—	120
Malaysia [10,17]	11.8	38	11	2.7	26	16.4	—	44	L	64 67	380
Philippines [10]	42.2	45	12	3.3	21	64.0	67	47	L	—	210
Portuguese Timor [11]	0.6	43	25	1.8	39	0.8	—	—	—	—38—	110
Singapore	2.3	23	5	2.2	32	3.0	21	39	L	—68—	920
Thailand [10]	39.9	43	10	3.3	21	57.7	—	43	L	—	200
Vietnam (Dem. Republic of)	22.5	—	—	—	—	28.2	—	—	—	—50—	100
Vietnam (Republic of)	19.1	—	—	—	—	23.9	—	—	—	—50—	200
EAST ASIA	978	29	12	1.7	41	1,182	—	35	4	—	—

China (People's Republic of)	799.3	30	13	1.7	41	964.6	—	—	—	—50—	160
Hong Kong [10,11]	4.5	20	5	2.4	29	6.0	19	38	L	67 73	970
Japan	107.3	19	7	1.2	58	121.3	13	24	7	69 74	1,920
Ryukyu Islands [11,14]	1.0	22	5	1.7	41	1.3	—	34	6	69 76	1,050
Korea (Dem. People's Rep. of)	15.1	39	11	2.8	25	20.7	—	40	—	—58—	330
Korea (Republic of)	34.5	31	11	2.0	35	45.9	—	40	L	60 64	250
Macau [11]	0.3	—	—	—	—	0.4	—	39	5	—	150
Mongolia	1.4	42	11	3.1	23	2.0	—	31	6	—58—	460
Taiwan (Rep. of China)	15.0	27	5	2.2	32	19.4	18	43	L	66 70	390
NORTH AMERICA	233	16	9	0.8	87	263	—	27	9	—	—
Canada	22.5	15.7	7.3	1.2	58	27.3	17.6	30	8	69 75	3,700
United States [15]	210.3	15.6	9.4	0.8	87	235.7	18.5	27	10	67 75	4,760
LATIN AMERICA	308	38	10	2.8	25	435	—	42	4	—	—
MIDDLE AMERICA [16]	75	43	11	3.2	22	112	—	46	3	—	—
Costa Rica	2.0	34	7	2.7	26	3.2	67	48	L	64 67	560
El Salvador	3.8	42	10	3.2	22	5.9	53	45	L	53 57	300
Guatemala	5.6	43	17	2.6	27	7.9	88	46	L	50 52	360
Honduras	3.0	49	17	3.2	22	4.6	—	47	L	47 51	280
Mexico [10]	56.2	43	10	3.3	21	84.4	69	46	L	61 64	670
Nicaragua	2.2	46	17	2.9	24	3.3	—	48	L	49 51	430
Panama	1.6	37	9	2.8	25	2.5	41	44	L	62 65	730
CARIBBEAN [16]	27	33	11	2.2	32	36	—	40	4	—	—
Bahamas [12]	0.2	28	6	4.6	16	0.2	37	43	L	—	2,300
Barbados	0.3	22	9	0.8	87	0.3	42	36	7	69 72	570
Cuba	8.9	27	8	1.9	37	11.0	36	31	6	65 69	530
Dominican Republic [10]	4.8	49	15	3.4	21	7.3	64	47	L	51 54	350
Guadeloupe [11]	0.4	30	8	2.2	32	0.5	45	43	5	67 70	760
Haiti	5.6	44	20	2.4	29	7.9	—	43	L	43 46	110
Jamaica [10]	2.1	35	7	1.5	47	2.6	39	46	5	67 70	670
Martinique [11]	0.4	27	8	1.6	44	0.5	35	43	L	67 70	910
Netherlands Antilles [11]	0.2	23	6	1.7	41	0.3	—	41	L	69 74	1,380
Puerto Rico [11]	2.9	25	7	1.4	50	3.4	25	37	7	70 73	1,650
Trinidad & Tobago [11]	1.1	24	7	1.1	63	1.3	40	41	L	65 69	860

Region or Country	Population Estimates Mid-1973 (millions) [2]	Birth Rate [3]	Death Rate [3]	Annual Rate of Population Growth (percent) [4]	Number of Years to Double Population [5]	Population Projections to 1985 (millions) [2]	Infant Mortality Rate [5]	Population under 15 Years (percent) [6]	Population over 64 Years (percent) [6]	Life Expectancy at Birth [7] M	Life Expectancy at Birth [7] F	Per Capita Gross National Product (US $) [8]
TROPICAL SOUTH AMERICA	165	40	10	3.0	23	236	—	43	3	—	—	—
Bolivia	5.0	44	19	2.4	29	6.8	—	42	L	44	46	180
Brazil	101.3	38	10	2.8	25	142.6	—	43	L	58	63	420
Colombia	23.7	45	11	3.4	21	35.6	76	47	L	57	60	340
Ecuador	6.7	45	11	3.4	21	10.1	91	48	L	56	59	290
Guyana	0.8	36	8	2.8	25	1.1	40	45	L	63	66	370
Peru	14.9	42	11	3.1	23	21.6	—	45	L	57	60	450
Surinam [11]	0.4	41	7	3.2	22	0.6	30	46	L	63	66	530
Venezuela	11.9	41	8	3.4	21	17.4	49	47	L	62	65	980
TEMPERATE SOUTH AMERICA	41	25	9	1.7	41	51	—	32	7	—	—	—
Argentina [10]	25.3	22	9	1.5	47	29.6	58	30	7	64	71	1,160
Chile [10]	10.4	26	9	1.7	41	13.6	88	39	5	58	64	720
Paraguay	2.7	45	11	3.4	21	4.1	—	46	L	57	61	260
Uruguay	3.0	23	9	1.4	50	3.4	43	28	8	66	72	820
EUROPE	472	16	10	0.7	99	515	—	25	12	—	—	—
NORTHERN EUROPE	82	15	11	0.4	175	90	—	24	13	—	—	—
Denmark	5.1	15.8	10.2	0.5	139	5.5	14.2	24	12	71	76	3,190
Finland	4.8	12.7	9.6	0.3	231	5.0	11.3	26	8	65	73	2,390
Iceland	0.2	19.7	7.3	1.2	58	0.3	13.2	33	9	71	76	2,170
Ireland	3.0	22.4	11.2	0.5	139	3.5	19.6	31	11	68	72	1,360
Norway	4.0	16.6	10.0	0.7	99	4.5	12.7	25	13	71	77	2,860
Sweden	8.2	13.8	10.4	0.3	231	8.8	11.1	21	13	72	77	4,040
United Kingdom	57.0	14.9	11.9	0.3	231	61.8	18.0	24	13	68	74	2,270

WESTERN EUROPE	151	14	11	0.4	175	163	—	24	13	—	—	—
Austria	7.5	13.8	12.6	0.1	700	8.0	25.1	24	14	67	74	2,010
Belgium	9.8	13.8	12.0	0.2	347	10.4	19.8	24	13	68	74	2,720
France	52.3	16.9	10.6	0.6	117	57.6	13.3	25	13	69	76	3,100
Germany (Federal Republic of)	59.4	11.5	11.7	0.0	—	62.3	23.2	25	13	68	74	2,930
Berlin, West [11]	2.1	9.1	19.0	-1.0	—	1.9	28.0	15	21	66	72	—
Luxembourg	0.4	11.8	11.9	0.0	—	0.4	13.6	22	12	—	—	2,890
Netherlands	13.4	16.1	8.5	0.8	87	15.3	11.4	27	10	71	77	2,430
Switzerland	6.5	14.4	8.7	1.0	70	7.4	14.4	23	11	69	74	3,320
EASTERN EUROPE	107	17	10	0.7	99	116	—	24	11	—	—	—
Bulgaria	8.7	15.3	9.8	0.6	117	9.4	25.8	23	9	69	73	760
Czechoslovakia	15.0	16.5	11.5	0.5	139	16.2	21.6	24	11	67	74	2,230
Germany (Dem. Republic of)	16.3	11.7	13.7	-0.2	—	16.9	17.7	24	15	69	74	2,490
Berlin, East [11]	1.1	13.4	16.2	-0.3	—	1.0	19.6	22	16	—	—	—
Hungary	10.4	14.7	11.4	0.3	231	11.0	32.7	21	11	62	72	1,600
Poland	34.0	17.4	8.0	0.9	77	38.2	28.5	28	8	67	73	1,400
Romania	21.0	19.6	9.5	1.0	70	23.3	42.4	26	8	66	70	930
SOUTHERN EUROPE	132	18	9	0.9	77	146	—	26	10	—	—	—
Albania	2.3	35.3	7.5	2.8	25	3.3	86.8	—	—	65	67	600
Greece	9.1	15.9	8.3	0.8	87	9.7	27.0	25	10	67	71	1,090
Italy	54.9	16.8	9.6	0.7	99	60.0	28.3	24	10	68	73	1,760
Malta [12]	0.3	16.8	9.1	-0.1	—	0.3	23.9	28	9	68	73	810
Portugal	9.8	21.3	11.1	1.0	70	10.7	49.8	29	9	65	71	660
Spain	34.2	19.4	8.2	1.1	63	38.1	27.9	28	9	67	72	1,020
Yugoslavia	21.2	18.2	9.1	0.9	77	23.8	48.8	28	7	64	69	650
USSR	250	17.8	8.2	1.0	70	286.9	22.6	28	8	65	74	1,790
OCEANIA [16]	21	25	10	2.0	35	27	—	32	7	—	—	—
Australia	13.3	20.5	8.5	1.9	37	17.0	17.3	29	8	68	74	2,820
Fiji	0.6	30	5	1.8	39	0.8	—	45	L	—68—		430
New Zealand	3.0	22.1	8.5	1.7	41	3.8	16.5	32	8	68	74	2,700
Papua-New Guinea [11]	2.6	42	18	2.4	29	3.6	—	43	L	—47—		300

World and Regional Population (Millions)

	WORLD	ASIA	EUROPE	USSR	AFRICA	NORTH AMERICA	LATIN AMERICA	OCEANIA
Mid-1973	3860	2204	472	250	374	233	308	21
UN Medium Estimate, 2000	6494	3777	568	330	818	333	652	35

GENERAL NOTES

Birth rate: Annual number of births per 1,000 population.

Death rate: Annual number of deaths per 1,000 population.

Population growth rate: Annual rate of natural increase combined with the plus or minus factor of net immigration or net emigration. (*Natural increase* is the birth rate minus the death rate in a given year.)

Infant mortality rate: Annual deaths to infants under one year of age per 1,000 live births.

World Population Data Sheets of various years should not be used as a time series. Because every attempt is made to use the most accurate information, data sources vary and apparently radical changes in rates from year to year may reflect improved source material, revised data, or a later base year for computation, rather than yearly rate changes.

Population figures are rounded to the nearest 100,000; thus increases amounting to less than that number do not appear on the *Data Sheet*.

Demographic data for most developing countries are often incomplete or inaccurate. In many cases, therefore, UN estimates are used.

For world urbanization data, see the *1972 World Population Data Sheet*.

FOOTNOTES

[1] The *Data Sheet* lists all UN members and all geopolitical entities with a population larger than 200,000.

[2] UN, *Total Population Estimates for World, Regions and Countries, Each Year, 1950–1985*, Population Division Working Paper No. 34 (October 1970).

[3] Latest available year. Except for North America, estimates are essentially those available as of April 1973 in UN, *Population and Vital Statistics Report*, Series A, vol. 25, no. 2 (1973). Because of deficient registration in some countries adjustments have been made where deemed necessary.

[4] Latest UN estimates, except for substantiated changes in birth rates, death rates, or migration streams.

[5] Assuming no change in growth rate.

[6] Latest available year. Derived from UN, *World Population Prospects, 1965–1985, As Assessed in 1968*, Population Division Working Paper No. 30 (December 1969); and UN, *Demographic Yearbook, 1970 and 1971.*

[7] Latest available year, in no case before 1960. Derived from UN, *Statistical Yearbook, 1972* (1973); and Centro Latinamericano de Demografía, *Boletín Demográfico*, vol. 4, no. 8 (Santiago, Chile, July 1971).

[8] International Bank for Reconstruction and Development, 1970 data. In some cases, figures are substantially different from those on the 1972 *Data Sheet* because of a different basis used for computing GNP.

[9] Total reflects UN adjustments for discrepancies in international migration data.

[10] UN estimates for this country differ from recent census figures by more than 3 percent but are used because of uncertainty about the completeness or accuracy of census data.

[11] Nonsovereign country.

[12] Kuwait has a rate of natural increase (births minus deaths) of 3.6 percent; Malta's is 0.8 percent, and the Bahamas' 2.2 percent. Their growth rates differ markedly from their rates of natural increase because of migration.

[13] Except for population, estimates for Pakistan include data for Bangladesh.

[14] Reverted to Japan May 15, 1972.

[15] U.S. figures are based on Series E population projections in Bureau of the Census, "Projections of the Population of the United States, by Age and Sex: 1972 to 2020," *Current Population Reports*, Series P-25, no. 493 (December 1972); and National Center for Health Statistics, *Monthly Vital Statistics Report*, vol. 21, no. 13 (June 27, 1973).

[16] Regional population totals take into account small areas not listed on the *Data Sheet*.

[17] Life expectancy for West Malaysia only. East Malaysia estimated to be 55.

Dashes indicate data are unavailable or unreliable.

L = Estimated to be less than 5 percent.

APPENDIX II

Nutritive value of the commonly eaten foods of animal and plant origin. These values have been based on 100 grams of the edible portion in its simplest form (i.e. without added salt, sugar, fats, fillers, mineral or vitamin enrichment).*

FOOD	Cals.	Water	Ash	Fat	Carb.	Prot.	Ca. (mg)	P (mg)	Fe (mg)	Na (mg)	K (mg)	Thiamine (mg)	Riboflavin (mg)	Nicotinic acid (mg)	Ascorbic acid (mg)	Vit. A I.U.
Animal Origin																
BACON, uncooked	665	19.3	2.0	69.3	1.0	8.4	13	108	1.2	680	130	0.36	0.11	1.8	......	0
BACON, broiled or fried, drained	611	8.1	6.3	52.0	3.2	30.4	14	224	3.3	1021	236	0.51	0.34	5.2	......	0
BEEF, chuck, 82% lean, 18% fat, raw	257	60.8	0.9	19.6	0	18.7	11	188	2.8	65	355	0.08	0.17	4.5	......	40
BEEF, chuck, 81% lean, 19% fat, braised or pot roasted	327	49.4	0.7	23.9	0	26.0	11	140	3.3	60	370	0.05	0.20	4.0	......	40
BEEF, sirloin, 73% lean, 27% fat, raw	313	55.7	0.8	26.7	0	16.9	10	155	2.5	65	355	0.07	0.15	4.1	......	50
BEEF, sirloin, 66% lean, 34% fat, broiled	387	43.9	1.1	32.0	0	23.0	10	191	2.9	60	370	0.06	0.18	4.7	......	50
BEEF, hamburger, lean, raw	179	68.3	1.0	10.0	0	20.7	12	192	3.1	......	......	0.09	0.18	5.0	......	20
BEEF, hamburger, lean, cooked	219	60.0	1.3	11.3	0	27.4	12	230	3.5	48	558	0.09	0.23	6.0	......	20
BRAINS, beef, cattle, hogs, sheep, raw	125	78.9	1.4	8.6	0.8	10.4	10	312	2.4	125	219	0.23	0.26	4.4	18	0

FOOD	Cals.	Water	Ash	Fat	Carb.	Prot.	Ca. (mg)	P (mg)	Fe (mg)	Na (mg)	K (mg)	Thia-mine (mg)	Ribo-flavin (mg)	Nico-tinic acid (mg)	Ascor-bic acid (mg)	Vit. A I.U.
BUTTERMILK, cultured from skim milk	36	90.5	0.7	0.1	5.1	3.6	121	95	trace	130	140	0.04	0.18	0.1	1	trace
CHEESE, American Pasteurized processed	370	40.0	4.9	30.0	1.9	23.2	697	771	0.9	1136	80	0.02	0.41	trace	0	1220
CHEESE, cottage creamed, natl.	106	78.3	1.0	4.2	2.9	13.6	94	152	0.3	229	85	0.03	0.25	0.1	0	170
CHEESE, Swiss, domestic, natl.	370	39.0	3.8	28.0	1.7	27.5	925	563	0.9	710	104	0.01	0.40	0.1	0	1140
CHICKEN, light meat, all classes, raw	117	73.7	1.0	1.9	0	23.4	11	218	1.1	50	320	0.05	0.09	10.7	.....	60
CHICKEN, light meat, all classes, roasted	166	63.8	1.2	3.4	0	31.6	11	265	1.3	64	411	0.04	0.10	11.6	.....	60
CHICKEN, dark meat, all classes, raw	130	73.7	1.0	4.7	0	20.6	13	188	1.5	67	250	0.08	0.20	5.2	.....	150
CHICKEN, dark meat, all classes, roasted	176	64.4	1.2	6.3	0	28.0	13	229	1.7	86	321	0.07	0.23	5.6	.....	150
EGGS, chicken, whole, fresh & frozen, raw	163	73.7	1.0	11.5	0.9	12.9	54	205	2.3	122	129	0.11	0.30	0.1	0	1180
EGGS, chicken, whole, hard cooked	163	73.7	1.0	11.5	0.9	12.9	54	205	2.3	122	129	0.09	0.28	0.1	0	1180
EGGS, chicken, whites, fresh & frozen, raw	51	87.6	0.7	trace	0.8	10.9	9	15	0.1	146	136	trace	0.27	0.1	0	0

EGGS, chicken, yolks, fresh, raw	348	51.1	1.7	30.6	0.6	16.0	141	569	5.5	52	98	0.22	0.44	0.1	0	3400
FISH FLOUR, from whole fish	336	2.0	19.7	0.3	0	78.0	4610	3100	41.0	170	430	0.07	0.62	2.2	.....	.....
FRANKFURTERS, all meat, raw	296	56.5	2.4	25.5	2.5	13.1	.....	.....	.....	.....	.....	.....	.....	.....	.....	.....
HEART, beef, lean, raw	108	77.5	1.1	3.6	0.7	17.1	5	195	4.0	86	196	0.53	0.88	7.5	2	20
HEART, beef, lean, braised	188	61.3	1.1	5.7	0.7	31.3	6	181	5.9	104	232	0.25	1.22	7.6	1	30
HEART, turkey, all classes, raw	171	71.3	1.1	11.2	0.2	16.2	.....	.....	.....	69	240	0.23	0.86	5.0	4	30
HEART, turkey, all classes, simmered	216	63.2	0.8	13.2	0.2	22.6	.....	.....	.....	61	211	0.25	0.98	5.7	4	30
LAMB, leg, 83% lean, 17% fat, raw	222	64.8	1.3	16.2	0	17.8	10	162	1.4	75	295	0.16	0.22	5.1	.....	.....
LAMB, leg, 83% lean, 17% fat, roasted	279	54.0	1.7	18.9	0	25.3	11	208	1.7	70	290	0.15	0.27	5.5	.....	.....
LIVER, beef, raw	140	69.7	1.3	3.8	5.3	19.9	8	352	6.5	136	281	0.25	3.26	13.6	31	43,900
LIVER, beef, fried	229	56.0	1.7	10.6	5.3	26.4	11	476	8.8	184	380	0.26	4.19	16.5	27	53,400
LIVER, lamb, raw	136	70.8	1.4	3.9	2.9	21.0	10	349	10.9	52	202	0.40	3.28	16.9	33	50,500
LIVER, lamb, broiled	261	50.4	2.1	12.4	2.8	32.3	16	572	17.9	85	331	0.49	5.11	24.9	36	74,500
MILK, whole, Pasteurized, raw	66	87.2	0.7	3.7	4.9	3.5	117	92	trace	50	140	0.03	0.17	0.1	1	150
MILK, dried	502	2.0	5.9	27.5	38.2	26.4	909	708	0.5	405	1330	0.29	1.46	0.7	6	1130
MILK, skim, Pasteurized, raw	36	90.5	0.7	0.1	5.1	3.6	121	95	trace	52	145	0.04	0.18	0.1	1	trace

FOOD	Cals.	Water	Ash	Fat	Carb.	Prot.	Ca. (mg)	P (mg)	Fe (mg)	Na (mg)	K (mg)	Thiamine (mg)	Riboflavin (mg)	Nicotinic acid (mg)	Ascorbic acid (mg)	Vit. A I.U.
MILK, nonfat solids, instant, dried	359	4.0	7.9	0.7	51.6	35.8	1293	1005	0.6	526	1725	0.35	1.78	0.9	7	30
MILK, evaporated, canned	137	73.8	1.6	7.9	9.7	7.0	252	205	0.1	118	303	0.04	0.34	0.2	1	320
PORK, ham, 74% lean, 26% fat, raw	308	56.5	0.7	26.6	0	15.9	9	178	2.4	70	285	0.77	0.19	4.1	……	0
PORK, ham, 74% lean, 26% fat, roasted	374	46.5	0.9	30.6	0	23.0	10	236	3.0	65	390	0.51	0.23	4.6	……	0
SAUSAGE, pork, raw	498	38.1	1.7	50.8	trace	9.4	5	92	1.4	740	140	0.43	0.17	2.3	……	0
SAUSAGE, pork, cooked	476	34.8	2.9	44.2	trace	18.1	7	162	2.4	958	269	0.79	0.34	3.7	……	……
SHRIMP, raw	91	78.2	1.4	0.8	1.5	18.1	63	166	1.6	140	220	0.02	0.03	3.2	……	……
SHRIMP, canned, solids & liquid	80	78.2	4.0	0.8	0.8	16.2	59	152	1.8	……	……	0.01	0.03	1.5	……	……
TUNA, canned in water, solids & liquid	127	70.0	1.2	0.8	0	28.0	16	190	1.6	41	279	……	0.10	13.3	……	……
TUNA, canned in oil, drained	197	60.6	2.0	8.2	0	28.8	8	234	1.9	……	……	0.05	0.12	11.9	……	80
Turkey, light meat all classes, raw	116	73.0	1.2	1.2	0	24.6	……	……	1.0	51	320	0.06	0.11	11.3	……	……
TURKEY, light meat, all classes, roasted	176	62.1	1.2	3.9	0	32.9	……	……	1.2	82	411	0.05	0.14	11.1	……	……

TURKEY, dark meat, all classes, raw	128	73.6	1.1	4.3	0	20.9	.....	.....	2.0	81	310	0.09	0.18	4.7	.....	.....
TURKEY, dark meat, all classes, roasted	203	60.5	1.2	8.3	0	30.0	.....	.....	2.3	99	398	0.04	0.23	4.2	.....	.....
VEAL, chuck, 86% lean, 14% fat, raw	173	70.0	1.0	10.0	0	19.4	11	199	2.9	90	320	0.14	0.26	6.5	.....	.....
VEAL, chuck, 85% lean, 15% fat, braised	235	58.5	0.8	12.8	0	27.9	12	151	3.5	80	500	0.09	0.29	6.4	.....	.....
YOGHURT, from whole milk	62	88.0	0.7	3.4	4.9	3.0	111	87	trace	47	132	0.03	0.16	0.1	1	140
YOGHURT, from partially skimmed milk	50	89.0	0.7	1.7	5.2	3.4	120	94	trace	51	143	0.04	0.18	0.1	1	70

Plant Origin

ALMONDS, dried	598	4.7	3.0	54.2	19.5	18.6	234	504	4.7	4	773	0.24	0.92	3.5	trace	0
APPLES, fresh picked, not pared, raw	56	84.8	0.3	0.6	14.1	0.2	7	10	0.3	1	110	0.03	0.02	0.1	7	90
APPLE JUICE, canned or bottled	47	87.8	0.2	trace	11.9	0.1	6	9	0.6	1	101	0.01	0.02	0.1	1	.....
APPLESAUCE, canned, unsweetened	41	88.5	0.3	0.2	10.8	0.2	4	5	0.5	2	78	0.02	0.01	trace	1	40
APRICOTS, raw	51	85.3	0.7	0.2	12.8	1.0	17	23	0.5	1	281	0.03	0.04	0.6	10	2700
APRICOTS, dried, uncooked	260	25.0	3.0	0.5	66.5	5.0	67	108	5.5	26	979	0.01	0.16	3.3	12	10,900
ASPARAGUS SPEARS, raw	26	91.7	0.6	0.2	5.0	2.5	22	62	1.0	2	278	0.18	0.20	1.5	33	900

FOOD	Cals.	Water	Ash	Fat	Carb.	Prot.	Ca. (mg)	P (mg)	Fe (mg)	Na (mg)	K (mg)	Thiamine (mg)	Riboflavin (mg)	Nicotinic acid (mg)	Ascorbic acid (mg)	Vit. A I.U.
ASPARAGUS SPEARS, boiled, drained	20	93.6	0.4	0.2	3.6	2.2	21	50	0.6	1	183	0.16	0.18	1.4	26	900
AVOCADOS, Calif., raw	171	73.6	1.2	17.0	6.0	2.2	10	42	0.6	4	604	0.11	0.20	1.6	14	290
AVOCADOS, Fla., raw	128	78.0	0.9	11.0	8.8	1.3	10	42	0.6	4	604	0.11	0.20	1.6	14	290
BAMBOO SHOOTS, raw	27	91.0	0.9	0.3	5.2	2.6	13	59	0.5	.....	533	0.15	0.07	0.6	4	20
BANANAS, common, raw	85	75.7	0.8	0.2	22.2	1.1	8	26	0.7	1	370	0.05	0.06	0.7	10	190
BARLEY, light, pearled	349	11.1	0.9	1.0	78.8	8.2	16	189	2.0	3	160	0.12	0.05	3.1	0	0
BEANS, white, dried, uncooked	340	10.9	3.9	1.6	61.3	22.3	144	425	7.8	19	1196	0.65	0.22	2.4	.....	0
BEANS, white, dried, cooked	118	69.0	1.4	0.6	21.2	7.8	50	148	2.7	7	416	0.14	0.07	0.7	0	0
BEANS, red, dried uncooked	343	10.4	3.7	1.5	61.9	22.5	110	406	6.9	10	984	0.51	0.20	2.3	.....	20
BEANS, red, dried, cooked	118	69.0	1.3	0.5	21.4	7.8	38	140	2.4	3	340	0.11	0.06	0.7	.....	trace
BEETS, common, raw	43	87.3	1.1	0.1	9.9	1.6	16	33	0.7	60	335	0.03	0.05	0.4	10	20
BEETS, greens, raw	24	90.9	2.0	0.3	4.6	2.2	119	40	3.3	130	570	0.10	0.22	0.4	30	6100
BEETS, greens, boiled, drained	18	93.6	1.2	0.2	3.3	1.7	99	25	1.9	76	332	0.07	0.15	0.3	15	5100

BLACKBERRIES, raw	58	84.5	0.5	0.9	12.9	1.2	32	19	0.9	1	170	0.03	0.04	0.4	21	200
BLUEBERRIES, raw	62	83.2	0.3	0.5	15.3	0.7	15	13	1.0	1	81	0.03	0.06	0.5	14	100
BROCCOLI SPEARS, raw	32	89.1	1.1	0.3	5.9	3.6	103	78	1.1	15	382	0.10	0.23	0.9	113	2500
BRUSSELS SPROUTS, raw	45	85.2	1.2	0.4	8.3	4.9	36	80	1.5	14	390	0.10	0.16	0.9	102	550
BUCKWHEAT, whole grain	335	11.0	2.0	2.4	72.9	11.7	114	282	3.1	......	448	0.60	......	4.4	0	0
BUCKWHEAT, flour dark	333	12.0	1.8	2.5	72.0	11.7	33	347	2.8	......	......	0.58	0.15	2.9	0	0
CABBAGE, common raw	24	92.4	0.7	0.2	5.4	1.3	49	29	0.4	20	233	0.05	0.05	0.3	51	130
CANTALOUPES or other netted varieties, raw	30	91.2	0.5	0.1	7.5	0.7	14	16	0.4	12	251	0.04	0.03	0.6	33	3400
CARROTS, raw	42	88.2	0.8	0.2	9.7	1.1	37	36	0.7	47	341	0.06	0.05	0.6	8	11,000
CARROTS, boiled, drained	31	91.2	0.6	0.2	7.1	0.9	33	31	0.6	33	222	0.05	0.05	0.5	6	10,500
CASHEW NUTS	561	5.2	2.6	45.7	29.3	17.2	58	373	3.8	15	464	0.43	0.25	1.8	......	100
CAULIFLOWER, raw	27	91.0	0.9	0.2	5.2	2.7	25	56	1.1	13	295	0.11	0.10	0.7	78	60
CAULIFLOWER, boiled, drained	22	92.8	0.6	0.2	4.1	2.3	21	42	0.7	9	206	0.09	0.08	0.6	55	60
CELERY, green & yellow, raw	17	94.1	1.0	0.1	3.9	0.9	29	28	0.3	126	341	0.03	0.03	0.3	9	270
CHERRIES, sour, red, raw	58	83.7	0.5	0.3	14.3	1.2	22	19	0.4	2	191	0.05	0.06	0.4	10	1000

FOOD	Cals.	Water	Ash	Fat	Carb.	Prot.	Ca. (mg)	P (mg)	Fe (mg)	Na (mg)	K (mg)	Thiamine (mg)	Riboflavin (mg)	Nicotinic acid (mg)	Ascorbic acid (mg)	Vit. A I.U.
CHICKPEAS, mature seeds, dried, uncooked	360	10.7	3.0	4.8	61.0	20.5	150	331	6.9	26	797	0.31	0.15	2.0	......	50
COCONUT, flesh, raw	346	50.9	0.9	35.3	9.4	3.5	13	95	1.7	23	256	0.05	0.02	0.5	3	0
COFFEE, dry powder, instant	129	2.6	9.7	trace	35.0	trace	179	383	5.6	72	3256	0	0.21	30.6	0	0
COLLARDS, raw	40	86.9	1.6	0.7	7.2	3.6	203	63	1.0	43	401	0.20	0.31	1.7	92	6500
CORN, kernels only, boiled & drained	83	76.5	0.5	1.0	18.8	3.2	3	73	0.8	1	184	0.09	0.06	1.5	5	350
CORN MEAL, white or yellow, unbolted	355	12.0	1.2	3.9	73.7	9.2	20	256	2.4	1	284	0.38	0.11	2.0	0	510
CORN STARCH	362	12.0	0.1	trace	87.6	0.3	0	0	0	trace	trace	0	0	0	0	0
CRANBERRIES, raw	46	87.9	0.2	0.7	10.8	0.4	14	10	0.5	2	82	0.03	0.02	0.1	11	40
CUCUMBERS, not pared, raw	15	95.1	0.5	0.1	3.4	0.9	25	27	1.1	6	160	0.03	0.04	0.2	11	250
DATES, domestic natural & dry	274	22.5	1.9	0.5	72.9	2.2	59	63	3.0	1	648	0.09	0.10	2.2	0	50
EGGPLANT, raw	25	92.4	0.6	0.2	5.6	1.2	12	26	0.7	2	214	0.05	0.05	0.6	5	10
FENNEL, common, raw	28	90.0	1.7	0.4	5.1	2.8	100	51	2.7	......	397	......	......	......	31	3500
FIGS, raw	80	77.5	0.7	0.3	20.3	1.2	35	22	0.6	2	194	0.06	0.05	0.4	2	80
GRAPEFRUIT, Calif. & Ariz., raw	44	87.5	0.4	0.1	11.5	0.5	32	20	0.4	1	135	0.04	0.02	0.2	40	10

GRAPES, slip skin, raw	69	81.6	0.4	1.0	15.7	1.3	16	12	0.4	3	158	0.05	0.03	0.3	4	100
HONEYDEW MELONS, raw	33	90.6	0.6	0.3	7.7	0.8	14	16	0.4	12	251	0.04	0.03	0.6	23	40
HORSERADISH, raw	87	74.6	2.2	0.3	19.7	3.2	140	64	1.4	8	564	0.07	.....	.....	81	.....
LEMONS, raw	27	90.1	0.3	0.3	8.2	1.1	26	16	0.6	2	138	0.04	0.02	0.1	53	20
LEMON JUICE, raw	25	91.0	0.3	0.2	8.0	0.5	7	10	0.2	1	141	0.03	0.01	0.1	46	20
LENTILS, mature seeds, dried, uncooked	340	11.1	3.0	1.1	60.1	24.7	79	377	6.8	30	790	0.37	0.22	2.0	.....	60
LENTILS, mature seeds, dried, cooked	106	72.0	0.9	trace	19.3	7.8	25	119	2.1	.....	249	0.07	0.06	0.6	0	20
LETTUCE, butter-head var., raw	14	95.1	1.0	0.2	2.5	1.2	35	26	2.0	9	264	0.06	0.06	0.3	8	970
LETTUCE, cos or romaine, raw	18	94.0	0.9	0.3	3.5	1.3	68	25	1.4	9	264	0.05	0.08	0.4	18	1900
LETTUCE, crisp head, raw	13	95.5	0.6	0.1	2.9	0.9	20	22	0.5	9	175	0.06	0.06	0.3	6	330
LIMA BEANS, immature seeds, raw	123	67.5	1.5	0.5	22.1	8.4	52	142	2.8	2	650	0.24	0.12	1.4	2.9	290
LIMA BEANS, immature seeds, boiled, drained	111	71.1	1.0	0.5	19.8	7.6	47	121	2.5	1	422	0.18	0.10	1.3	17	280
LIMES, acid type, raw	28	89.3	0.3	0.2	9.5	0.7	33	18	0.6	2	102	0.03	0.02	0.2	37	10
LIMES, juice, raw	26	90.3	0.3	0.1	9.0	0.3	9	11	0.2	1	104	0.02	0.01	0.1	32	10
MANGOS, raw	66	81.7	0.4	0.4	16.8	0.7	10	13	0.4	7	189	0.05	0.05	1.1	35	4800

FOOD	Cals.	Water	Ash	Fat	Carb.	Prot.	Ca. (mg)	P (mg)	Fe (mg)	Na (mg)	K (mg)	Thiamine (mg)	Riboflavin (mg)	Nicotinic acid (mg)	Ascorbic acid (mg)	Vit. A I.U.
MUNG BEANS, mature seeds, dried, uncooked	340	10.7	3.5	1.3	60.3	24.2	118	340	7.7	6	1028	0.38	0.21	2.6	.....	80
MUSHROOMS, raw	28	90.4	0.9	0.3	4.4	2.7	6	116	0.8	15	414	0.10	0.46	4.2	3	trace
MUSTARD GREENS, raw	31	89.5	1.4	0.5	5.6	3.0	183	50	3.0	32	377	0.11	0.22	0.8	97	7000
MUSTARD GREENS, boiled, drained	23	92.6	0.8	0.4	4.0	2.2	138	32	1.8	18	220	0.08	0.14	0.6	48	5800
OKRA, raw	36	88.9	0.8	0.3	7.6	2.4	92	51	0.6	3	249	0.17	0.21	1.0	31	520
OKRA, boiled, drained	29	91.1	0.6	0.3	6.0	2.0	92	41	0.5	2	174	0.13	0.18	0.9	20	490
ONIONS, young, green, entire, raw	36	89.4	0.7	0.2	8.2	1.5	51	39	1.0	5	231	0.05	0.05	0.4	32	2000
ONIONS, mature, raw	38	89.1	0.6	0.1	8.7	1.5	27	36	0.5	10	157	0.03	0.04	0.2	10	40
ORANGES, Calif., navels, raw	51	85.4	0.5	0.1	12.7	1.3	40	22	0.4	1	194	0.10	0.04	0.4	61	200
PARSLEY, common & curled leaf, raw	44	85.1	2.2	0.6	8.5	3.6	203	63	6.2	45	727	0.12	0.26	1.2	172	8500
PARSNIPS, raw	76	79.1	1.2	0.5	17.5	1.7	50	77	0.7	12	541	0.08	0.09	0.2	16	30
PEACHES, raw	38	89.1	0.5	0.1	9.7	0.6	9	19	0.5	1	202	0.02	0.05	1.0	7	1330
PEANUTS, with skins, raw	564	5.6	2.3	47.5	18.6	26.0	69	401	2.1	5	674	1.14	0.13	17.2	0	.....
PEANUTS with skins, roasted	582	1.8	2.7	48.7	20.6	26.2	72	407	2.2	5	701	0.32	0.13	17.1	0	.....

PEANUT FLOUR, defatted	571	7.3	4.1	9.2	31.5	47.9	104	720	3.5	9	1186	0.75	0.22	27.8	0	......
PEARS, not pared, raw	61	83.2	0.4	0.4	15.3	0.7	8	11	0.3	2	130	0.02	0.04	0.1	4	20
PEAS, edible pod, raw	53	83.3	1.1	0.2	12.0	3.4	62	90	0.7	......	170	0.28	0.12	......	21	680
PEAS, edible pod, boiled, drained	43	86.6	0.8	0.2	9.5	2.9	56	76	0.5	......	119	0.22	0.11	......	14	610
PEAS, green, immature seeds, raw	84	78.0	0.9	0.4	14.4	6.3	26	116	1.9	2	316	0.35	0.14	2.9	27	640
PEAS, green, immature seeds, boiled, drained	71	81.5	0.6	0.4	12.1	5.4	23	99	1.8	1	196	0.28	0.11	2.3	20	540
PECANS	687	3.4	1.6	71.2	14.6	9.2	73	289	2.4	trace	603	0.86	0.13	0.9	2	130
PEPPERS, hot chili, green, raw	37	88.8	0.6	0.2	9.1	1.3	10	25	0.7	......	......	0.09	0.06	1.7	235	770
PINEAPPLE, raw	52	85.3	0.4	0.2	13.7	0.4	17	8	0.5	1	146	0.09	0.03	0.2	17	70
PINEAPPLE, canned in juice	58	84.0	0.4	0.1	15.1	0.4	16	8	0.4	1	147	0.10	0.03	0.3	10	60
PINEAPPLE JUICE, canned	55	85.6	0.4	0.1	13.5	0.4	15	9	0.3	1	149	0.05	0.02	0.2	9	50
PISTACHIO NUTS	594	5.3	2.7	53.7	19.0	19.3	131	500	7.3	......	972	0.67	......	1.4	0	230
PLUMS, Damsom, raw	66	81.1	0.6	trace	17.8	0.5	18	17	0.5	2	299	0.08	0.03	0.5	......	300
POTATOES, raw	76	79.8	0.9	0.1	17.1	2.1	7	53	0.6	3	407	0.10	0.04	1.5	20	trace
POTATOES, not pared, baked	93	75.1	1.1	0.1	21.1	2.6	9	65	0.7	4	503	0.10	0.04	1.7	20	trace
POTATOES, not pared, boiled	76	79.8	0.9	0.1	17.1	2.1	7	53	0.6	3	407	0.09	0.04	1.5	16	trace

FOOD	Cals.	Water	Ash	Fat	Carb.	Prot.	Ca. (mg)	P (mg)	Fe (mg)	Na (mg)	K (mg)	Thiamine (mg)	Riboflavin (mg)	Nicotinic acid (mg)	Ascorbic acid (mg)	Vit. A I.U.
PRUNES, dehydrated, uncooked	344	2.5	2.4	0.5	91.3	3.3	90	107	4.4	11	940	0.12	0.22	2.1	4	2170
PRUNE JUICE, canned or bottled	77	80.8	0.5	0.1	19.0	0.4	14	20	4.1	2	235	0.01	0.01	0.4	2	......
PUMPKIN, raw	26	91.6	0.8	0.1	6.5	1.0	21	44	0.8	1	340	0.05	0.11	0.6	9	1600
RADISHES, common, raw	17	94.5	0.8	0.1	3.6	1.0	30	31	1.0	18	322	0.03	0.03	0.3	26	10
RAISINS, unbleached, cooked	289	18.0	1.9	0.2	77.4	2.5	62	101	3.5	27	763	0.11	0.08	0.5	1	20
RASPBERRIES, black, raw	73	80.8	0.6	1.4	15.7	1.5	30	22	0.9	1	199	0.03	0.09	0.9	18	trace
RICE, brown, raw	360	12.0	1.2	1.9	77.4	7.5	32	221	1.6	9	214	0.34	0.05	4.7	0	0
RICE, brown, cooked	119	70.3	1.1	0.6	25.5	2.5	12	73	0.5	282	70	0.09	0.02	1.4	0	0
RICE, white, raw	363	12.0	0.5	0.4	80.4	6.7	24	94	0.8	5	92	0.07	0.03	1.6	0	0
RICE, white, cooked	109	72.6	1.1	0.1	24.2	2.0	10	28	0.2	374	28	0.02	0.01	0.4	0	0
RYE, whole grain	334	11.0	1.8	1.7	73.4	12.1	38	376	3.7	1	467	0.43	0.22	1.6	0	0
SESAME SEEDS, dried	563	5.4	5.3	49.1	21.6	18.6	1160	616	10.5	60	725	0.98	0.24	5.4	0	30
SOYBEANS, immature seeds, raw	134	69.2	1.6	5.1	13.2	10.9	67	225	2.8	......	......	0.44	0.16	1.4	29	690
SOYBEANS, immature seeds, boiled, drained	118	73.8	1.2	5.1	10.9	9.8	60	191	2.5	......	......	0.31	0.13	1.2	17	660

SOYBEANS, mature seeds, dried, uncooked	403	10.0	4.7	17.7	33.5	34.1	226	554	8.4	5	1677	1.10	0.31	2.2	......	80
SOYBEANS, mature seeds, dried, cooked	130	71.0	1.5	5.7	10.8	11.0	73	179	2.7	2	540	0.21	0.09	0.6	0	30
SOYBEAN FLOUR, full fat	421	8.0	4.6	20.3	30.4	36.7	199	558	8.4	1	1660	0.85	0.31	2.1	0	110
SOYBEAN FLOUR, low fat	356	8.0	5.3	6.7	36.6	43.4	263	634	9.1	1	1859	0.83	0.36	2.6	0	80
SOYBEAN MILK, fluid	33	92.4	0.5	1.5	2.2	3.4	21	48	0.8	......	......	0.08	0.03	0.2	0	40
SOYBEAN MILK, powder	429	4.2	5.7	20.3	28.0	41.8	275	......	......	......	......	......	......	......	......	......
SPINACH, raw	26	90.7	1.5	0.3	4.3	3.2	93	51	3.1	71	470	0.10	0.20	0.6	51	8100
SPINACH, boiled, drained	23	92.0	1.1	0.3	3.6	3.0	93	38	2.2	50	324	0.07	0.14	0.5	28	8100
SQUASH, summer, crook & straight neck, raw	20	93.7	0.6	0.2	4.3	1.2	28	29	0.4	1	202	0.05	0.09	1.0	25	460
SQUASH, Zuccini & Cocozelle, raw	17	94.6	0.5	0.1	3.6	1.2	28	29	0.4	1	202	0.05	0.09	1.0	19	320
STRAWBERRIES, raw	37	89.9	0.5	0.5	8.4	0.7	21	21	1.0	1	164	0.03	0.07	0.6	59	60
SUGAR, beet or cane, brown	373	2.1	1.5	0	96.4	0	85	19	3.4	30	344	0.01	0.03	0.2	0	0
SUGAR, beet or cane, granulated	385	0.5	trace	0	99.5	0	0	0	0.1	1	3	0	0	0	0	0

FOOD	Cals.	Water	Ash	Fat	Carb.	Prot.	Ca. (mg)	P (mg)	Fe (mg)	Na (mg)	K (mg)	Thiamine (mg)	Riboflavin (mg)	Nicotinic acid (mg)	Ascorbic acid (mg)	Vit. A I.U.
SUNFLOWER SEEDS, dried	560	4.8	4.0	47.3	19.9	24.0	120	837	7.1	30	920	1.96	0.23	5.4	.....	50
SWEET POTATOES, not pared, baked	141	63.7	1.2	0.5	32.5	2.1	40	58	0.9	12	300	0.09	0.07	0.7	22	8100
SWEET POTATOES, not pared, boiled	114	70.6	1.0	0.4	26.3	1.7	32	47	0.7	10	243	0.09	0.06	0.6	17	7900
SYRUP, cane	263	26.0	1.5	0	68.0	0	60	29	3.6	.....	425	0.13	0.06	0.1	0	0
SYRUP, maple	252	33.0	0.7	.....	65.0	.....	104	8	1.2	10	176	.....	.....	.....	0	.....
TANGERINES, Dancy, raw	46	87.0	0.4	0.2	11.6	0.8	40	18	0.4	2	126	0.06	0.02	0.1	31	420
TANGERINE JUICE, canned	43	88.8	0.3	0.2	10.2	0.5	18	14	0.2	1	178	0.06	0.02	0.1	22	420
TAPIOCA, dried	352	12.6	0.2	0.2	86.4	0.6	10	18	0.4	3	18	0	0	0	0	0
TOMATOES, green, raw	24	93.0	0.5	0.2	5.1	1.2	13	27	0.5	3	244	0.06	0.04	0.5	20	270
TOMATOES, ripe, raw	22	93.5	0.5	0.2	4.7	1.1	13	27	0.5	3	244	0.06	0.04	0.7	23	900
TOMATO JUICE, canned or bottled	19	93.6	1.1	0.1	4.3	0.9	7	18	0.9	200	227	0.05	0.03	0.8	16	800
TURNIPS, raw	30	91.5	0.7	0.2	6.6	1.0	39	30	0.5	49	268	0.04	0.07	0.6	36	trace
TURNIPS, boiled, drained	23	93.6	0.5	0.2	4.9	0.8	35	24	0.4	34	188	0.04	0.05	0.3	22	trace

TURNIP GREENS, raw	28	90.3	1.4	0.3	5.0	3.0	246	58	1.8	......	......	0.21	0.39	0.8	139	7600
WATERMELONS, raw	26	92.6	0.3	0.2	6.4	0.5	7	10	0.5	1	100	0.03	0.03	0.2	7	590
WHEAT, whole meal, dry	338	10.4	1.8	2.0	72.3	13.5	45	398	3.7	2	370	0.51	0.13	4.7	0	0
WHEAT, whole meal, cooked	45	87.7	0.8	0.3	9.4	1.8	7	52	0.5	212	48	0.06	0.02	0.6	0	0
WHEAT FLOUR, all purpose	364	12.0	0.43	1.0	76.1	10.5	16	87	0.8	2	95	0.06	0.05	0.9	0	0
WHEAT FLOUR, whole	333	12.0	1.7	2.0	71.0	13.3	41	372	3.3	3	370	0.55	0.12	4.3	0	0
WHEAT GERM, crude	363	11.5	4.3	10.9	46.7	26.6	72	1118	9.4	3	827	2.01	0.68	4.2	0	0
YEAST, Brewers	283	5.0	7.1	1.0	38.4	38.8	70–760	1753	17.3	121	1894	15.61	4.28	37.9	trace	trace

P. L. Altman, and D. S. Dittmer, (Eds.): "Metabolism," Federation of American Societies for Experimental Biology, pp. 9–47, 1968.

APPENDIX III

COMPOSITION OF MILK *

(Values are grams per 100 grams mature whole milk)

	Human	Cow	Goat	Buffalo
Water	87.3	87.3	87.2	82.1
Ash	0.25	0.72	0.81	0.78
Fat	3.7	3.7	4.0	7.89
Carbohydrate	6.6	4.8	4.5	4.7
Protein	1.63	3.3	3.6	5.9
Amino [g/16g Acids total N]				
Alanine	3.6	3.4	3.7	
Arginine	3.4	3.5	3.0	
Aspartic Acid	8.4	7.9	8.6	
Cystine	1.7	0.8	1.1	
Glutamic Acid	15.5	21.9	19.0	
Glycine	2.3	2.0	2.0	
Histidine	2.3	2.7	3.0	
Isoleucine	4.4	5.9	5.3	
Leucine	8.6	9.7	10.0	
Lysine	6.5	8.1	8.6	
Methionine	1.7	2.6	2.8	
Phenylalanine	3.4	4.9	5.5	
Proline	7.3	9.9	10.9	
Serine	4.6	5.6	5.8	
Threonine	4.5	4.6	5.9	
Trypotophan	1.7	1.4	1.6	
Tyrosine	3.7	5.1	5.1	
Valine	4.8	6.6	7.6	
MINERALS:				
Calcium, g/100g.	0.032	0.12	0.14	
Chlorine, g/100g.	0.042	0.11	0.15	
Magnesium, g/100g.	0.004	0.01	0.02	
Phosphorsu, g/100g.	0.015	0.10	0.12	
Potassium, g/100g.	0.054	0.15	0.17	
Sodium, g/100g.	0.015	0.05		
Aluminum, ppm.	0.33	0.008		
Boron, ppm.		0.5–1.0	0.18	
Bromine, ppm.		0.18–0.24		
Cobalt, ppm.	0.001	.0002–.0011		
Copper, ppm.	0.04	0.05–0.45	0.2	
Fluorine, ppm.		0.2		
Iodine, ppm.	0.007	.0007–.05		
Iron, ppm.	0.15	0.15–0.7	0.02	
Manganese, ppm.	0.01	.037–0.37		
Molybdenum, ppm.		0.05–0.15		
Silicon, ppm.	0.34	1		

454

Silver, ppm.		.015–.037	
Strontium, ppm.		.0075–.075	
Zinc, ppm.	0.53	.22–5.0	
VITAMINS-FAT SOL.:			
A, ug/g fat	14	8	8
Carotenoids, ug/g fat	3.5	7	Trace
D, I.U./100g	0.4	1.8	2.3
E, mg/100g	1.1	0.08	
K, Dam-Glavind units/100g	26	100	
VITAMINS-WATER SOL.:			
Thiamine, ug/100g	14	45	49
Riboflavin, ug/100g	51	180	140
Nicotinic Acid, ug/100g	190	75	250
B_6, ug/100g	4	40	60
Biotin, ug/100g	1.1	2.5	3.8
Pantothenic Acid, ug/100g	260	320	360
Folic Acid, ug/100g	5.3	6.3	0.4
p-Aminobenzoic A.		10	
Inositol, mg/100g	40	18	
B_{12}, ug/100g	0.02	0.35	0.07
Choline, mg/100g	9	20	
Ascorbic Acid, mg/100g	4.3	2.0	2.0

* P. L. Altman, and D. S. Dittmer, (Eds.): "Metabolism," Federation of American Societies for Experimental Biology, pp. 5–8, 1968.

SUBJECT INDEX

You Will Be Interested Also In These . . .

Eldon M. Boyd — PROTEIN DEFICIENCY AND PESTICIDE TOXICITY 480 pp., 106 il. (1 in full color), 129 tables, $29.50

William D. Hurley — ENVIRONMENTAL LEGISLATION. 96 pp., $6.50

Sylvan J. Kaplan & Evelyn Kivy-Rosenberg — ECOLOGY AND THE QUALITY OF LIFE. 308 pp., 23 il., 11 tables, $17.50

Norman Kiell — THE PSYCHOLOGY OF OBESITY: Dynamics and Treatment. 480 pp. (6 3/8 x 9 5/8), 41 tables, $13.95

Laura P. Krawitt & Emily K. Weinberger — PRACTICAL LOW PROTEIN COOKERY. 128 pp., 1 il., 3 tables, $6.75, paper

Francis K. V. Leh & Richard K. C. Lak — ENVIRONMENT AND POLLUTIONS: Sources, Health Effects, Monitoring and Control. 308 pp., 25 il., 71 tables, $14.75

Sohan L. Manocha — MALNUTRITION AND RETARDED HUMAN DEVELOPMENT. 400 pp., 20 il., 8 tables, $19.75

Jean Mayer — HUMAN NUTRITION: Its Physiological, Medical and Social Aspects. A Series of Eighty-Two Essays. 2nd Ptg., 740 pp., 5 il., $12.95

H. C. Meng & David H. Law — PARENTERAL NUTRITION: Proceedings of an International Symposium, Vanderbilt University School of Medicine, Nashville, Tennessee. 616 pp., 219 il., 86 tables, $24.75

Theron G. Randolph — HUMAN ECOLOGY AND SUSCEPTIBILITY TO THE CHEMICAL ENVIRONMENT. 4th Ptg., 160 pp., 1 il., $7.50

Sheldon J. Segal, Ruth Crozier, Philip A. Corfman & Peter G. Condliffe — THE REGULATION OF MAMMALIAN REPRODUCTION. 614 pp. (7 x 10), 260 il., 91 tables, $44.50

Helen M. Wallace, Edwin M. Gold & Edward F. Lis — MATERNAL AND CHILD HEALTH PRACTICES: Problems, Resources and Methods of Delivery. 1,400 pp., 49 il., 170 tables, $37.50

Charles G. Wilber — THE BIOLOGICAL ASPECTS OF WATER POLLUTION. 2nd Ptg., 308 pp. (7 x 10), 54 il., 85 tables, $23.75

Marion N. Wood — DELICIOUS AND EASY RICE FLOUR RECIPES: A Sequel To Gourmet Food On A Wheat-Free Diet. 160 pp., $5.50, paper

Marion N. Wood — GOURMET FOOD ON A WHEAT-FREE DIET. 2nd Ptg., 128 pp. (5 3/4 x 8 3/4), $5.95

CHARLES C THOMAS • PUBLISHER • SPRINGFIELD • ILLINOIS